Oxford Medical Publications

Nature and narrative

International Perspectives in Philosophy and Psychiatry

Series editors

Bill (KWM) Fulford
Katherine Morris
John Z Sadler
Giovanni Stanghellini

Published volumes in this series:

Mind, Meaning and Mental Disorder, 2e
Bolton and Hill

Forthcoming volumes in the series:

Handbook of Philosophy and Psychiatry
Radden (ed)

Values and Psychiatric Disorders
Sadler

The Philosophical Understanding of Schizophrenia
Chung, Fulford and Graham (eds)

Disembodied Spirits and Deanimated Bodies
Stanghellini

The Vulnerable Self: The Clinical Phenomenology of the Schizophrenic and Affective Spectrum Disorders
Parnas, Sass and Stanghellini

Concise Oxford Textbook of Philosophy and Psychiatry
Fulford, Thornton and Graham

Postpsychiatry
Bracken and Thomas

Nature and narrative

An introduction to the new philosophy of psychiatry

Edited by

Bill (KWM) Fulford
Katherine Morris
John Z Sadler
Giovanni Stanghellini

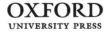
OXFORD
UNIVERSITY PRESS

*This book has been printed digitally and produced in a standard specification
in order to ensure its continuing availability*

OXFORD
UNIVERSITY PRESS

Great Clarendon Street, Oxford OX2 6DP

Oxford University Press is a department of the University of Oxford.
It furthers the University's objective of excellence in research, scholarship,
and education by publishing worldwide in

Oxford New York

Auckland Cape Town Dar es Salaam Hong Kong Karachi
Kuala Lumpur Madrid Melbourne Mexico City Nairobi
New Delhi Shanghai Taipei Toronto
With offices in
Argentina Austria Brazil Chile Czech Republic France Greece
Guatemala Hungary Italy Japan South Korea Poland Portugal
Singapore Switzerland Thailand Turkey Ukraine Vietnam

Oxford is a registered trade mark of Oxford University Press
in the UK and in certain other countries

Published in the United States
by Oxford University Press Inc., New York

© Oxford University Press, 2003

Not to be reprinted without permission
The moral rights of the author have been asserted
Database right Oxford University Press (maker)

Reprinted 2006

All rights reserved. No part of this publication may be reproduced,
stored in a retrieval system, or transmitted, in any form or by any means,
without the prior permission in writing of Oxford University Press,
or as expressly permitted by law, or under terms agreed with the appropriate
reprographics rights organization. Enquiries concerning reproduction
outside the scope of the above should be sent to the Rights Department,
Oxford University Press, at the address above

You must not circulate this book in any other binding or cover
And you must impose this same condition on any acquirer

ISBN 0-19-852611-3

Printed and bound by CPI Antony Rowe, Eastbourne

Foreword

Paul Appelbaum

As we welcome this initial volume in the series on International Perspectives on Philosophy and Psychiatry, it seems fair to ask why psychiatric clinicians and researchers should care about philosophic approaches to their field. Philosophers can hardly be faulted for seeking to apply their methods to whatever area of human endeavor catches their fancy. But psychiatrists, psychologists, and members of other mental health disciplines, whether practitioners or researchers — in what way might philosophical explorations, such as those collected here, be of help to them?

Without attempting to catalogue fully the answers to this fundamental question, let me sketch some possible responses. One of the things that philosophers do well is to force us to clarify the concepts with which we deal. In the press of everyday clinical work, and even in the routine of clinical investigation, it is remarkably easy to elude the broader issues. Where are the borders between mental illness and mere idiosyncrasy? How ought we to think about causal influences in mental life and hence in the mental disorders? Are our diagnostic categories constructed with a rigor that permits them to withstand close conceptual examination? Philosophy should matter to the mental health professions not least because it may help us to refine the ideas and notions that lie at the core of what we do.

There is, moreover, an important thread in philosophical inquiry that has involved close observation of mental function — normal and deviant — from, as it were, the inside. Phenomenology, a methodologic approach linked to a number of philosophical schools, has put philosophy at the forefront of empirical investigation of psychological and psychopathological processes by the examination of subjective experience. This was true even during a time when psychiatry itself had retreated from empiricism, spinning itself a theoretical web from which it has only recently broken free. And it remains true today, when psychiatric empiricism, now resurgent, routinely slights the lived experience of people with mental disorders in favor of more 'objective' sources of data. The phenomenological tradition not only promises to sharpen our approaches to diagnosis and allow us better to understand the effects of treatment. By bringing mental health professionals closer to the experience of their patients, a reinvigorated phenomenology also holds the key to strengthening the alliance between treaters and the people whom they treat.

Perhaps the area of philosophical work most familiar to clinicians is ethics: the systematic examination of the behavior of practitioners in relation to their patients, with the goal of identifying morally preferable options. Even to list the major issues in psychiatric ethics today is to encapsulate the day-to-day experience of the clinician. Under what circumstances is the use of coercion legitimate? When may patients' confidences be breached? What obligations does society have to provide care and treatment for persons with mental disorders and how can they be balanced with competing needs? Absolute and universal answers to these dilemmas are vanishingly rare. However, it is not rules that clinicians need most from philosophical ethics, but ways to think about these problems, knowledge of pitfalls to avoid, and at best help in identifying those options that may be morally suspect.

In an era in which clinical work threatens to sink into a routine of unexamined practice, an endless cycle of diagnosis and prescription, divorced from genuine human interaction and performed at an unsustainable pace dictated by economic concerns, philosophy can remind those of us in the clinical disciplines of what attracted us to the mental health professions in the first place. It can immerse us in the resources of diagnosis, expose us to the felt experience of illness, and help us navigate the ethical challenges we face along the way. Philosophical examination shows the mind and its afflictions in all their complexity, encouraging us to reject reductionism of all sorts and fostering our will to sustain a critical and inquisitive attitude toward practice and research.

It may be that philosophy too benefits from this endeavor, learning methods from psychiatry and cognitive science and finding ground on which to test approaches and theories of broader applicability. Others, though, are better suited to opine on that matter, and I will leave it to them to do so. For me, I have no doubt that psychiatry is enriched by its involvement with the philosophic enterprise, and I am grateful for it. May this series grow from strength to strength, bringing our fields ever closer together.

Foreword

Baroness Mary Warnock

The philosopher, J. L. Austin, once remarked that the task of philosophy was to speculate about those subjects which had not, or not yet, become science. The history of the presocratic Greek philosophers who theorized about the true hidden composition of the universe before the birth of physics as an empirical science seems to confirm this view. It may therefore seem surprising that as psychiatry seems, to the lay person at least, at last to be becoming more scientific, it should at the same time be more and more closely interlocked with philosophy. *Nature and Narrative* explores the reasons for this apparently indissoluble marriage.

One superficial place where psychiatry and philosophy may seem to overlap, and where psychiatrists might be thought to need the service of philosophers, is in Ethics. But in my view Medical Ethics is a somewhat overrated subject, and in any case is in danger of getting into a rut. If this is so, then ethicists have more to learn from psychiatrists than the other way round. For example the idea of Informed Consent, a central building block in medical ethics, surely needs to be further-examined in a context of mental illness.

At a much more interesting level, philosophy has much to learn from psychiatry. Ever since Descartes, philosophers have been obsessed with the relation between what we experience and what there is. Having divided the mind from the body, and thus from sensory input, Descartes was at a loss to provide any satisfactory answer to the question whether or not the outside world exists. He had to rely on faith in a fair-minded non-deceiving God to reassure sceptics. But the great empiricist Hume had no such faith to fall back on, and was bound to remain sceptical, taking his mind off the problem only by forgetting it in social life. He had no answer to the question how, if all my impressions are my own and momentary, I can communicate them to you. Kant's effort in the *Critique of Pure Reason* to explain a priori how the human mind is bound to conceive of the perceived world, and why it is, therefore, that we agree about the world of perception, about space, time, causation, and the other categories of understanding, was magnificent and impressive. But it was a priori nevertheless. It was not, though he hoped it was, capable of proof. Nor did it purport to tell us about the real world, but only about the world as it appears.

The beginning of phenomenology, which brought the existing outside world into consciousness by the definition of what consciousness was, came with the publication in 1874 of Franz Brentano's book *Psychology from an Empirical Point of View*. He defined consciousness as essentially Intentional, that is, as consciousness *of* something. You could not describe your awareness of a tree without mentioning two things, yourself and the tree. Hitherto, there had been three parts to the description, you, your idea or impression, and the (putative) tree. In his early days, Edmund Husserl took over this simple principle, and from then onwards the philosophical problem of the relation between the inner and the outer was radically transformed. When Sartre came back in 1939 from visiting Germany to learn about Husserl's work, he was in a state of high excitement about the revolution he had found. In particular he delighted in the thought that perception can no longer be separated from emotions: consciousness of things is not limited to knowledge of them. 'It is things that reveal themselves to us as hateful, sympathetic, horrible, lovable . . . Husserl has restored things to their horror and their charm.' Wittgenstein denied that he had read Husserl, but whether or not he had, his new insistence that language is essentially and not inexplicably for communication, is certainly a part of the same philosophical history.

From the moment of entering the world we are caught up in a network of interpretations and communications. Nowhere does this become more obvious than in Karl Jaspers' descriptions of anomalies of perception in *General Psychopathology* (not published in England until 1963). We may be in danger of being so respectful of the objectivity of science that we forget the element of imagination which we necessarily bring to the world that we, however objectively, try to explore. Philosophers will welcome and benefit from the series of books now to be launched. The books will be right up their street.

Preface

Celebrating the remarkable renewal of interest in cross-disciplinary work between philosophy and psychiatry in the final decade of the 20th century, *Nature and narrative* is the launch volume for a new international book series, *International Perspectives in Philosophy and Psychiatry*.

We say 'renewal' because in many respects the new philosophy of psychiatry has taken up where Karl Jaspers, the first philosopher of psychiatry and the founder of modern psychopathology, left things at the start of the twentieth century. The title of this first volume, *Nature and narrative*, indeed directly reflects a central theme of Jaspers' work, viz., the need for both scientific ('nature') and experiential ('narrative') accounts of psychopathology. It is a mark of the maturity of the new philosophy of psychiatry that our contributors, although representing a very wide variety of disciplines and points of view, both philosophical and practical, provide us with a well-integrated story line around Jaspers' theme. Cross-talk abounds. Each chapter, though, illustrates how recent developments — respectively in philosophy, in ethics, in psychology, and in phenomenology — have contributed, separately and together, to a new rapprochement between nature and narrative in mental health.

It is a mark of the vigour of the new philosophy of psychiatry, on the other hand, that each of the contributors to *Nature and narrative* has something distinctive and fresh to say. Here you will find no recycled material! There is new light, from Wittgenstein's *Diktat fur Schlick*, only recently translated into English, on the remarkable similarities in aims and methods between philosophy and psychoanalysis (Baker, Chapter 3). There are novel methodologies, from hermeneutics (Widdershoven and Widdershoven-Heerding, Chapter 6), from empirical linguistics (van Staden and Kruger, Chapter 16) and from philosophical systems theory (Glas, Chapter 15); there is a new slant on citizenship and the dangers of "political" psychiatry (Robinson, Chapter 5); and there are no less than three contrasting "takes" on the concept of mental disorder, cognitivist (Bolton, Chapter 7), discursive (Harré, Chapter 8, and Gillett, Chapter 9) and from Merleau-Ponty's phenomenology (Matthews, Chapter 4). Here, too, phenomenology is used in a fine-grained way to illuminate specific kinds of psychopathology — delusion (Musalek, Chapter 10), body dysmorphophobia (Morris, Chapter 11), schizophrenia (Depraz, Chapter 12), and depression (Kraus, Chapter 13). There is also thoughtful work on the *limits* of understanding in psychosis and its implications for practice (Heinimaa, Chapter 14). Finally, there are pointers to the future of the philosophy of psychiatry from the history of ideas, respectively of the twentieth century (Meares, Chapter 2) and of the scientific renaissance (Rossi, Chapter 17).

In launching *International Perspectives in Philosophy and Psychiatry* we owe a considerable debt to the organisers of the many meetings and conferences, national and international, that have played a key role in building up the new philosophy of psychiatry. The series was conceived at the 4th International Conference for Philosophy and Psychiatry, convened under the Presidency of Arnaldo Ballerini, on behalf of the Italian and British groups, in Florence in the millennial year, 2000. The Florence meeting built on groundbreaking international conferences, in Spain, organised by the British and American groups, and in France — Jean Naudin's conference in Nice, and the conference organised by Dominic Pringuey and Franz Sammy-Kohl in Marseille. The momentum has since been wonderfully maintained with a record-breaking conference organised by Bernard Granger in Paris; a first conference specifically for trainees organised by Tanja Suomela and Markus Heinimaa in Finland; and, most recently, the launch of the International Network for Philosophy and Psychiatry (INPP), hosted by Tuviah Zabow and Werdie van Staden during the biennial meeting of the South African Society of Psychiatrists in Cape Town on Heritage Day in September 2002.

During the twentieth century both philosophy and psychiatry were too-often diminished by splits and factional infighting. This was counterproductive academically for philosophy. For mental health, though, it was nothing short of a disaster. Divided amongst ourselves, we contributed, unwittingly, to the stigmatization, exclusion and prejudice, to which, notwithstanding the many positive achievements of the twentieth century, users and providers of services alike remain subject.

The new philosophy of psychiatry, by contrast, has been remarkable for its strongly collegial spirit. We have had our differences! But the hallmark of the new philosophy of psychiatry has been the openness and generosity with which everyone involved has reached out, across disciplines, across national and cultural boundaries, and between language groups. This is why we were so particularly honoured and delighted that the INPP could be launched from the new South Africa. No community is safe from the renewed fanaticism that we face at the start of the twenty-first century. But whatever happens in the future, the unique achievements of the new South Africa to date stand as a symbol of what can be done when we put our efforts into building bridges rather than putting up walls.

The Editors
2003

Contents

List of contributors

Gordon Baker died in 2002. He had for many years been a Fellow in Philosophy at St. John's College, Oxford. He was the co-author, with P. M. S. Hacker, of many books and articles on Wittgenstein and Frege including *Wittgenstein, understanding and meaning* (Oxford: Blackwell, 1980), and, with Katherine Morris, of *Descartes' dualism* (London: Routledge, 1996). He wrote extensively on Wittgenstein, Frege, Waismann, and Russell, and oversaw the English translation of Waismann's dictations to Wittgenstein (forthcoming from Routledge under the title, *The voices of Wittgenstein*). **Chapter 3**

Derek Bolton read philosophy at Cambridge and following doctoral research published on Wittgenstein. Subsequently he pursued a career in clinical psychology involving empirical and philosophical research. Recent publications include *Problems in the definition of mental disorder* (*The Philosophical Quarterly* (2001), **51**: 182–199) and *Knowledge in the human sciences*, in *What is evidence in mental health care?* edited by S. Priebe and M. Slade (London: Wiley, 2002). **Chapter 7**

Natalie Depraz is a Professor in the Philosophy Department, University of the Sorbonne, Paris, with a longstanding interest both in German and French phenomenology and in existential psychiatry. Among her recent publications are *Transcendance et incarnation. Le statut de l'intersubjectivité comme altérité à soi chez Husserl* (Vrin, 1995), *La conscience. Approches croisées des Classiques aux Sciences cognitives* (A. Colin, 2001) and *Lucidité du corps. De l'empirisme transcendantal en phénoménologie* (Kluwer, Phaenomenologica, 2001). **Chapter 12**

Bill (K. W. M.) Fulford is Professor of Philosophy and Mental Health in the Department of Philosophy, University of Warwick, where he runs Masters, PhD, and research programmes in *Philosophy, Ethics and Mental Health Practice*. He is also an Honorary Consultant Psychiatrist in the Department of Psychiatry, University of Oxford; Visiting Professor in Psychology, The Institute of Psychiatry and King's College, London University; Visiting Professor in Philosophy and Professional Practice Skills in the Centre for Professional Ethics, University of Central Lancashire; and Visiting Professor, Kent Institute of Medicine and Health Sciences, University of Kent. He is the Founder Chair of the Philosophy Special Interest Group in The Royal College of Psychiatrists. He is a Fellow of both the Royal College of Psychiatrists and The Royal College of Physicians (London). He is the Editor of the first international journal for philosophy and mental health, *PPP – Philosophy Psychiatry and Psychology*. He has published widely on philosophical and ethical aspects of mental health, in particular *Moral theory and medical practice* (1989, paperback 1995, reprinted 1999, second edition forthcoming from Cambridge University Press). **Chapter 1**

Grant Gillett is a Professor of medical Ethics at the University of Otago in Dunedin, New Zealand. He is also a practising neurosurgeon. His main philosophical work is in the philosophy of mind and psychiatry though he also writes on topics in bioethics. His most recent books are *The mind and its discontents* (OUP) and *Consciousness and intentionality* (with John McMillan). He is interested in the overlap between postmodern and traditional analytic approaches to mind and language and their relevance to psychiatry. **Chapter 9**

Gerrit Glas is psychiatrist and philosopher. He is currently developing a psychiatric residency training program in Zwolse Poort (NL). He has a special chair for Christian philosophy at the University of Leiden (NL). He wrote a dissertation on anxiety and anxiety disorders, in which theories of anxiety were analysed from a conceptual point of view. He recently published a book on the anthropological aspects of anxiety. He has written on epistemological, anthropological, and ethical topics in (mental) health care. He is (a.o.) chairman of the Section Psychiatry and Philosophy of the Dutch Association for Psychiatry and of the Dutch Foundation for Psychiatry and Religion, and member of the Board of the Social Sciences Council of the Dutch Academy of Sciences and Arts. **Chapter 15**

Rom Harré began his academic career in mathematics and physics, teaching in New Zealand and Pakistan. After graduate work at Oxford under J. L. Austin he turned to philosophy and psychology. After many years in Oxford he now works in Washington, DC. His recent publications include *Great scientific experiments, Varieties of realism, The singular self, One thousand years of philosophy*, and most recently, *Cognitive Science: a philosophical introduction*. **Chapter 8**

Markus Heinimaa has degrees in both medicine and philosophy from the University of Helsinki. After specialising in psychiatry he has been working in Turku area both as a clinician and as a research psychiatrist in the field of early detection of psychosis. His main research interest is conceptual problems in psychiatry. A recent publication is: *Ambiguities in the psychiatric use of the concepts of the person: an analysis. (Philosophy, Psychiatry, Psychology* (2000), **7**: 125–36). **Chapter 14**

Alfred Kraus is a Professor at the Psychiatric University Clinic of Heidelberg, Germany. His main interest is psychopathology: phenomenological-anthropological and role-theoretical approach. Among recent publications: *Phenomenological-anthropological psychiatry*. In: *Contemporary Psychiatry, Volume 1. Foundations of Psychiatry*. (Berlin: Springer; New York: Heidelberg, 2001). *Role performance,* *identity structure and psychosis in melancholic and manic-depressive patients.* In: Mundt Ch., Goldstein M. J., Hahlweg K., Fiedler P. (eds.). *Interpersonal factors in the origin and course of affective disorders.* London: Gaskell, pp. 31–47. **Chapter 13**

Christa Krüger is senior lecturer and senior consultant psychiatrist, Department of Psychiatry, University of Pretoria, South Africa. She was awarded an MD (Warwick) for her study of concurrent electro-encephalographic correlates of dissociation and the development of the State Scale of Dissociation, published in *Psychology and Psychotherapy: Theory, Research and Practice* (2002, **75**: 33–51). **Chapter 16**

Eric Matthews is a Professor in the Philosophy Department, University of Aberdeen, Scotland, with a longstanding interest both in the philosophy of psychiatry and in modern French Philosophy. Among his recent publications are *Twentieth-Century French philosophy* (OUP, 1996) and *The Philosophy of Merleau-Ponty* (Acumen Publishing, 2002). **Chapter 4**

Russell Meares is Professor of Psychiatry at Sydney University and Academic Head of Psychiatric Services at Westmead Hospital and the Western Area of Sydney Mental Health Services. He has over 200 scientific publications in the fields of psychotherapy, child development, and psychosomatic medicine. He is also a published poet and has a continuing interest in literature and art. His most recent book is *Intimacy and alienation: memory, trauma and personal being* (Routledge, 2000; paperback 2002). **Chapter 2**

Katherine Morris is a lecturer and supernumerary fellow in philosophy at Mansfield College, Oxford. She is the co-author, with Gordon Baker, of *Descartes' dualism* (London: Routledge, 1996) and has written extensively on Descartes, Wittgenstein, Sartre, and Merleau-Ponty. She is on the editorial board of PPP – *Philosophy, Psychiatry and Psychology.* **Chapter 1, 11, 12(trans.)**

Michael Musalek is a Psychiatrist and Psychotherapist. He is Professor of Psychiatry, University of Vienna, and Head (Medical Director) of a Department for Alcohol and Drug Addiction at the Anton Proksch Institute Vienna. He is Vice-Chairman, WPA Section Clinical Psychopathology and Secretary, AEP Section Psychopathology. He is an Honorary Member of the Società Italiana di Psicopatologia, Member of the AEP Board, and President-elect, European Society for Dermatology and Psychiatry (ESDAP). He is co-editor of the journal *Psychopathology* and Associate Editor of the journal *Dermatology and Psychosomatics.* **Chapter 10**

Daniel N. Robinson is Distinguished Research Professor Emeritus, Georgetown University, Adjunct Professor of Psychology at Columbia University, and a member of the Philosophy faculty at Oxford. He is past-President of the Division of the History of Psychology and of The Division of Theoretical and Philosophical Psychology of the American Psychological Association. His most recent book is *Praise and blame: moral realism and its applications,* published in 2002 by Princeton University Press. **Chapter 5**

Paolo Rossi is Emeritus Professor of History of Philosophy at Florence University. Among his publications in English are: *Philosophy, technology and the arts in the early modern era* (New York: Harper and Row, 1970); *Francis Bacon: from magic to science* (London: Routledge and Kegan Paul, 1968); *The dark abyss of time: the history of the Earth and the history of Nations from Hooke to Vico* (Chicago: The University of Chicago Press, 1984); *Logic and the art of memory: a quest for a universal language* (Chicago: The University of Chicago Press, 2001); *The birth of modern science* (Oxford: Basil Blackwell, 2001). In 1985 he was awarded the *Sarton Medal* for the history of science by the History of Science Society (USA). In 1988 he was appointed member of the *Accademia dei Lincei and of Academia Europaea*. In 2002 he was awarded the Médaille Marc-Auguste Pictet by the Societé de Physique et d'Histoire Naturelle de Genève. **Chapter 17**

John Z. Sadler, M.D. is Professor of Psychiatry and Director of Undergraduate Psychiatric Education at the University of Texas Southwestern Medical Center and co-editor of the journal *Philosophy, Psychiatry, and Psychology*. His work in the philosophy of psychiatry has focused on the value aspects of psychiatric diagnosis and classification. An edited volume on this topic, *Descriptions and prescriptions: values, mental disorders, and the DSMs*, was published by the Johns Hopkins University Press in 2002. **Chapter 1**

Giovanni Stanghellini, psychiatrist, University Lecturer in Psychopathology, Florence University, has written extensively on the philosophical foundations of psychopathology, especially from a phenomenological and anthropological viewpoint. He is co-editor of the Series *International Perspectives in Philosophy and Psychiatry*, and of the journal, *Psychopathology*. He is co-chair of the World Psychiatric Association (WPA) Section on the Humanities, and secretary to the WPA Section of Clinical Psychopathology and to the Italian Association for Psychopathology. **Chapter 1, 12(trans.)**

Werdie (C. W.) van Staden is senior lecturer and senior consultant psychiatrist, Department of Psychiatry, University of Pretoria, South Africa. He holds a Master's in Medicine (MMed(Psych)) cum laude, a MD in Philosophy (Warwick), a Fellowship of the Trinity College of Music (London), and a Licentiate in Music (University of South Africa). He directs training and research programmes for undergraduate medical students and registrars in psychiatry. He is the Founder Chair of the Philosophy of Psychiatry Special Interest Group in the South African Society of Psychiatrists. His most recent work is on incapacity to give informed consent owing to mental disorder, published in the *Journal of Medical Ethics*. **Chapter 16**

Guy Widdershoven is a philosopher and social scientist. He is Professor of Ethics of Healthcare at Maastricht University (The Netherlands). His research interests are hermeneutic ethics, ethics of care, and empirical ethics. He has published articles in various international journals and contributed to books on ethics of chronic care, especially care for the elderly and psychiatric care. He is currently president of the European Association of Centres of Medical Ethics (EACME). **Chapter 6**

Ineke (C.) Widdershoven-Heerding is a philosopher. She wrote a PhD-thesis on the concepts of disease and clinical judgement in the history of medicine. For 16 years she worked as a philosopher at the Open University in The Netherlands and published courses on ethics and philosophy of science. Recently she has taken up a position as co-ordinator of the working group on Ethics and Social Aspects of the Commission on Genetic Modification (COGEM), advisory body of the Ministry of Housing, Spatial Planning and Environment (VROM) in The Netherlands. **Chapter 6**

Oxford University Press makes no representation, express or implied, that the drug dosages in this book are correct. Readers must therefore always check the product information and clinical procedures with the most up to date published product information and data sheets provided by the manufacturers and the most recent codes of conduct and safety regulations. The authors and the publishers do not accept responsibility or legal liability for any errors in the text or for the misuse or misapplication of material in this work.

1 Past improbable, future possible: the renaissance in philosophy and psychiatry

K. W. M. (Bill) Fulford, Katherine J. Morris, John Z. Sadler, and Giovanni Stanghellini

Introduction

As recently as the late 1980s it would have seemed highly improbable that the closing decade of the twentieth century, although at the time eagerly anticipated as the 'decade of the brain',[1] would turn out to be the decade in which the philosophy of psychiatry was to make a dramatic international come-back. With hindsight, there were early signals of the coming renaissance. In the United States, for example, sessions on philosophical psychopathology organized by George Graham at meetings of the Society for Philosophy and Psychology, were already attracting growing interest; and Division 24 of the American Psychological Association (for Theoretical and Philosophical Psychology) regularly included relevant sessions in its convention programming. In the UK, Alec Jenner and Tim Kendall had established the first Masters Programme, in *Philosophy, Psychiatry and Society*, at Sheffield University. And by the end of the 1980s, building on these and similar initiatives, new academic groups for philosophy and psychiatry had been launched in Britain and America. Yet few could have anticipated that the 1990s would witness:

1. rapid expansion of both the American and British groups to a combined membership totalling over 2500 (the Royal College Philosophy Group is now the second largest section of the College);

2. other similar groups springing up in many parts of the world, including Australia, Denmark, Finland, France, Germany, Italy, Japan, The Netherlands, New Zealand, Norway, Romania, Russia, Scotland, South Africa, South America, Sweden and Turkey;

---

[1]The 'decade of the brain' motto was coined by an American psychiatrist, Lewis L. Judd (Judd, 1990).

3. the launch of a new international journal, *PPP – Philosophy, Psychiatry, and Psychology*, by the British and American groups through The Johns Hopkins University Press. Supported by a strong Editorial Board representing many of the national groups and chaired by Baroness Mary Warnock, *PPP* is now in its ninth year;[2]

4. the first 'chair' of *Philosophy and Mental Health* established at Warwick University in the UK. There have been a number of other teaching and research initiatives at several universities around the world;

5. the Royal College of Psychiatrists adding to its curriculum for higher specialist training a substantial section on philosophy (covering relevant areas of conceptual analysis, value theory, philosophy of science, philosophy of mind, and phenomenology);

6. the 'philosophy of psychiatry' being adopted as a distinct citation category by the premier bibliographical index for philosophical publications, the *Philosopher's Index*;

7. a series of international conferences, in Spain, France, and Italy, attracting several hundred delegates from all parts of the world.

For those wedded to an exclusively 'brain disease' model of biological psychiatry, these developments may seem not only improbable but retrogressive, a back-sliding to pre-scientific ways of thinking (Fulford 2000a).[3] There is, though, a clear historical precedent for the emergence of philosophy of psychiatry at a time of rapid advances in the neurosciences, in the work of no less a figure than one of the founders of modern scientific psychiatry, and the guiding spirit of this book, the great German philosopher-psychiatrist, Karl Jaspers (Fig. 1.1).

Recycling history

The historical back-drop to Jaspers' work, and of its significance for psychiatry, is provided by our first contributor, the Australian psychiatrist Russell Meares. In an account that draws deeply on art and literature as well as philosophy, Meares charts the shifting *Zeitgeist* of the twentieth century against

---

[2]A number of edited books have made important contributions to the modern development of philosophy of psychiatry, including *Psychopathology and Philosophy* (Spitzer *et al.* 1988), *Philosophy and Psychopathology* (Spitzer and Maher 1990), *Phenomenology, Language and Schizophrenia* (Spitzer *et al.* 1992), *Philosophy, Psychology and Psychiatry* (Phillips Griffith 1994), *Exploring The Self* (Zahavi 2000), and *Anger and Fury, Philosophy and Psychopathology* (Stanghellini 2000a). Authored volumes that were influential include Flew (1973), Glover (1988), Wilkes (1988), Fulford (1989), Hundert (1989), and Reznek (1991).

[3]A commitment to the 'brain disease' model is, of course, itself an expression of what at base is a *philosophical* commitment, grounded in (unexpressed) theories of explanation, causation, etc.

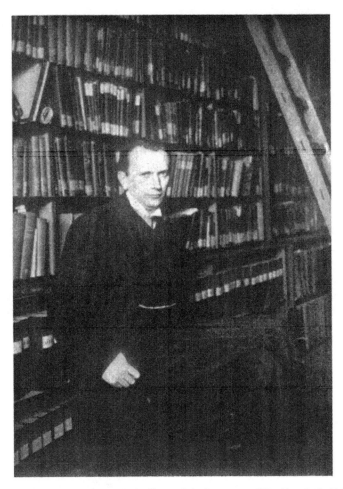

Fig. 1.1 Karl Jaspers as a young man in the library of the Department of Psychiatry in the University of Heidelberg.

which developments in psychology and psychiatry should be understood. We will briefly outline Jaspers' place in the modern history of psychiatry and then return to Meares' cultural insights.

Jaspers has a central place in the development of psychiatry. As a young doctor in Heidelberg in the early 1900s, he was at the centre of a revolution in biological psychiatry no less radical than our own. This period, with advances in neuropathology and discoveries such as neurosyphilis and Alzheimer's disease, has become known by analogy with the present period, as psychiatry's 'first biological phase'. As a philosopher, though, Jaspers was perhaps more aware than many of his colleagues of the danger of biology collapsing to biologism. Thus, in 1913, he published two seminal papers, one arguing for attention to meanings as well as causes in psychopathology (Jaspers 1913a),[4] and the other for the role of phenomenology as a rigorous 'science' of subjective experience to stand alongside the empirical sciences employed in the study of the brain (Jaspers 1913b). These papers were the foundation for the first edition of his *Allgemeine Psychopathologie* (Jaspers 1912), or *General Psychopathology*, which, through several subsequent editions, was to become the basis of the psychopathology used in all areas of psychiatry right up to the present day.

Psychiatry, though, in building on Jaspers' work, has cherry-picked. It has run with the empirical science in his psychopathology while neglecting the phenomenology; it has run with causes while neglecting meanings. And Meares' shows us why. For, as he describes in the first part of his article, 1913 — the very year of Jaspers' seminal publications — was also the year in which the American psychologist, John Watson, published his behaviourist manifesto.[5] It was the year, too, in which the first 'Model T' rolled off the production lines in Henry Ford's Detroit. In literature and in philosophy, in art and in architecture, as Meares' illustrates, 1913 was the year in which Western culture underwent a subtle but ultimately seismic shift from a concern with what Meares (Chapter 2) calls 'personal being', the rich and varied content of subjective experience, to a machine-dominated view of human beings — spare, objective, and impersonal.

Small wonder, then, that in psychiatry, even psychoanalysis, although ostensibly concerned with meanings, consolidated on Freud's machine model of the psyche, 'laborious and clanking' (Chapter 2, p. 48); small wonder that descriptive categories of mental disorder were to triumph over Adolf Meyer's psychobiology of the individual; small wonder that British empiricism, building on the now well-established (if disputed) disease model of mental disorder through the Maudsley 'school' and the Institute of Psychiatry, was to pave the way for post-Second World War positivism in Anglo-American psychiatry; small wonder that the World Health Organization (WHO)'s ICD-8 (WHO, 1967), following Stengel's recommendations (see below), moved decisively to a descriptive (symptom based) classification, which, in turn, through ICD-9 (WHO, 1978) and the introduction of 'operational' criteria in DSM-III (American Psychiatric Association, 1980), developed into the current ICD-10 (WHO, 1992) and DSM-IV (American Psychiatric Association, 1994) classifications; small wonder that the descriptive categories in these classifications

---

[4]In this, Jaspers represents a link in a long chain of champions battling the reductive tendencies of medicine and biology. This chain reaches back at least to Goethe, whose *Farben Lehre* declares that the Newtonian theory of light explains everything except *what we see*! It includes many significant figures in the German movement — Fichte and Hegel to mention only two. Within psychiatry, though, it is above all Jaspers who maintains the importance of meanings in psychopathology while at the same time recognizing the importance of causal explanations.

[5]The Manifesto aimed to liberate psychology from biologism as well as metaphysics.

were envisaged as a preliminary to the identification of causal 'disease categories', the psychiatric equivalents of the causal disease categories of such
medical disciplines as gastroenterology and cardiology; small wonder that the
early successes of drug treatments in the 1950s and 1960s (lithium, the anti-
depressants, and the neuroleptics) were hailed as proving the precedence of
this 'medical' model; and small wonder, finally, that with the emergence of the
'new' neurosciences in the late 1980s, it seemed to many psychiatrists that
with the coming 'decade of the brain', psychiatry would finally become, as the
American philosopher of science, Christopher Boorse (1975), anticipated, a
branch of applied biological science no different in principle from any other
area of medicine.

There are exceptions to this overview, of course. In a number of European
countries, in particular,[6] the distaff side (as it had become) of Jaspers' psychopathology was energetically sustained. Consistent with Meares' general
thesis that psychology reflects culture, this was especially so in countries
where philosophers held out most strongly against positivism, notably
Germany (Straus, K. Schneider, von Gebsattel, von Weizsaeker, Tellenbach
and more recently Blankerburg, Kraus, and Mundt), France (Minkowski,
Ey, Tatossian, Lanteri–Laura), Italy (Cargnello, Barison, Callieri and more
recently A. Ballerini and Borgna), and Switzerland (Binswanger, Wyrsch
Kuhn, Boss).[7] In these countries, contrary to the tide of Anglo-American analytical philosophy, phenomenology, along with existentialism and hermeneutics, continued to thrive — so much so that these disciplines became known,
collectively, as 'Continental Philosophy'.[8] Thus, in Germany in the 1920s and
1930s, even as Kurt Schneider was delineating his descriptive 'first rank'
symptoms of schizophrenia (which were to become the basis of our current
descriptive diagnostic criteria), and emphasizing the precedence of statistical
over ideal norms for psychiatric science (paving the way for reliably identifiable symptoms and syndromes), the 'Heidelberger Schule' (see Mundt 1992)
maintained the flame of phenomenology in psychopathology, a flame that
indeed burns bright in the modern renaissance of philosophical psychopathology. In France, similarly, psychoanalysis took a very different direction
from its counterparts in Britain and America, through the work of Jean-Paul
Sartre, Jaques Lacan, and the group founded by Eugène Minkowski, L'Evolution
Psychiatrique, culminating in Paul Ricoeur's scholarly reframing of the
subject essentially as a hermeneutic (meaning driven) rather than empirical

---

[6]Although also in Japan (Kimura Bin) and in the Americas (Sass, Dörr-Zegers, Schwartz,
Wiggins, and Rovaletti).

[7]There are important exemplars in other countries, of course, for example in Denmark (Parnas),
England (Laing), Holland (Buytendijk), and Spain (Lopez-Ibor).

[8]The analytical/continental distinction has (rightly) been contested, but it was, and for many
decades of the twentieth century remained, widely adopted in academic philosophy.

discipline (Ricoeur 1970).[9] But these exceptions notwithstanding, empiricism grew in influence in psychiatry through the twentieth century, until, by the 1990s, even in continental Europe the final triumph of 'biological psychiatry' seemed secure.

And then along came the renaissance in philosophy of psychiatry! Exactly how and why this happened is a history still to be explained. Meares' account of how psychology and psychiatry follow the *Zeitgeist* of the time is clearly relevant. There is current concern, in psychiatry's second biological phase as in its first, that biological psychiatry, understood in the image of brain imaging as *brain* psychiatry, and reflecting widespread fears about the impact of science and technology in our society, is at risk of a dehumanizing reduction of experience to brain processes. There is a renewed fear, similarly, that reductionist and statistical modes of impersonal enquiry will eclipse idiographical approaches that are centred on the lived experience of individuals. To this extent, then, as with psychiatry's first *philosophical* phase, as it were, so with its second. But what of the future? The new philosophy of psychiatry is more widely based than in Jaspers' day. But even so, will it go the same way?

There are differences between Jaspers' time and our own, which, we will suggest in the remainder of this introductory chapter, amount to a strong case for believing that the new philosophy of psychiatry is no blip, still less a back-sliding, but a permanent and positive shift in the intellectual climate of psychiatry.

A new kind of philosophy

Philosophy constantly reconceives its own aims; one might almost say (para-phrasing Heidegger) that philosophy is the discipline whose being is such that its being is always in question. In Jaspers' time, at the beginning of the twentieth century, philosophy was widely understood to be concerned with foundations.[10]

---

[9]We neglect here, of course, in this overview, the work of many significant figures, such as Taine, Binet, and Janet.

[10]Descartes is popularly viewed as a paradigm 'foundationalist', seeking the foundations of knowledge in what he called 'clear and distinct perception'. Recent scholarship throws this conception into serious doubt. First, it presents him as primarily focused on epistemology (what is knowledge? what can be known? etc.), when he saw his own focus as 'first philosophy' or metaphysics (what is there? what is the essence of the things which exist? etc.), as the title of his most famous work, *Meditations on First Philosophy*, stresses (see, for example, Garber 1992; Baker and Morris, forthcoming). Second, foundationalism is usually understood as the attempt to build all knowledge on ground-level, axiomatic *beliefs*; although Descartes famously employs a metaphor of 'the foundations of a building' in his *Meditations*, it is not at all to be understood in this way. The issue he addresses is which cognitive faculty, the senses or the intellect, is the most reliable, and his target is certain bad *habits* of forming judgements — bad *because* they give preference to the less reliable cognitive faculty. This bears little resemblance to what is today called 'foundationalism', and modern critiques of foundationalism seem irrelevant to *his* conception. See Baker and Morris (forthcoming).

Gottlob Frege's *The Foundations of Arithmetic* was hugely influential; so too was the monumental work of the English philosophers Bertrand Russell and A. N. Whitehead, *Principia Mathematica*, which sought to establish a secure foundation for mathematics in logic. Jaspers, working as a philosopher at this time, had similar objectives. In seeking to define the boundary between the realm of causes and that of meanings, and to distinguish between explanation (the method of natural science), interpretation (the method of psychoanalysis and hermeneutical disciplines), and understanding (the method of phenomenological psychopathology), Jaspers sought to provide a secure foundation for psychopathology.[11,12]

By the end of the twentieth century, few philosophers saw their own enterprise as foundational, although there remained little consensus on how that enterprise *is* to be conceived. A pivotal figure in this twentieth century shift was the Austrian-born Cambridge philosopher, Ludwig Wittgenstein.[13,14] Wittgenstein's idiosyncratic, aphoristic style has meant that there is a multiplicity of

---

[11]Recent attempts to combine these different methods and their corresponding disciplines have had the express aim of developing phenomenological psychopathology as an empirical science (see Sadler 1992; Stanghellini and Mundt 1997).

[12]The term 'psychopathology' has many meanings that cover a multitude of empirical and theoretical approaches (Berrios 1989, 1992). In psychiatry, the term generally refers to the precise description of psychiatric symptoms. This 'descriptive psychopathology' emphasizes the exact naming of experiences and behaviours elicited by the psychiatric examination. In the United States, the tradition rooted in William James, Morton Prince, and Adolf Meyer defined 'psychopathology' as the 'scientific study of abnormal behaviour', establishing a clear parallel between psychopathology and psychiatry, and neuropathology and neurology. In this perspective psychopathology, having no prevailing interpretative paradigm, had a clear aetiological purpose and was also much involved with diagnostic classification. In continental Europe, psychopathology, rooted in Jaspers' work, has developed as the discipline that (1) isolates mental phenomena, and (2) classifies groups of phenomena according to their phenomenological affinities. This builds on Jaspers' view that phenomenology is equivalent to empathic understanding, and that its purpose is to gather *subjective* mental phenomena and to distinguish and rank them according to *semantic* categories. Jaspers' project of developing a 'conceptual, communicable and systematic thought' is aimed at making psychopathology the *common language* of psychiatry (Rossi Monti and Stanghellini 1996). In this regard, most authors consider Jaspers to have been influenced mainly by Husserl's project of establishing a rigorous discipline dealing with subjective phenomena (see the debate in *Philosophy, Psychiatry, and Psychology,* Walker 1994*a,b*, 1995*a,b*; Wiggins and Schwartz 1995). Jaspers' categories also reflect Weber's concept of *ideal types* as heuristic devices that 'create a conceptual order that, when imposed on reality, merely permits inquiry to begin' (Rossi Monti and Stanghellini 1996).

[13]For an authoritative biography, see Monk (1990).

[14]The Austrian logician, Kurt Gödel, was also influential. Gödel's theorems, as they are now called, showed that any system of mathematics sufficiently complex to allow the basic procedures of addition, subtraction, multiplication, and division will contain within itself statements that are fully meaningful within that system, and yet the truth or falsehood of which can be decided only within a more complex system; but this more complex system will in turn contain Gödel-undecidable statements; and so on, *ad infinitum*. Even mathematics, then, contrary to the Russell and Whitehead project (above), cannot be completed. And if mathematics cannot be completed, it might be held, what chance philosophy? (although, of course, the inference can be resisted).

interpretations of his own philosophical aims and methodology. One consequence of this has been that, although few late twentieth-century and early twenty-first century philosophers can claim to be wholly uninfluenced by him, even self-styled 'Wittgensteinians' may disagree fundamentally with one another.

Wittgenstein's methodology is standardly viewed as one of 'dissolving' philosophical problems by clearing up conceptual confusions, this being accomplished by reminding philosophers of the ordinary use of words. Thus understood, Wittgenstein's method has much in common with the so-called 'ordinary-language philosophy' of, for example, Gilbert Ryle and J. L. Austin, whose way of doing philosophy so dominated Oxford in the middle of the century that it became known as 'Oxford philosophy' or 'the Oxford school'. Austin's *tour de force, Sense and Sensibilia*, for example, tackled the Argument from Illusion. This argument began from the idea that many 'appearances' are 'delusory' (e.g. straight sticks that appear to be bent in water), and argued that we must be seeing *something* in such cases that has the properties it appears to have. These things were called 'sense-data' (or 'sensibilia'). Thus, in the case described, what we were seeing was an immaterial sense-datum that really was bent. Some versions of the argument concluded that even in 'non-delusory' perception we must also be seeing 'sense-data', distinct from 'material objects'. Against this apparently bizarre conclusion, Austin marshalled the forces of ordinary language, reminding us of the ordinary use of such expressions as 'seems', 'looks', 'appears', 'illusion', and 'delusion'. If we use words correctly, he suggested, we will not be tempted to assent to the Argument from Illusion.[15]

The standard reading of Wittgenstein often goes along with a picture of the philosopher as a kind of police officer, patrolling the borders between between 'what we do say' (= 'sense') and 'what we don't say' (= 'nonsense') and arresting philosophers — and others — who transgress 'the bounds of sense'.[16] Our next two contributors respond to this view in two very different ways. Gordon Baker argues that Wittgenstein sees himself less as a policeman than as

---

[15]Ordinary-language philosophy, to the extent that it encourages careful attention to language use as a guide to meanings, has a wide range of applications in psychiatry (Fulford 1990). Combined with empirical methods derived from the social sciences, it has been used to characterize the often very different models of disorder implicit in the perspectives of different stakeholders in mental health: users, carers, nurses, doctors, social workers, etc. With renewed interest in the importance of diversity of values in mental health, ideas and examples derived from Oxford analytical philosophers such as R. M. Hare (in, for example, his *The Language of Morals*; Hare 1952) are finding their way into practical training programmes for healthcare professionals, including social workers and psychiatric nurses, working in such challenging areas as assertive outreach (Fulford *et al.* 2002).

[16]The English philosopher, Mary Midgley (1996), writes of the modern philosopher, at least in her connections with practice, as being somewhat like a plumber. Our concepts, then, in the terms of this metaphor, are the pipes and taps and washers of the plumbing in our houses. As such, they remain largely unnoticed so long as they remain problem-free. DIY is an option when things go wrong, but at some stage we may need to call in the plumber — a skilled artisan with a bag of specialized tools — if we are to avoid flooding the sitting room!

a psychotherapist attempting to cure individuals of their mental unease, and that concomitantly what matters is not *that* someone says something that we would not ordinarily say, but what *motivates* him to do so (and there may be perfectly non-pathological reasons). Eric Matthews challenges, not so much the standard reading of Wittgenstein, as the efficacy of the methodology thus conceived. He argues that so-called conceptual confusions may, in a sense, reflect confusions or ambiguities in the reality to which the concepts refer, so that 'clearing up conceptual confusions' leaves the real problem untouched.

Wittgenstein certainly draws analogies between his own philosophical method and psychoanalysis, although they are seldom taken fully seriously; philosophers are deeply reluctant to give up the idea that philosophy is in the business of discovering truths, even if the truths it is now supposed to discover are more mundane than those of earlier generations. Gordon Baker (Chapter 3), drawing on previously unpublished materials from Wittgenstein's *Diktat für Schlick*, spells out the analogies in detail. A philosopher, like a patient undergoing psychoanalysis, may feel *driven* to say things that are odd or bizarre (e.g. Heidegger's 'Das Nicht nichtet', 'Nothing noths'); he cannot but be aware of the oddity of what he feels driven to say. Indeed, he is in a state of *conflict*: whatever it is that drives him to say the strange thing he wants to say makes him think that it *must* be like that, but his awareness of its strangeness makes him think that it *can't* be like that. Consequently, he is not to be 'cured' merely by having the oddity pointed out to him, as the standard interpretation would seem to presuppose — he knows full well that it is odd! What is required is therapeutic help in uncovering the *unconscious motives* that drive him to say such strange things, and a criterion for their being *his* motives is his own *acknowledgement*, once *resistance* is overcome. Very often the 'motive' is the unconscious adoption of a picture or analogy. It is *not* that these pictures or analogies are 'wrong' or 'false' (how, indeed, *could* a picture or an analogy be 'false'?). It is that, because they operate unconsciously, the philosopher is unable to recognize that they are *only* pictures or analogies, i.e. ways of looking at things to which there are alternatives. If he recognized that there are alternatives, they would be harmless, because he would no longer be *driven* to say the things that he says — and might no longer wish to. The acknowledgement that one has adopted such a picture *as a picture* may require one to be persuaded that there are *other* ways of looking at things.

Baker's target audience here is philosophers, who might find not only that his interpretation of Wittgenstein's method is illuminating, but that it requires them to think afresh about their *own* methods as practising philosophers. Unconscious analogies can easily influence the thinking of other professionals, however, including practising psychotherapists or psychiatrists. If they find themselves feeling the sort of *philosophical* unease that expresses itself as 'It must be like that — but it can't be', they might try to practise Wittgenstein's method on themselves.

This particular way of expressing unease about concepts may not be familiar outside philosophy, but difficulties about concepts, broadly construed, are certainly familiar enough in mental health practice and research. Indeed, as

Eric Matthews (Chapter 4) suggests, psychiatry is unique among medical disciplines in that its central concepts, 'mental illness', 'mental disorder', and so forth, are not only difficult to define (the medical concept of disease is no less difficult[17]), but also problematic in day-to-day use in clinical work and research. Other concepts are causing increasing difficulty in all areas of medicine: 'consent', 'capacity', 'confidentiality', 'risk', and 'best interests', for example, are all increasingly problematic concepts in connection with the new philosophical discipline of bioethics (to which we return in a moment). But it is only in psychiatry that difficulties about concepts in day-to-day practice and research run right through to the very concept of 'disorder' itself.

Matthews tackles a particular aspect of the difficulty attaching to the concept of mental disorder: its equivocal status as between moral (value-laden) and medical (scientific) categories. This is not a new difficulty. Some recent commentators have argued that a medical understanding of 'madness' (the so-called 'medical model' of mental disorder) is a new invention; the French philosopher and historian, Michel Foucault, believed it to be a product of the industrial revolution, driven by the work ethic of the day (Foucault 1973). We shall see later that there are important insights here. However, as the Oxford classicist and philosopher, Anthony Kenny (1969), has argued, the equivocal status of mental disorder in this respect was evident over 2000 years ago in Plato's political and psychological work, *The Republic*. Another of our contributors, Daniel Robinson, in a work of wide-ranging scholarship, has traced the swings between medical and moral constructions of mental disorder as reflected particularly in the fluctuating fortunes of the insanity defence, from classical times to the present day (Robinson 1996). These swings came to a head in the 1960s and 1970s in the so-called 'debate about mental illness'. In this debate moral and medical interpretations became sharply polarized,[18] with a range of other models — psychological, social labelling, family, etc. — strung out between them.[19]

Our difficulty here, Matthews argues, reaches an *impasse*. It is not just that 'mental disorder' is equivocal as between moral and medical interpretations: mental disorder does really have to be understood in *both* ways. This will certainly be a familiar experience for any mental health professional asked to make judgements of responsibility by the courts — and corresponding judgements are

---

[17]Indeed as one of us has shown elsewhere, much of the debate about the concept of mental illness has been driven by disagreements, often unrecognized for what they are, about the meaning of *physical* illness (see Fulford 1989, Chapter 1). And, of course, the concept of physical illness is not *wholly* unproblematic in use: the early debate about concepts of disorder was prompted by difficulties over the use of the concept of disease in respiratory medicine (Campbell *et al.* 1979). The difference, then, in this respect, between mental illness and physical illness, is one of degree rather than kind.

[18]In the work, for example, of Thomas Szasz and R. E. Kendell. Szasz (1960) argued that mental disorders are, really, moral problems; Kendell (1975*a*), by contrast, argued that they are no different in principle from any other kind of medical disease.

[19]See Clare (1979) for an early review and Fulford (1998) for an update. Tyrer and Steinberg (1993) describe the variety of models evident in clinical work. A still valuable collection of canonical articles is found in Caplan *et al.* (1981).

called for daily in all areas of mental health practice in relation to issues of involuntary treatment. In practice, a judgement *has* to be made. This implies, as Matthews describes, an either/or choice. It implies that the person concerned either *is* responsible in law (hence subject to civil or criminal sanction, but also, and crucially, free to choose what is or is not done to them by way of treatment), or they are *not* responsible (hence relieved of legal responsibility, but, by the same token, subject to treatment if necessary against their wishes). Yet this often feels like a false antithesis. No doubt there are instances where a person is clearly not responsible for their actions. But why should a person not be both 'mad and bad'? Moreover, the whole thrust of the 'user empowerment' movement is towards recognizing not merely the responsibility but the authority of people with mental disorders, as being no less than that of people with physical disorders.

The *impasse*, Matthews suggests, arises from mistaken assumptions about the relationship between mind and body. It arises, indeed, from what are widely thought of as 'Cartesian' mistaken assumptions. Cartesianism, as popularly understood, requires us to think of experiences and behaviour as *either* bodily (hence medical/not free) *or* mental (hence moral/free).[20] But this, Matthews says, drawing particularly on the work of the French philosopher, Maurice Merleau-Ponty, is mistaken. Merleau-Ponty's notion of 'embodied experience' allows, instead, for what Matthews describes as a pluralistic view of mental disorder, one in which it encompasses a range of different but related concepts.

The problem, then — and it is a very *practical* problem in this instance — is a philosophical one; to borrow Wittgenstein's term, it is an 'unease' about the concept of mental illness. The origin of this unease, consistently with Baker's interpretation of Wittgenstein, is an underlying but unarticulated picture of the relationship between mind and body. This picture Mathews' analysis suggests, is a dualistic one. The 'cure' for our unease, furthermore, combining Baker's and Matthews' insights, is to recognise that dualism is indeed *only* a picture, and, hence, that there *are* alternatives. And the practical corollary of this conclusion is that there are legitimately *different* models of

---

[20]Again, recent Descartes scholarship would distance Descartes himself from 'Cartesianism' as popularly understood. Experiences, in so far as this term covers, say, feeling pain, seeing light, or feeling heat, may be either 'bodily' or 'mental', because the *terms* 'feeling pain', 'seeing light', and so on are, Descartes held, multiply ambiguous and these meanings are commonly confused in ordinary usage. In one sense, 'feeling pain' refers to something purely bodily, shared by non-rational animals and human beings; in another, it refers to the thought or judgement that one is feeling pain in this animal sense (and hence is purely mental because thoughts are mental); in its usual usage, it confusedly refers to both at once. Note that certain descriptions of 'experience' cannot refer to something purely bodily, because animals cannot coherently be ascribed them, for example 'feeling Weltschmerz', 'seeing a Rembrandt (as a Rembrandt)'. Parallel ambiguities beset 'behaviour': 'moving one's leg' or 'baring one's teeth' may refer to something purely bodily, purely mental (e.g. the judgement that one ought now to move one's leg), or — in its usual, confused usage — both at once. Again, many descriptions of 'behaviour' cannot refer to something purely bodily, such as 'smiling ironically', 'signalling the waiter', and, of course, 'speaking'. See Baker and Morris (1996).

mental disorder, legitimately *different* ways in which a given experience of mental distress and disorder may be understood.

It will be worth pausing on this conclusion for a moment because it illustrates one of the ways in which philosophy is important for modern mental health practice. In the psychiatry/antipsychiatry debate of the 1960s, and 1970s, as we noted earlier, opinion was openly divided between mutually exclusive, often mutually hostile, models — moral, medical, psychological, family, social labelling, and so forth. The position nowadays is that the different models are still there but more implicit than explicit (Fulford, 2000a). The open hostilities of the 1960s and 1970s have thus been replaced with, at best, inexplicable failures of shared decision-making in multi-disciplinary teams (Colombo *et al.*, forthcoming), at worst covert 'turf wars' between different healthcare disciplines.

Baker and Matthews, then, in the new conceptual degrees of freedom they open up for mental health policy and practice, offer us a framework for collaboration rather than competition between models. Where this takes us is, of course, not solely a matter for philosophy. It takes us into the role of communication skills, for example; it makes central the organizational, political and managerial contributions to establishing the processes, at national, local, and clinical levels, that support shared decision-making; it brings in sociology and anthropology; it connects mental health practice with literature and with a range of other resources for helping us to understand the different perspectives that bear on clinical decision-making in our diverse, and often multicultural, communities (Fulford *et al.*, 2002, chapter 1). The Baker/Matthews framework, then, is not sufficient to dissolve, still less resolve, the difficulties associated with the concept of mental disorder in individual cases, but it provides a basis for engaging positively with the range of further knowledge and skills required to act effectively in the complexities of real-life clinical encounters.

This is no minor achievement. In mental health practice, the difficulties associated with the concept of mental disorder are considerable. They amount, indeed, not so much to an unease (Wittgenstein's term) as to a *disease*, in the sense that in many instances difficulties about concepts put mental health practice at risk of becoming highly dysfunctional. Mental health practitioners feel increasingly demoralized by what they and others perceive to be the muddle they are in. This is reinforced by the stigmatizing attitudes of their peers in other healthcare professions, and of the public. Faced, then, not only with all the burdens of clinical overload and the impossible targets of increasingly budget-driven services, mental health practitioners have the added burden of self-perceived failure. The risks of burn-out and demotivation, the difficulties of recruiting and retaining staff, are obvious enough. For users of services, similarly, the consequences are entirely dysfunctional. Demoralized professionals will ill-serve their clients and patients in any area of health care. But in mental health, users of services (patients and carers) share with professionals the burdens of stigmatization, exclusion, and discrimination, generated, in part but importantly, by a failure to distinguish between *deficiencies* in the conceptual structure of psychiatry and plain *difficulties*.

The first and perhaps key step in the 'cure' suggested Wittgenstein's work is thus to see that mental health, far from being deficient, is a good deal more difficult, conceptually speaking, than other areas of health care. 'Cartesian' dualism, even if one thinks it a flawed model of the mind–body relationship, is good enough for the conceptually simple areas of bodily health. In cardiology and gastroenterology, a model of mind and body as distinct substances is sufficient for most clinical purposes. Or, at any rate, it is sufficient so long as the concerns of these disciplines are focused on acute life-threatening situations — such as heart attacks and appendicitis — where bodily interventions are the priority. Even here, dualism is arguably not really a *good* model, for it is a model in which the patient-as-a-person tends to drop out of sight (Fulford 2000*b*).

But in mental health, the pathology is by definition 'in the mind'. Hence there is no possibility, in mental health practice and research, of hiding behind naive dualism. The hegemony of physical medicine, however, has meant that those working in mental health have sought to resolve their difficulties by identifying with the traditional 'medical' model. But this, we can now see, is like taking a set of carpenter's chisels to do neurosurgery. A set of concepts that works well enough in the conceptually simple areas of bodily medicine will not be fine enough for the conceptually more demanding work required in mental health. Hence we should understand the frustration of those working in mental health as arising, not simply from an unarticulated model, but from the fact that this model works well enough in areas of health care that in the public (and indeed professional) estimate are taken to be paradigmatic.

In mental health, then, rendering our difficulties about the concept of mental illness harmless really could be part of curing the ills experienced by those concerned practically with mental health. Just the recognition that we — professionals and users alike — are not deficient in finding our subject difficult involves a critical paradigm shift. Our subject really *is* conceptually more difficult than areas such as cardiology and gastroenterology.

But there is a further and still more positive twist to the practical implications of the Baker/Matthews account: it shows, not merely that mental health is more *difficult* (rather than deficient) compared with other areas of health care, but that, once the difficulties are articulated, in tackling them we are tackling issues that, although more deeply hidden, are indeed important for all areas of health care. There are reasons for believing, moreover, that the importance of these conceptual issues in all areas of medicine will increase, rather than decrease, with future advances in the medical sciences. And, if this is right, then psychiatry, in tackling these difficulties, is leading the way for all other areas of health care in twenty-first century medicine.

The arguments supporting this 'psychiatry first' interpretation of the role of philosophy in medicine have been set out by one of us in detail elsewhere (Fulford 2000*a* and *c*). These arguments turn centrally on the point that science opens up choices. For much of the twentieth century, medical science focused on acute life-threatening situations in which the problems were, largely, empirical rather than conceptual. Such problems will remain important clinically, of course, but as science advances so the range and kinds of problem with which medicine is concerned will become ever wider. Reproductive medicine is a case in point. Even 20 years ago, reproductive medicine was concerned almost entirely with conditions, like infertility, spontaneous abortion, and so forth, where the problems, from a medical point of view, are primarily empirical. But recent advances in 'assisted reproduction' have opened up a range of choices — about gamete donation, foetal selection, and so forth — in which the key clinical variables involve, as they have always involved in mental health, such *conceptually* difficult areas as emotion, desire, volition and belief. Again, empirical considerations will remain important. But in reproductive medicine, and eventually in all other medical disciplines, the new choices made possible by advances in medical science mean that conceptual issues will become increasingly important as well.

Mental health, then, once the origins of its conceptual 'unease' are identified in an overly restrictive underlying conceptual model, and once this model is rendered harmless by the extra conceptual degrees of freedom opened up by Baker's and Matthews' interpretations of Wittgenstein, emerges, not merely on an equal footing with supposedly more 'scientific' areas of bodily medicine, but as leading the medical field.

A new kind of ethics

A first change, then, in philosophy, between the beginning and the end of the twentieth century, supporting our belief that psychiatry's second philosophical phase will not go the way of its first, is the shift in the aims of philosophy from the search for foundations to the more modest objective of tackling conceptual difficulties. As we have seen, this objective connects directly with the practical difficulties faced by those at the clinical, managerial, and research coal-faces — professionals and users of services alike. To this extent, then, the new philosophy of psychiatry, just in being a *philosophy*, connects directly with the concerns of practice.

A second change in philosophy, speaking to the likelihood that the new philosophy of psychiatry is no blip, is the growth in importance, over the last quarter of the twentieth century, of what has become known as bioethics. The British philosopher, Bernard Williams, has reminded us that there is a good deal more to ethics than, just, philosophy (Williams 1985). But, to the extent that bioethics is a philosophical discipline, it is perhaps the premier case-in-point of the re-engagement of philosophy with practical disciplines over this period.[21] We return to this re-engagement, and to what it means for the future of philosophy of psychiatry, towards the end of this introductory chapter. For

---

[21]For, of course, philosophy of psychiatry is not alone in this respect. It follows the philosophy of physics, the philosophy of psychology, and so forth (see Fulford 1995).

the present, it is enough to note that this is one area, at least, where a new connection between philosophy and practice shows no sign of running out of steam. To the contrary, bioethics emerged originally (in the 1960s) in direct response to the growing power of medical technology (Fulford *et al.* 2002); and the need for ethical debate and reflection, and for a framework of ethical regulation complementing that of law, has continued to expand even as medical technology has continued to expand.

Psychiatry has been a relative latecomer to bioethics (Fulford and Hope 1993).[22] Given that technology has been the main driver of bioethics, this may at first glance seem not too surprising. But there were, after all, technological issues in psychiatry over the period when bioethics was starting up. Indeed, in the debate about mental illness (noted above), which was running in parallel with the emergence of bioethics, many of those ranged against the medical model were concerned precisely by the growing power of high-tech interventions in psychiatry: new drugs, electroconvulsive therapy, and even neurosurgical interventions. So psychiatry had its own range of technology-driven ethical issues. And, to the extent that ethical issues are at lease as pervasive, and in some respects deeper, in psychiatry than in other areas of health care, it turns out to be very surprising indeed that psychiatry was for so long neglected by bioethics (Dickenson and Fulford 2000).

So why was psychiatry neglected? One reason, we believe, is that the ethical problems arising in psychiatry are in general a lot more difficult than in other areas of health care. This is because the problems with which psychiatric ethics is concerned arise in part from, and indeed are an aspect of, the conceptual difficulties, noted above, by which psychiatry itself is characterized. In respect of these difficulties, one might say, psychiatric ethics often starts where bioethics stops. Consider involuntary treatment, for example. In other areas of health care, involuntary treatment of a fully conscious adult and in their own interests, rather than for the protection of others, is prohibited. This is because in such cases the patient, however unwise their refusal of treatment may appear to the practitioners concerned, is assumed to be rational and hence capable of choosing for themselves. But it is precisely the rationality, or otherwise, of the patient that is at the heart of the ethical dilemmas raised by involuntary treatment in psychiatry. These dilemmas thus import into psychiatry, at

---

[22]Trail-blazing volumes on psychiatric ethics included *Psychiatric Ethics* (Bloch and Chodoff 1981) and *Law and Psychiatry: Rethinking the Relationship* (Moore 1984). Sidney Bloch was one of the founders of the Philosophy Group in the Royal College of Psychiatrists; now at Melbourne University, he was at the time a lecturer in the Department of Psychiatry in Oxford. *Psychiatric Ethics* is currently in its third edition as Bloch *et al.* (1999). See also a sister volume to *Psychiatric Ethics*, in the form of a case book with philosophical analyses and practitioner commentaries (Dickenson and Fulford 2000). For other materials, including review articles on ethical issues in psychiatry, see in particular *Philosophy, Psychiatry, and Psychology* and the *History and Philosophy Section* of *Current Opinion in Psychiatry*. Volume 16(5) of *Bioethics* (September, 2002) is a special issue on psychiatric ethics.

the very cutting edge of practice, the whole range of deep conceptual issues explored in philosophical work on the nature of rationality.[23]

For ethical difficulty, then, in psychiatry, read (in part) conceptual difficulty. And for psychiatric ethics, correspondingly, read (in part) a philosophically turbo-charged bioethics.[24] Our next two contributors, Daniel Robinson (introduced above) and the Dutch husband and wife team, Guy Widdershoven and Ineke Widdershoven-Heerding, illustrate the value of this philosophical turbo-charging respectively for policy and for practice in mental health.

Robinson (Chapter 5) draws on his work on the meaning of citizenship to tackle an issue of perennial importance in psychiatry: the boundary between (medical) care and (social) coercion, between psychiatry's role as a medical discipline, concerned with treating patients with mental disorders, and its role as an agent of society concerned with controlling deviance. Much has been written on this issue. It is, indeed, an aspect of the equivocal status of mental disorders, as between moral and medical categories, discussed by Matthews. Robinson approaches it by the novel route of comparing and contrasting the roles of therapy and law. Adopting a broadly Aristotelian approach, he argues for citizenship as a condition of flourishing. But citizenship does not mean conformity. To the contrary, he argues, by the test of history, citizens flourish where '. . . law is part of a larger political context respectful of the dignity of the person' (Chapter 5, p. 95); and *authentic* respect is '. . . measured by the degree to which the individual person is valued, even at the expense of the wishes of the collective . . .' (p. 96).

Robinson is perhaps uniquely qualified to warn of the dangers of the erosion of the principle of respect for individual persons by a biologistic psychiatry in which causes are allowed to eclipse meanings. As a psychologist, he has contributed many papers to the cannon of scientific approaches to understanding human experience and behaviour. As a historian and philosopher, and the author of a major book on the insanity defence (Robinson 1996), he is all too well aware of the dangers of converting the citizen into a patient. Robinson, however, is not among those who argue that there is no place for therapy. To the contrary, he follows no less a libertarian than the nineteenth century British philosopher, John Stuart Mill, in including people with mental disorders among those who may need help to protect both themselves and others.[25] But the role

---

[23]See, for example, Beauchamp and Childress (1989) for a careful treatment of these issues in a 'classic' of bioethics; see also Gardner (1993) and Hinshelwood (1995, 1997) for work by a philosopher and psychiatrist respectively. Some of the deepest philosophical problems about rationality in relation to the ethical issues raised by involuntary psychiatric treatment are connected with the psychopathological concept of delusion (see Fulford 1989, Chapter 10).

[24]See Dickenson and Fulford (2000, Chapter 1) for a more detailed account of the special features of psychiatric ethics.

[25]John Stuart Mill, 1806–1873, British moral philosopher and philosopher of science; argued for utilitarianism ('the greatest good of the greatest number') and developed much of the political philosophy underpinning modern democratic forms of government. In his *On Liberty*, published in London in 1859, Mill included (by implication) people with mental disorders among those whose liberty might sometimes be curtailed for their own good or the good of society.

of therapy and law alike, Robinson argues, must always be to enlarge '. . . the possibilities for what is finally the good in life' (Chapter 5, p. 95).

The potential abuse of psychiatry for purposes of social control is a concern in the UK at the present time. Notoriously, such abuses occurred in the former Soviet Union, where tens of thousands of political dissidents were diagnosed as 'suffering' from 'delusions of reformism' and 'treated' in mental hospitals (Bloch and Reddaway 1997). There is current concern about similar political abuses developing in China (Human Rights Watch 2002). But, in the UK, a proposed new Mental Health Act, if it is enacted, risks making dangerousness the responsibility of mental health professionals.[26] Ostensibly, the proposed legislation is limited to those cases where dangerousness is or is a consequence of a mental disorder. However, the disorder in question is defined in the draft legislation by reference to dangerous behaviour or the propensity for such behaviour. Dangerousness, therefore, as conceived within this legislation, is equated with mental disorder, much as, in the former USSR, political dissidence was equated with psychosis. The 'disease of dangerousness', indeed, was dignified in an early draft of the legislation by an acronym, DSPD — or dangerously severe personality disorder.

The aim of the proposed legislation is not to make psychiatry an agent of the State, but all the hazards identified by Robinson are evident here: a lowering of the barriers against abuse (some of the protections afforded individuals in current legislation are being watered down or dropped); an aura of friendly persuasion (there has been much talk of it being in the interests of the persons concerned to accept 'treatment'); and the extension of powers of coercion to what Robinson calls 'prior restraint', the power (even the obligation) on the part of health professionals to intervene where there is no more than a risk of dangerous behaviour (i.e. whether or not such behaviour has actually been displayed).

Where Robinson's chapter is relevant particularly at the level of policy, the next chapter (Chapter 6), by Widdershoven and Widdershoven-Heerding, brings us back to the day-to-day concerns of clinical practice. Widdershoven (a philosopher and social scientist) and Widdershoven-Heerding (a philosopher and historian of medicine) start from a case history illustrating the problems raised by the sometimes strange utterances and behaviours of people with dementia. In interpreting such strangeness, they suggest, hermeneutics offers a third way between the Jaspersian alternatives of explanation and understanding. Explanation discounts it: strange utterances and behaviour are assumed to be caused by

---

[26]Part II of the proposed new Mental Health Act is concerned with people with mental disorders who pose a risk of harm to themselves or others (this expanded category replaced what in the White Paper that preceded the bill, was called Dangerously Severe Personality Disorder, or DSPD). The intention of this legislation is to ensure that people who are at risk of harming themselves or others are offered help by psychiatric services. However, taken with new powers of compulsion introduced in the generic Part I of the legislation, many are concerned that the effect of Part II, if the legislation is introduced in its present form, will be to equate risk of harm with mental disorder and to make mental health professionals responsible for 'treating' it.

pathological changes (by neurofibrillary tangles and plaques) in the person's brain, and, hence, to be no more meaningful than the 'fizz' of electrical interference on the radio. Understanding, by contrast, takes strangeness *too* seriously: in starting from an assumption of meaningfulness, it seeks an interpretation of strange utterances and behaviours relative to the patient's subjective world.

Hermeneutics, Widdershoven and Widdershoven-Heerding's third way, offers what they call a 'dialogical' approach. Derived from the work of the German philosopher, Hans-George Gadamer, the dialogical approach takes strangeness to be a wake-up call of the need for a new or wider perspective. Then, instead of 'waving away the perspective of the person with dementia as irrelevant (as happens in the explanatory approach), or of treating it as the only relevant point of view (as in the interpretative approach), the hermeneutic approach claims that the confrontation of perspectives may lead to a new and better (shared) perspective' (Chapter 6, p. 106).

Hermeneutics, as Widdershoven and Widdershoven-Heerding go on to show, is not in itself enough to achieve this. Skills of good communication are required to understand and to balance the often very different perspectives of those concerned — the patient, informal carers, and professionals. This, in turn, depends on what Aristotle called *phronesis*: practical wisdom achieved through work-based learning. Like Robinson, then, Widdershoven and Widdershoven-Heerding find an Aristotelian concept apt to the requirements of good clinical practice.[27] But the key step, the adoption of a mind-set that is learning ready for new interpretive possibilities, a mind-set that in Robinson's terms could be said to be constantly ready to widen the horizons of citizenship, is provided by hermeneutics.

A new kind of psychology

The four contributors to our next section are all concerned with what has become known as the cognitive revolution. Over the last three decades of the twentieth century, psychology, and to a lesser extent neuroscience and Anglo-American philosophy of mind, rediscovered meanings. We say *re*discovered, because of course this process has been the reverse of the behaviourist denial of meanings, from about 1913, described by Meares (Chapter 2). Behaviourism sought to delete meanings from psychology.[28] The cognitive revolution has brought them back.[29]

---

[27]The moral philosopher, Bernard Williams, was among the first to point practical ethics back to the riches of pre-Christian philosophy (Williams 1985). A number of authors have started to explore these riches in connection with psychiatry (see, for example, Megone 1998; Nordenfelt 1997).

[28]Or at any rate to ground them in what Daniel Robinson has called their 'behavioural instantiations' (D. Robinson, personal communication).

[29]For a philosophical review of cognitivism in psychology and the sciences, see Bechtel, Abramson, and Graham, 1998. For an account of cognition in the philosophy of mind, see Thornton, 1998, Chapter 1.

Psychiatry, perhaps because of the continuing influence of the medical model (see above), has been somewhat slow to join the cognitive revolution, although the influence of the revolution on psychiatry is evident (if in no other ways) in the recent spread of cognitive–behavioural therapies (CBTs). CBTs differ from behaviour therapies just in starting from personal meanings, from the values and beliefs, of the persons concerned. The Cs in CBTs, then, just are the meanings that behaviourism sought to abolish.[30]

Derek Bolton (Chapter 7), formerly a lecturer in philosophy and now Professor of Philosophy and Psychopathology and Head of Clinical Psychology at the Institute of Psychiatry in London, opens his chapter with a masterly overview of the connections between the cognitive revolution and Jaspers' work. Jaspers' psychopathology, as Bolton describes, did not come out of the blue. It built on nearly a century of debate about whether the human sciences could be pursued with precisely the same methods as the natural sciences. From this debate, the 'Methodenstreit' as it came to be called, Jaspers derived his view that psychopathology, being a human science, had to be concerned with meanings as well as causes, and pursued by the methods of phenomenology as well as empirical science. As described earlier (in relation to Meares' Chapter 2), psychiatry ran with the causal/scientific side of Jaspers' psychopathology. However, the cognitive revolution, understood against the *Methodenstreit* as the back-drop to Jaspers' work, is no more and no less than a return to the other (the meanings) side of Jaspers' agenda.

With a psychiatrist, Jonathan Hill, Bolton has developed a detailed cognitivist model for abnormal psychology and psychiatry (Bolton and Hill 1996). Drawing on ideas from evolutionary biology and developmental psychology as well as philosophy, Bolton and Hill argue that meanings, encoded as information in the brain, may have causal power. In this model, then, meanings *are* a species of cause.[31] That is to say, just as information encoded in a computer can cause things to happen where the computer is wired up to, say, a machine tool or an aeroplane, so meanings encoded as information in a brain can make things happen where the brain is wired up to a body.

In his chapter, Bolton summarizes some of the main features of the Bolton–Hill account, he responds to some of their critics (including Harré and Gillett; see below), and he shows how the model can be applied across a range of psychopathologies. The latter include not only obvious candidates for meaningful explanation, such as post-traumatic stress disorder (PTSD),[32] but also

---

[30]For a detailed guide to these therapies, see Hawton *et al.* (1989).

[31]Bolton and Hill call this 'intentional causation'. Whether meanings can be reduced to causes in this way remains an open question; see, for example, the English philosopher, Tim Thornton (1997), for a careful Wittgensteinian argument against the Bolton and Hill claim that what they call 'intentional causation' bridges the gap between causes and meanings; see also Thornton (1998).

[32]PTSD has, by definition, to be related to events that are perceived as stressful by the person concerned. Theories of PTSD involve the effects of severe stress as destroying the taken-for-granted meaningfulness of the world around us (see Bracken, forthcoming).

psychotic disorders, both functional (schizophrenia) and organic (dementia). Bolton also makes the novel suggestion that, while information is pervasive in biology, the term 'meaning' might be reserved for those biological systems, like our brains, that are capable of second-order thoughts, or thoughts about thoughts. Other authors have suggested that such thoughts are the mark of true consciousness (e.g. Frankfurt 1971). This could be important, particularly for our understanding of psychotic disorders, because a number of key psychotic symptoms are possible only for a being who is capable of second-order thoughts. Thought insertion, for example, a first-person thought that is experienced as the thought of someone else, is impossible except for beings capable of thoughts about their own thoughts.[33]

Rom Harré (Chapter 8), Emeritus Fellow of Linacre College, Oxford, and Adjunct Professor of Psychology at Georgetown University in the States, is one of Bolton and Hill's critics. The basis of his criticism is that the cognitive revolution itself, of which Bolton and Hill are part, has not gone far enough. The rediscovery of meanings in psychology, he has argued (Harré and Gillett 1994), was only the first cognitive revolution. More important has been the discovery — and this really is something new — that meanings are not 'in the head' but interpersonal. Cognitivism in psychology, and indeed in philosophy, conceives of the mind as a series of specialized subsystems. Operating together 'in the head', much as the subsystems of a computer operate, these subsystems produce outputs that are goal-directed and in other ways information-driven. What Harré calls the 'second' cognitive revolution, by contrast, is the discovery that meanings are created, not by inner subsystems within each individual, but discursively, by communications between people.

Harré outlines one of the sources of discursive psychology in Wittgenstein's work on the philosophical 'problem of other minds'. This is the puzzle about how we know, or can even come close to knowing, what is in someone else's mind. It is an important problem for psychiatry, both for its bearing on certain particular kinds of psychopathology, such as autism (see Hobson 1991, 2002), and for its wider significance for a profession that, as Harré points out, claims expertise in knowing what is in other people's minds. Wittgenstein, characteristically, argued that the philosophical problem of other minds arises from a grammatically induced false model. Thus, there is a grammatical similarity between 'he has a pound in his pocket' and 'he has a pain in his foot'. We could learn the meaning of 'a pound', in this context, by looking in his pocket. But, despite the grammatical similarity, there is no corresponding way that we could learn the meaning of the word 'pain'. Wittgenstein's great insight was that, in such cases,

---

[33]See, for example, Stephens and Graham (2000); also a number of articles in a double issue of *Philosophy, Psychaitry, and Psychology*, edited by the Warwick philosopher, Christoph Hoerl (Special issue: On Understanding and Explaining Schizophrenia. *Philosophy, Psychiatry and Psychology*, **8**(2/3): 2001).

there are logically holistic 'public expression–private feeling' complexes, and that we learn the words for experiences via their public expressions.

This somewhat abstract Wittgensteinian point has a rich crop of consequences for psychiatry.[34] In particular, Harré argues, there is now no (philosophical) problem of other minds, for meanings are no longer hidden in a private space behind other people's eyes. They are out there in the public space of discourse. There are no, as Wittgenstein put it, 'private languages'. Combine this relocation of meaning, moreover, as Harré and others have done, with discursive and other kinds of social psychology, and you have a new and powerful set of tools for exploring meanings, both normal and (as in psychopathology) abnormal. Elsewhere, Harré has applied these tools to forensic psychopathology, to the pathological autobiography of a serial killer (Harré 1997), and, with the American psychologist, Steven Sabat, to the problems of communication in Alzheimer's disease (Sabat and Harré 1997). Sabat has since gone on to produce a series of papers culminating in a major book that is rich with practical insights (Sabat 2001). In Chapter 8, Harré is concerned mainly with the theory underpinning discursive psychology. He gives a careful and clear account of Wittgenstein's central insights into the priority of the public over the private space of meaning; he connects this with social psychological concepts, such as 'positioning', in the work particularly of feminist writers on personal identity; and he signals the implications of all this for studies of personal pronoun use in psychopathology (to which we return below; see Chapter 16).

Grant Gillett, a long-term collaborator of Harré,[35] carries the discursive story deeper into psychiatric territory in Chapter 9.[36] Gillett, who did a doctorate in the philosophy of mind with Kathleen Wilkes in Oxford, now holds what we believe is a unique split post between neurosurgery and philosophy, at Otago University in New Zealand. Arguing against Bolton and Hill, he draws, like Harré, on Wittgenstein's demonstration of the priority of public over private, to resist the reduction of meanings to causes. He reminds us of Wittgenstein's example of a game of chess as being, irreducibly, a 'shared project of meaning' (Chapter 9, p. 146). The brain, then, he insists, 'does not provide a level of basicness for psychiatric explanation . . .'. On the contrary '. . . discursive explanation has an epistemically and metaphysically coeval status' (p. 143).

As a neurosurgeon–philosopher, Gillett brings a particular authority to the claim that neurons and synapses cannot be, as it were, the basic atoms of meaning. This is not an antiscientific view, however. It is rather a view of human nature that incorporates culture on an equal basis with biology.

---

[34]Although there are, of course, empirical problems aplenty (e.g. of deception).

[35]See, for example, their book *The Discursive Mind* (Harré and Gillett 1994).

[36]See Gillett (1999) for a full working out of the implications of the discursive approach for psychiatry.

Indeed, Gillett suggests that neural nets provide a 'hard science' model of how cultural processes — discursively created values, beliefs, and meanings — may 'shape . . . the microprocessing structure of the brain . . . ' (Chapter 9, p. 145). Gillett would be the first to warn against over-simple models of the brain, but his point is that Jaspers' insistence on the importance of meanings, alongside causes, and of related concepts such as empathy, are given new and heuristically powerful shape by developments in computing and the neurosciences. He concludes his chapter with an illustrative discursive psychology of anorexia nervosa, showing that cultural processes, including those involved in and among healthcare practitioners, shape not only the content but the form of this condition — and that anorexia nervosa is no less real for that!

Bolton argues that the gap between the first and the second cognitive revolutions is not as wide as the critics of cognitivism — including Harré and Gillett — have suggested. Bolton is surely right that cognitivism has never claimed to put meanings exclusively 'in the head'.[37] Its guiding idea is rather that meanings (whether derived from inside or outside) are *encoded* (as information) in the brain. Our fourth contributor to this section of the book, however, the Austrian psychiatrist Michael Musalek (Chapter 10), shows that the difference of emphasis, if this is all it is, between the first and second cognitive revolutions, between the private and the public spheres of meaning, could still be important for psychopathology. Harré and Gillett illustrate the insights from discursive psychology for overtly meaningful conditions such as psychopathy and anorexia, and for conditions, like dementia, in which we are too ready to discount meanings. Musalek, although writing here in a different philosophical tradition (phenomenology), shows the importance of interpersonal processes for our understanding of delusions, a symptom traditionally regarded, even by Jaspers, as being (in some cases) meaning-less.

Delusions, as Jaspers pointed out, have a central place in psychopathology. Traditionally the hallmark of 'madness', they are identifiable across many cultures and over much of recorded history; they are, furthermore, at least as reliably identifiable as any of the symptoms of physical illness (including 'measurable' signs such as raised blood pressure);[38] and they are the paradigm case both of mental illness as an excuse in law and of the corresponding

---

[37]In philosophy of content the standard distinction is between wide and narrow content where the latter is fixed by what is in the head. Fodor (1981), for example, argues that wide content depends on narrow content plus context.

[38]See Clare (1979) for an early but still relevant review of the evidence on this point.

[39]Although CBT has been well established since the 1970s, it was not until the 1990s that the 'cognitive revolution' really reached the psychoses, and the first randomized controlled trials have appeared only within the last few years. For a recent review of cognitive theories of delusions, see Garety and Freeman (1999); for an excellent overview of contemporary CBT for psychosis, see Morrison (2001); and for an overview of the psychological approach generally to psychosis, see British Psychological Society (2000).

loss of responsibility underpinning involuntary psychiatric treatment. Yet, just as psychiatry has been a late recruit to the cognitive revolution, so delusions, and the psychotic disorders of which they are characteristic, have been late recruits to CBT.[39]

Again, we can see the influence of the medical model at work here. It has seemed to many that the psychoses, unlike, say, anxiety disorders and depression, are good candidates for a straightforwardly causal disease model of mental illness and, correspondingly, for medical (drug) treatment. After all, with the organic psychoses (like dementia), we already know some of the causal processes involved. The similarities, then, between the organic and the functional psychoses such as schizophrenia (in particular their many shared symptoms) suggest that it will not be long, with the tools of modern neuroscience, before we understand the causal processes at work in such conditions. It was for this reason that Thomas Szasz, one of those who since the 1960s has argued most vigorously against the medical model, famously called schizophrenia 'the sacred symbol of psychiatry' (Szasz 1976). And delusion, we might now add in similar vein, is the 'sacred *symptom*' of psychiatry. For delusion, to the extent that it may seem wholly irrational, is readily perceived as what Widdershoven and Widdershoven-Heerding (Chapter 6) call 'fizz', as meaningless interference caused by brain lesions. Even Jaspers, as we noted above, took this line, arguing that with delusion we reach the limit of the comprehensible (also discussed below by Heinimaa in Chapter 14). And recent authors, although acknowledging that the content of delusional beliefs may be meaningful, continue to assume that their form is determined solely by causal (pathological) processes operating in the brain.

Wrong, says Musalek. Causal processes — genetic, biochemical, infective, etc. — may well be involved, but both empirical and phenomenological research suggest that meanings may also be crucial, not only to the content but also to key aspects of the form of delusional beliefs. Consider 'persistence', for example, a key feature of the form of delusional psychopathology. Delusions may persist, often for years, and in the face of apparently incontrovertible evidence and argument against them. In a causal-lesion model, this is taken to be evidence that delusions are the product of a pathological process, driving along out of control. But Musalek shows how the meaning of a delusion for the person concerned may evoke responses in others, verbal and non-verbal, the meanings of which reinforce the delusion, and so on in a vicious cycle.[40] Importantly, these 'pathology maintaining factors', as Musalek calls them, may include the reactions of doctors and other professionals. This is consistent, then, with the otherwise somewhat surprising observation that schizophrenia has a better prognosis in so-called developing countries (i.e. in countries that are more hospitable to psychotic experiences), and with the growing evidence that delusions are indeed modifiable through cognitive–behavioural (meaningful) approaches to management (Gould *et al.* 2001).

---

[40]Delusions of persecution, for example, or of infidelity, may well be self-fulfilling.

Musalek's work, like that of Harré and Gillett, is not, of course, exclusive of the brain. The point is rather that their respective disciplines, phenomenology, and discursive psychology, bring new resources to the scientific study of psychopathology. In the case of delusions, the 'sacred symptom' of psychiatry as we described it above, these resources could be decisive. Cognitivist psychologists, working broadly with a subsystems-inside-the-brain model of meaning, have sought for more than 20 years, without success, to identify one or more components of cognitive functioning (i.e. components of the internal cognitive machinery of the mind) that are characteristically impaired in delusional thinking.[41] But, as one of us has argued elsewhere (Fulford 1989, Chapter 10), the very logical structure of delusions, the variety of forms they take in practice, suggests that delusional thinking is or involves an impairment, not of one or more cognitive *sub*systems, but of practical reasoning — the reasoning that is characteristic of persons *as a whole*.[42] The work of Harré and Gillett, and of Musalek, extends this line of argument. Cognitive psychology, then, seeks delusions in failures of *subsystems* of the brain; the logical forms of delusion suggest that they are located rather in the reasoning of *whole persons*; discursive psychology adds to this the suggestion that such reasoning may be meaningful only in *inter*personal space; and Musalek's *phenomenological and empirical* work on delusions suggests that, at least in some cases, this is indeed so.

A new kind of phenomenology

As empirical psychology rediscovered meanings in the closing years of the twentieth century, so phenomenology rediscovered its links with empiricism. Through much of the twentieth century, phenomenology, despite its central role in the early development of psychology and psychiatry, became increasingly indifferent (and sometimes openly hostile; e.g. Heidegger 1962; Husserl 1970) to the natural sciences. As the science of subjectivity, it came to see itself as antithetical to the sciences of objectivity. This was perhaps a reaction to behaviourism. At all events, as the cognitive revolution has brought meanings back into psychological science, so a new 'naturalized phenomenology' has started to emerge (Petitot *et al.* 2000).

---

[41]For a careful overview, see Garety and Freeman (1999). Philippa Garety, with David Hemsley, came close at one point to identifying a cognitive impairment specific to delusions in their work on probabilistic reasoning. People with delusions, they showed, tended to jump to conclusions, but this turned out to be true only of *some* people with delusions; these subjects, moreover, inconsistently with the *persistence* of delusional beliefs, were equally ready to give up their beliefs (see Hemsley and Garety 1986).

[42]Thus, delusions, like the reasons of practical reasoning, may take the form either of value judgements (positive or negative) or of judgements of fact (true or false). This remarkable match, together with the existence of the paradoxical 'delusion of mental illness', leads to a theory of delusional thinking in which, consistently with the central place of delusion in psychopathology (see above), disturbances of practical reasoning emerge as a central case of the experience of illness generally as loss of agency (Fulford 1989, Chapter 10).

Phenomenology, Katherine Morris reminds us in Chapter 11, the opening chapter in this section, encompasses a number of different subdisciplines. The brain child, originally, of the German philosopher, Edmund Husserl, phenomenology was taken up and developed through the work of several of the major mid-twentieth century philosophers of continental Europe, notably Heidegger, Sartre, Scheler, and Merleau-Ponty. Each of these has contributed, directly or indirectly, to modern phenomenological psychopathology (represented here by Depraz and Kraus; see below). What unites these approaches, though — what makes them all *phenomenological* — is the attempt to identify what Morris calls the 'essence' of an experience, including, centrally, its meaning to the person concerned.[43]

Morris's article illustrates, directly, the value of phenomenology, so defined, as a resource for psychiatry. She draws on the French philosopher and novelist Jean-Paul Sartre's phenomenology of the body to explore the diagnostic concept of 'body dysmorphic disorder' (BDD). Sartre distinguished a number of different ways in which a person's experience of their body may be meaningful to themselves or others. Drawing on these distinctions, Morris shows that many cases of BDD involve a disturbance specifically of what Sartre characterized as the 'lived-body-for-others'. This carefully precise identification, within the Sartrean framework, allows Morris: (1) to distinguish BDD (of this kind, for, as she says, there could be more than one kind) from other kinds of psychopathology involving changes in how one's body is experienced (obsessive–compulsive disorder, hypochondriasis, eating disorders, social phobia, and schizophrenia), and (2) to draw on other Sartrean concepts (invisibility, nausea, alienation, shame, etc.), each with a substantive theoretical content, to characterize further the experience of (this kind of) BDD itself.

Morris's phenomenology of BDD is important practically at a number of levels. It is relevant, first, for classification. As Morris indicates, BDD is categorized as a somatoform disorder in DSM-IV, as a type of hypochondriasis in ICD-10, and as a social phobia in the corresponding Japanese manual. Her

---

[43]There is a sense in which any psychology is concerned with the essence of experience: behaviourism identified the essence in observable behaviours; cognitive science treats mental subsystems as essential; in psychoanalysis the essence is unconscious counterparts of conscious experiences. Phenomenology differs from these in being concerned with the precise description of subjective experience (first-person perspective) as organized around meanings. The 'search for purity' in describing an experience is a priority for phenomenology, and for phenomenological psychopathology (see Parnas and Zahavi 2000). In relation to psychopathology, phenomenology can be thought of as identifying what one of us has called elsewhere 'psychopathological organisers' (Rossi Monti and Stanghellini 1996). These are synthesizing schemes of comprehension aimed at connecting different pathological experiences to a unitary core of meaningfulness. They seek to provide a framework within which common denominators can be identified among the heterogeneous components of pathological experiences. They are complementary to empirically defined categories, (1) in emphasizing validity rather than reliability, (2) in focusing on internal experience rather than behaviours, and (3) in defining specific psychopathological units (e.g. verbal–acoustic hallucinations) rather than nosographical syndromes (e.g. schizophrenia). See also below, Chapter 13, the distinction between phenomena and symptoms in psychopathology.

Sartrean analysis suggests that none of these is wholly appropriate. Of course, classifications in psychiatry, as in other areas of science, are open and contestable. But, as Morris points out, to the extent that psychiatric classification is based on phenomenology, it should be based on *accurate* phenomenology. Then, second, her analysis, particularly in the further characterization it offers of BDD, is important for improved understanding and communication. This in turn is a basis, *inter alia*, for deeper insight into the values and beliefs on which CBT approaches to therapy depend. Third, her analysis could be important for neuroscience research. In such research, precisely because it is concerned with the brain basis of experience and behaviour, it is essential that work on the brain is paired with accurate characterizations of the content of consciousness. As a philosopher, then, Morris derives potentially fruitful ideas about BDD from phenomenology.[44] However, the trade, it is important to add, between phenomenology and psychiatry is not all one way. If phenomenology informs our understanding of BDD, BDD also informs phenomenology; Morris, here, extends Sartre's analysis in two key respects guided by her work on BDD.[45]

The two-way trade between philosophy and psychiatry is further illustrated by the French philosopher and phenomenologist, Natalie Depraz, in her work on schizophrenia (Chapter 12).[46] Like Morris, Depraz examines the experiences of people with schizophrenia primarily from her perspective as a

---

[44]For an example of potentially important insights from Merleau-Ponty's phenomenology for empirical research on dyslexia, see Philpott (1998), with commentaries by Komesaroff and Wiltshire (pp. 21–24), Rippon (pp. 25–28), and Widdershoven (pp. 29–32), and the authors' response to the commentaries (pp. 33–36).

[45]The Oxford philosopher, Kathleen Wilkes (1988), was one of the first to make a detailed case for the importance of psychopathology as a resource for philosophy. This was anticipated by one of the founders of Oxford linguistic philosophy, J. L. Austin (see the end of his key methodological paper; Austin 1956–7), and in the early work of two important contributors to the renaissance in philosophy of psychiatry, Jonathan Glover (1970, 1988) and Stephen Clark (1996), the latter with commentaries by M. Bavidge (pp. 29–30) and T. Sprigge (pp. 31–36). The new MIT Series, Philosophical Psychopathology, edited by Owen Flanagan and George Graham, is premised on the importance of this two-way trade (Graham and Stephens, 1994).

[46]The preliminary step for phenomenological enquiry to begin is 'bracketing' (or suspending) one's preconceptions about a given phenomenon. Preconception in this context refers to our common sense or taken-for-granted knowledge of the world and other people, including scientific knowledge. This preliminary attitude, as it is sometimes called, although imported into psychopathology from the phenomenological tradition (*époché*) and hermeneutics, is also reflected in Wittgenstein's work: 'The difficulty of renouncing all theories: one has to regard what speaks so obviously incomplete as something complete' (*Philosophische Untersuchungen*). To do this in psychopathology, one has to depart from the meaning that both common sense and medical science give to psychopathological phenomena. The difference between symptoms and phenomena in psychopathology is discussed further in Stanghellini (2000*b*). The aim of psychopathological enquiry, disclosed by this attitude, is obtaining a *uebersichtlich Darstellung* (Wittgenstein's term), that is a clear representation and a panoramic view, i.e. seeing phenomena directly as they present to us, connecting them with one another, and obtaining a meaningful whole. Renouncing all theories and obtaining a panoramic view are the cornerstones of the psychopathological enquiry.

philosopher. The main thrust of her argument in this paper is the extent to which a key aspect of schizophrenic experience (*l'époché schizophrénique*) illuminates a key concept of phenomenological philosophy (*l'époché transcendentale*) (see also Stanghellini 1997). The phenomenological method employs empathy with the aim of achieving a clear and complete understanding of a given person's experience. The '*époché*' is the aim of this process — the understanding that comes when prejudice and presupposition have been stripped away[47] and we perceive the phenomenon as the other person perceives it. But can this process ever be completed? Or is the *époché* always beyond our reach (hence transcendental, a guiding ideal rather than an actual or actualisable state)? Depraz argues that the changes in consciousness experienced by people with schizophrenia show the extent to which *époché* is indeed, through *praxis*, achievable.

Depraz's chapter makes a further and important point about the relationship between what might broadly be characterized as Western and Eastern philosophy. Western philosophy, even within the phenomenological tradition, has developed mainly as a theoretical discipline. Eastern philosophy, by contrast, has developed essentially as a *practice*. In the final section of her chapter, Depraz shows how the *praxis* of the *époché*, guided by the experiences of people with schizophrenia, follows, in a number of key respects, the meditative practices of Eastern philosophy, particularly as illustrated by the work of Yuasa (1987) and Yamaguchi (1997).

Eastern philosophy is not highlighted in this introductory volume, but the connection drawn by Depraz through phenomenology and the experience of schizophrenia to meditation suggests possible new approaches, not only to phenomenology, but also to research and treatment in the area of the psychoses. Cognitive–behavioural approaches, in particular, might be complemented by such techniques. Similarly, the positive associations with personal growth and development in Eastern philosophy relate directly to the growing 'recovery movement' in mental health (Ralph 2000). The connections drawn, then, in this area by Depraz, provide a powerful illustration of the potentially rich resources available to research and practice in mental health from an openness to cross-cultural and interdisciplinary perspectives.

Alfred Kraus (Chapter 13) moves the phenomenological agenda on from its relevance for specific syndromes and symptoms to psychiatric classification. Writing from his perspective as a psychiatrist and phenomenologist, he is concerned with the extent to which modern classifications of mental disorders may have sacrificed validity for reliability. He introduces a distinction, which is important for us in thinking about psychopathology, between 'symptom' and 'phenomenon'. Symptoms are what we are familiar with in psychiatry as

---

[47]Through a three-stage process, described by Depraz.

a medical discipline: they are medically relevant general aspects of experience and/or behaviour that are reliably identifiable;[48] they are capable of criterio-logical description (e.g. by explicit inclusion and exclusion criteria, as in DSM); and they carry implications for aetiology, prognosis, and treatment. Phenomena, on the other hand, are individual and personal, in that they are inseparable from the meaning of an experience for the person concerned. As the characteristic 'datum' for phenomenological enquiry in psychopathology, a phenomenon, as Kraus puts it, 'is limited to that which, in our lived experi-ence, is revealed or disclosed by itself without any theoretical presupposi-tions' (Chapter 13, p. 200).[49]

Jaspers, Kraus suggests, despite his skills as a philosopher, failed to maintain the distinction between symptoms and phenomena. His *Allgemeine Psychopathologie*, although ostensibly a product of phenomenological enquiry (and hence about phenomena), is actually more about symptoms. And psychopathology, as we noted in the first section of this chapter, certainly moved strongly in this direction in post-Second World War Western psych-iatry: the WHO moved explicitly to a symptom-based classification with ICD-8; the American Psychiatric Association followed with DSM-III, introducing (under Robert Spitzer's guidance) clear inclusion and exclusion criteria; reliable mental state interview schedules were introduced over this period (such as the PSE[50]); and this whole development was the direct result of recommendations made to the WHO by Stengel (1959) that psychiatry should model itself more firmly on other branches of medical science,[51] recommendations that, in turn, reflected the insights of the American philoso-pher of science, Carl Hempel.[52]

This process has been in many respects salutary. The terminology of psychiatric classification is nowadays considerably more transparent; and the reliability of psychiatric diagnosis is greatly improved. Kraus' point, though,

---

[48]That is, identifiable consistently from one occasion to the next ('test–retest reliability'), and between different observers on the same occasion ('inter-observer reliability').

[49]Recall Depraz's account of the phenomenological method as involving, *inter alia*, 'bracketing' (i.e. the stripping away of preconceptions); see above.

[50]Present State Examination: developed by a group at the Institute of Psychiatry in London, and accompanied by a glossary of terms, the PSE showed that many psychiatric symptoms can be identified clinically with the same degree of reliability as the corresponding symptoms of physical illness. The PSE is published as Wing *et al.* (1974); the glossary to the PSE is a resource of clear definitions of all the main psychiatric symptoms.

[51]Modelling itself on physical medicine, psychiatry aims to develop categories of disorder defined by symptoms, on the basis of which, eventually, causal disease processes would be discovered. This is consistent with Jaspers' (and the phenomenological) approach, but differs from it crucially, as Kraus argues, in emphasis.

[52]Hempel made these recommendations in a paper given originally at a conference convened by Stengel at the request of the WHO, to consider the future of psychiatric classification (Hempel, 1961). It was from this conference that Stengel's decisive report emerged (Stengel 1959). See also Kendell (1975*b*), Fulford (1989, Chapter 9), Fulford (1994), and the introduction to Sadler *et al.* (1994).

is not that we should, somehow, abandon empirical scientific approaches in psychiatry; it is rather that empirical approaches need to be balanced by the phenomenological. We need symptoms, certainly, and we need generalizable criteria; but we also need phenomena, and the personal meanings by which phenomena are (in part) defined. Like Morris, Kraus argues that in letting our approach to psychopathology get out of balance, in focusing on symptoms to the exclusion of phenomena, we have cut ourselves off from a potentially important resource for classification in psychiatry.[53]

Kraus illustrates how attention to phenomena might enrich our classifications with examples from three areas of psychopathology: depression, mania, and hysterical personality disorder. The limitations of our current classifications are evident, however, across a far wider range of problems in psychiatry: the growing rejection of psychiatric categories by users of services (who find that these categories too often fail to make sense in terms of their own experiences); the difficulty experienced by practitioners in 'fitting' their patients to these categories; the managerial misuse of categories (the 'managed care' syndrome of payment-led diagnoses); the lack of connection of our categories with CBT approaches to therapy; the split between 'scientific' and ethical/legal uses of diagnostic categories (the DSM explicitly proscribes the use of its diagnostic categories for legal determinations; American Psychiatric Association 1994, pp. xxiii–xxiv); and, not least, their failure to specify coherent and relevant groups for study in scientific research programmes, including the neurosciences (see Jackson and Fulford 1997, and several articles in Sadler *et al.* 1994).

Kraus, then, reinforces Jaspers' own message — and the message of this book — that in psychiatry meanings as well as causes are essential to good clinical care. As we noted earlier, this message is more, not less, important with advances in neuroscientific understanding, even in supposedly 'causal' conditions such as dementia. We must be careful, though, not to swing the balance too far the other way: instead of throwing out meanings in the pursuit of causes, to end up throwing out causes in the pursuit of meanings. Are there,

---

[53]The difference, then, between phenomenological psychopathology and current approaches to psychiatric classification (or nosography) based on descriptively defined symptoms is, again, one of emphasis. In the phenomenological tradition, diagnosis — as Jaspers wrote — is the last point to be considered in the comprehension of a psychiatric case, because what matters most is that the 'chaos of phenomena' should not be buried under a diagnostic label, but rather 'stand out in an evident way and in multiple connections'. Jaspers thus warned us to beware of a hasty marriage between psychopathology and nosography. Other influential figures in the history of psychiatry have taken a different view. Thus the German psychiatrist, Kurt Schneider, in the preface to the fourth edition of his *Clinical Psychopathology*, argued that psychopathology aims at becoming the 'doctrine of symptoms and diagnosis', because it deals with the 'psychically abnormal looking for clinical unities' (Rossi Monti and Stanghellini 1996). It is the latter, more descriptive, approach that is currently dominant in psychiatry. Kraus argues for the need to balance this with the phenomenological approach.

then, limits to the meaningful interpretation of psychopathology? Is there a point at which meaningful communication, however strange (as Widdershoven and Widdershoven-Heerding put it in Chapter 6), runs out, where words and behaviours really are meaningless, the byproducts of failures of causal processes in the brain?

Jaspers certainly believed that meanings do run out.[54] Indeed, as the Finnish psychiatrist, Markus Heinimaa, reminds us in the final contribution to this section (Chapter 14), Jaspers based a key distinction in his psychopathology on just this point: he distinguished the 'primary' delusions of schizophrenia from the 'secondary' delusions of other conditions, such as depression, precisely in their incomprehensibility. The former, in Jaspers' view, are the product of a meaning-*less* disease process, the latter of a meaning-*ful* psychological reaction. Delusions of guilt in depression, for example, are understandable as being secondary to lowered mood, but the delusion that one has a nuclear reactor in one's abdomen, in a patient with schizophrenia, is, in Jaspers' terms, not understandable as a psychological reaction to other pathology; it is thus 'primary'.

The distinction between primary and secondary delusions, as drawn by Jaspers, has been much criticized in recent years. Psychiatrists on both sides of the Atlantic have pointed out the extent to which delusions, even if apparently incomprehensible, may turn out to have clearly understandable meanings in terms of a particular patient's background and experiences (e.g. Roberts 1991). Heinimaa cites the claim of the British historian and philosopher of psychiatry, German Berrios (1991), that a delusion that is incomprehensible today may be comprehensible tomorrow.[55] So understood, the concept of incomprehensibility is little more than provisional on the state of development of psychological science. Heinimaa, though, drawing particularly on the work of the Finnish philosopher, Lars Hertzberg, argues that psychopathology, and the 'grammar' of psychosis in particular, necessarily implies a concept of incomprehensibility.[56] The line between the comprehensible and incomprehensible may not come where Jaspers drew it. Also, we should never finally give up the search for meaning. Certainly, we should never assume that our incomprehension is a product of the other's incomprehensibility![57] But there is, none the less, bound to be a point at which, at least

---

[54]Berrios (1991) has made a similar claim, arguing that delusions should be understood as empty speech acts.

[55]Berrios has produced major histories of the symptoms and (with Roy Porter) of the syndromes currently employed in psychiatry (Berrios 1996, and Berrios and Porter, 1995).

[56]Heinimaa distinguishes, in fact, two concepts: a positive and a negative concept of incomprehensibility.

[57]A point given extra weight by Harré and Gillett's work — the discursive creation of meaning implies that comprehension is *always* a two-way process. Sabat's work on dementia shows the importance of this even where pathology affecting the brain has been demonstrated unequivocally (Sabat 2001).

in individual cases, meaning runs out. And accepting this, as Heinimaa shows in the last part of his chapter, may have important practical implications, implications that could be crucial particularly for recent work on prodromal psychotic symptoms and on the advantages and hazards of strategies for early detection of and intervention in these conditions.

A new kind of scientific psychiatry

The developments outlined in the last two sections, although entirely to be welcomed, open up deep questions of methodology. Or, perhaps we should say, again, *re*-open. For the confluence of meanings and causes in psychiatry, empirical psychology rediscovering meanings and phenomenology rediscovering empiricism, reopens the debate about methodology in the human sciences, the *Methodenstreit*, which, as we noted above, ran and ran through much of the nineteenth century. The question at the heart of the *Methodenstreit* was whether the methods that had proven so successful in the natural sciences could be adopted, direct and unchanged, in the human sciences. Behaviourism was an attempt to do just that. Phenomenology is an attempt to do the opposite: to create a (human) science of subjectivity, equal to but distinct from the (natural) sciences of objectivity.

The contributions to the penultimate section of this book illustrate two rather different responses to the methodological issues raised by taking seriously the need for meanings as well as causes in psychiatry, one ontological, the other linguistic. Gerrit Glas (Chapter 15) is, as it were, our 'ontologist'. A psychiatrist at the Zwolse Poort in Zwolle, Glas also has a post in the Department of Philosophy at the University of Leiden. In his chapter he brings the two sides of his split post together in an exploration of the conceptual issues raised by research on anxiety. Anxiety, as Glas shows, nicely spans meanings and causes. On the one hand it is 'an *existential* phenomenon, expressing the meaning of universal facts of life such as . . . the threat of absurdity, isolation, and/or imminent non-being' (Chapter 15, p. 231). As such, anxiety has been the focus of philosophical and literary scholarship. On the other hand, though, anxiety is '. . . a primarily *biological* reaction, which is built into the hardware of the brain' (p. 231). And, as a biological reaction, anxiety has been the focus of scientific research, in biology, psychology, and medicine. There are thus two discourses on anxiety. Both are *prima facie* important in psychiatry. Yet, such is the gap between meanings and causes, narrative and nature, that the two discourses have largely ignored each other. So, how to bring them together?

Glas draws on both sides of his expertise to introduce some of the concrete detail of the two discourses on anxiety. This makes clear the depth of the divide. On the one side there are neuroendocrines, behavioural paradigms, physiological responses, and clinical–diagnostic criteria; on the other side, there are richly detailed personal accounts of the 'fundamental' anxieties

(Glas sets out a novel typology of these; see Table 15.1, p. 236). Working *either* as scientists *or* as philosophers/novelists, we might be content to stay on one or other side of the divide. In psychiatry, though, we do not have this luxury. For, as Glas shows, the two discourses come together in the clinical situation. Noting the dangers of reification (highlighted by the portrayal of magnetic resonance images of the brain as 'pictures of anxiety'), he draws on the work of a Dutch philosopher, Herman Dooyeweerd,[58] to develop a theoretical framework in which the biological precursors of existential anxiety can, in principle, be studied without reducing meanings to causes. This broadly 'systems theory' approach is consistent with the innovative ideas of neuroscience-oriented researchers such as Antonio Damasio, Gerald Edelman, and Giulio Tononi. It adds to the work of these authors the novel concept of 'opening up', which, in Dooyeweerd's ontology, accommodates a developmental model of existential anxieties as evolving from biological precursors in animal reactions.

Ontology, as the study of what kinds of things there are, approaches the problem of combining meanings with causes from a theoretical 'ground-up' perspective. Linguistic approaches, by contrast, exploit meanings empirically in relation to particular research questions, without seeking to resolve the general theoretical problem of reconciling meanings with causes. Thus, in Chapter 16, the South African psychiatrists, Werdie van Staden and Christa Kruger (our second husband and wife team), describe the results of an empirical linguistic study of changes in personal pronoun use in the course of psychotherapy.[59] The importance of personal pronouns as 'variables' in research in psychiatry is signalled in this book by Rom Harré, towards the end of his Chapter 8 on the discursive origins of meaning. Van Staden and Kruger note a further reason for studying personal pronoun use in psychotherapy and psychoanalysis, in the significance of self, ego, and other personal concepts in the theories underpinning these disciplines. Yet, as these authors indicate, remarkably little empirical work has been reported in this area.

Van Staden and Kruger's methodology turns on the distinction between semantic (meaning driven) and syntactical (grammatical) uses of the first personal pronouns (I, we, me, etc.). Van Staden derived this distinction originally in his MD thesis. Drawing particularly on the semantic theory of the German

---

[58]Herman Dooyeweerd (1894–1977) was Professor of Philosophy at the Free University in Amsterdam. Criticizing traditional substantialist and metaphysical conceptions of human beings and nature, he developed a phenomenology of functional modes and a theory of the structural interconnections between these modes in 'entitary' structures. He anticipated many of the criticisms of positivism in the 1960s. Dooyeweerd was convinced that the sterility of the philosophical debates of his time resulted from avoidance of the religious 'depth dimension'.

[59]This study was started by Van Staden during his time as an MD student in the Department of Philosophy at Warwick University, and has since continued with Kruger at the University of Pretoria.

mathematician and philosopher, Gottlob Frege,[60] and his logic of relations, van Staden defined two specific semantic variables, called here 'alpha' and 'omega' positions. Defined in this way, these variables, although meaningful, can be operationalized in a form suitable for empirical research. Van Staden and Kruger applied them to a series of *verbatim* psychotherapy transcripts. The results showed that, in the course of good-outcome psychotherapy, while syntactical uses of the personal pronouns showed no significant changes, semantic (meaning-driven) uses showed clear and statistically significant changes (an increase in alpha and corresponding decrease in omega positions).

There are other empirical approaches to combining meanings with causes. Qualitative methods, after all, as developed in the social sciences, are concerned with meanings. Combined with philosophical theory, such methods have proven value for psychiatry.[61] Van Staden and Kruger's work, as they note, needs to be repeated using other source materials, different diagnostic groups, and so on. But if their results hold up then their study is, we believe, the first empirical study of personal pronoun usage to examine both semantic and syntactic variables in psychotherapy; and to show that semantic (meaning-driven) variables, derived from philosophical logic, can be employed reliably in a quantitative research paradigm from which results with clear implications for practice can be derived.

Future possible?

We opened this introductory chapter by asking whether the current renaissance in philosophy of psychiatry, impressive as its vital statistics may be, is a blip. The themes now outlined, and which will be illustrated further in the individual chapters of this book, amount to five good reasons why it is not a blip, why the renaissance in philosophy of psychiatry is likely to develop into a long-term partnership between the two disciplines.

Working backwards, the reasons are:

1. that philosophy is a resource of both ontological and linguistic approaches for empirical research on meanings in psychiatry;

---

[60]Gottlob Frege (1848–1925) was Professor of Mathematics at Jena University (Germany) and the founding father of contemporary mathematical logic, philosophy of mathematics, and philosophy of language. One of his major works, *Die Grundlagen der Arithmetic*, was translated by the Oxford philosopher, J. L. Austin, as *The Foundations of Arithmetic*. His general project was to explore the similarities between mathematical language and ordinary language. For example, he observed that (1) sentences of ordinary language and (2) mathematical expressions are both logical ways of expressing functions and relations.

[61]See, for example, drawing on linguistic analytical philosophy, Tony Colombo and Bill Fulford's work at Warwick University on the different models of disorder implicit in the community care of people with long-term schizophrenia (Colombo *et al.*, forthcoming, Fulford, 2001), and, drawing on continental philosophy, Philpott (1998).

2. that phenomenology, the main philosophical source of Jaspers' psychopathology, and now developed through a century of scholarship (mainly) in continental Europe, amounts to a 'science of subjectivity' capable of standing alongside and complementing the sciences of objectivity;

3. that psychology, having excluded meanings (along with all other aspects of subjectivity) from the black box of behaviourism, is now actively re-engaged with them in both private (cognitivist) and public (discursive) spaces;

4. that ethics, although largely regulative in other areas of health care, is centrally concerned in psychiatry with some of the deepest issues of philosophical theory;

5. that philosophy itself, although at the start of the twentieth century still in pursuit of foundations, is now engaged, centrally, with conceptual difficulties (Wittgenstein's 'unease' about concepts), i.e. with difficulties of precisely the sort by which the defining concepts of psychiatry itself — mental disorder, mental illness, and so forth — are characterized.

A further reason for believing that the future relationship between philosophy and psychiatry will be one of ongoing partnership is that, if philosophy has changed in the course of the twentieth century, so too has science. In the early twentieth century, when Jaspers was at work on his psychopathology, science was understood, as it had been understood since the scientific renaissance, to be engaged in revealing an ever more accurate picture of reality by the accumulation of observations which, although constrained practically by the limits of available instrumentation, were in principle theory-free. The paradigm science in this respect was physics. But this model of science is now known to be over-simple.[62] There are no 'theory-free' observations. Even in physics, what we see is constrained not only by what we see *with* (our instruments) but by the framework of ideas — the concepts — by which we structure and give meaning to *what* we see.

From the point of view of psychiatry there are both pluses and minuses to be had from this change in our understanding of the nature of science. On the plus side, the natural sciences, now that they are recognized to be concept as well as data driven, are more hospitable to the human sciences. There is no longer a stark objective–subjective divide between them. The 'view from nowhere', as the American philosopher of science, Thomas Nagel (1986), famously characterized the aim of the natural sciences traditionally understood, has turned out to be always a view from somewhere.

---

[62]The American philosopher and historian of science, Thomas Kuhn, for example, drew this conclusion from his important observation that sciences proceed, not continuously, but in a series of jumps or 'paradigm shifts', separated by periods of 'normal science' (Kuhn 1970). The Hungarian philosopher, Imre Lakatos, linked these shifts of paradigm more or less explicitly to changes in the underlying concepts guiding the interpretation of evidence (Lakatos 1974).

On the minus side, though, the theory-ladenness of observation carries the risk of an unacceptable relativization of knowledge, that variant of the 'post-modern' stance according to which all perspectives are equal. The fear of relativism, we believe, is exaggerated. The fact that there may be more than one way of understanding a given set of observations in no way implies that all ways of understanding it are equal. Even in psychiatric ethics, in which a legitimate diversity of human values is a given, human values are not chaotic (Dickenson and Fulford 2000). Historically, indeed, psychiatry has been more at risk from absolutism than from relativism. Things have tended to go wrong in psychiatry, that is to say, where a plan or policy or an approach to treatment has been adopted, with all-too-genuine enthusiasm, but to the exclusion of all others.[63] And one proper role of philosophy is to provide a sceptical super-ego, helping us, if not to find 'the' right answer, at least to avoid premature closure on wrong answers!

The greater danger, though, for psychiatry in the twenty-first century is perhaps neither relativism nor absolutism, but obscurantism. It is to this danger that our final contributor, the Italian philosopher and historian of science, Paolo Rossi, points in Chapter 17. Writing from the birthplace of the renaissance, in Florence, Rossi provides a vivid and richly illustrated picture of the struggles of the new natural sciences in fourteenth- and fifteenth-century Europe, to escape from the thraldom of received authority. His point is that it really *was* a struggle. Nowadays we take the pre-eminence of the natural sciences for granted. But, as Rossi shows, for a long time it was touch-and-go whether science (open to all people) or magic (reserved to the select) would prevail. And there are worrying signs, as Rossi goes on to describe, of a return to magical thinking at the present time.

In developing the new philosophy of psychiatry, then, in bringing together causes and meanings as Jaspers envisaged, in combining empirical science with phenomenology, biology with culture, nature with narrative, we should heed Rossi's warning words (Chapter 17, p. 263):

'The history of science, and more explicitly the history of the first scientific revolution, can help us to understand how logical rigour, experimental control, the public character of results and methods, and the very structure of scientific knowledge are not perennial facts of the history of humankind, but historical advances that can easily be lost.'

Acknowledgements

The authors are grateful to Professor Christoph Mundt and to Dr Peter Schoenknecht in the Department of Psychiatry, University of Heidelberg, for the picture of Karl Jaspers as a young man. We are grateful to our contributors and to many other colleagues for their advice and help with this chapter.

---

[63]The extremes of the psychoanalytical movement, the political excesses of 'community care', and the current dominance of 'biological' psychiatry, are all cases in point (see Fulford 2000*a*).

References

American Psychiatric Association (1980). *Diagnostic and statistical manual of mental disorders (third edition)*. Washington, DC: American Psychiatric Association.

American Psychiatric Association (1994). *Diagnostic and Statistical Manual of Mental Disorders*, 4th edn. Washington, DC: American Psychiatric Association.

Austin, J. L. (1956–7). A plea for excuses. *Proceedings of the Aristotelian Society*, **57**: 1–30. (Reprinted in White, A. R. (ed.) (1968). *The Philosophy of Action*. Oxford: Oxford University Press.)

Baker, G. and Morris, K. J. (1996). *Descartes' Dualism*. London: Routledge.

Baker, G. and Morris, K. J. (forthcoming). *Descartes' Meditations: First Philosophy*.

Beauchamp, T. L. and Childress, J. F. (1989). *Principles of Biomedical Ethics*, 3rd edn. Oxford: Oxford University Press.

Bechtel, W., Abrahamson, A., and Graham, G. (1998). The Life of Cognitive Science. In: *A Companion to Cognitive Science* (ed. W. Bechtel, and G. Graham), pp. 1–104. Oxford: Blackwell.

Berrios, G. E. (1989). What is phenomenology? *Journal of the Royal Society of Medicine*, **82**: 425–8.

Berrios, G. E. (1991). Delusions as 'wrong belief': a conceptual history. *British Journal of Psychiatry*, **159**(Suppl. 14): 6–13.

Berrios, G. E. (1992). Phenomenology, psychopathology and Jaspers: a conceptual history. *History of Psychiatry*, **3**: 303–28.

Berrios G. E. and Porter R. (1992) Eds. *A History of Clinical Psychiatry: the Origin and History of Mental Disorders*. London: The Athlone Press.

Berrios, G. E. (1996). *The History of Mental Symptoms*. Cambridge: Cambridge University Press.

Bloch, S. and Chodoff, P. (eds) (1981). *Psychiatric Ethics*, 1st edn. Oxford: Oxford University Press.

Bloch, S. and Reddaway, P. (1977). *Russia's Political Hospitals: The Abuse of Psychiatry in the Soviet Union*. Southampton: Camelot Press.

Bloch, S., Chodoff, P., and Green, S. A. (1999) *Psychiatric Ethics*, 3rd edn. Oxford: Oxford University Press.

Bolton, D. and Hill, J. (1996). *Mind, Meaning and Mental Disorder: The Nature of Causal Explanation in Psychology and Psychiatry*. Oxford: Oxford University Press.

Boorse, C. (1975). On the distinction between disease and illness. *Philosophy and Public Affairs*, **5**: 49–68.

Bracken, P. (forthcoming). *Meaning and Trauma in the Post-Modern Age: Heidegger and a New Direction for Psychiatry*. London: Whurr Publishers.

British Psychological Society (2000). *Recent Advances in Understanding Mental Illness and Psychotic Experiences*. Leicester: British Psychological Society, Division of Clinical Psychology.

Campbell, E. J., Scadding, J. G., and Roberts, R. S. (1979). The concept of disease. *British Medical Journal*, **ii**: 757–62.

Caplan, A. L., Engelhardt, T., and McCartney, J. J. (eds) (1981). *Concepts of Health and Disease: Interdisciplinary Perspectives*. Reading, MA: Addison-Wesley.

Clare, A. (1979). The disease concept in psychiatry. In: *Essentials of Postgraduate Psychiatry* (ed. P. Hill, R. Murray, and A. Thorley), pp. 55–76. New York: Grune & Stratton, and London: Academic Press.

Clark, S. R. L. (1996). Minds, memes and multiples. *Philosophy, Psychiatry and Psychology*, **3**: 21–8.

Colombo A., Bendelow, G., Fulford K. W. M., and Williams, S. (forthcoming). Evaluating the influence of implicit models of mental disorder on processes of shared decision-making within community-based multi-disciplinary teams. *Social Science and Medicine*.

Dickenson, D. and Fulford, K. W. M. (2000). *In Two Minds: A Casebook of Psychiatric Ethics*. Oxford: Oxford University Press.

Flew, A. (1973). *Crime or Disease?* New York: Barnes and Noble.

Fodor, J. A. (1980). Methodological solipsism considered as a research strategy in cognitive psychology. *The Behavioral and Brain Sciences*, **54**: 63–72.

Foucault, M. (1973). *Madness and Civilization: A History of Insanity in the Age of Reason*. New York: Random House.

Frankfurt, H. G. (1971). Freedom of the will and the concept of a person. *Journal of Philosophy*, *LXVIII*(1): 15–20.

Fulford, K. W. M. (1989; reprinted 1995, 1999). *Moral Theory and Medical Practice*. Cambridge: Cambridge University Press.

Fulford, K. W. M. (1990). Philosophy and medicine: the Oxford connection. *British Journal of Psychiatry*, **157**: 111–15.

Fulford, K. W. M. (1993). Value, action, mental illness and the law, pp. 279–310. In: *Action and Value in Criminal Law* (ed. S. Shute, J. Gardner, and J. Horder), pp. 279–310. Oxford: Oxford University Press.

Fulford, K. W. M. (1994). Closet logics: hidden conceptual elements in the DSM and ICD classifications of mental disorders, pp. 211–32. In: *Philosophical Perspectives on Psychiatric Diagnostic Classification* (ed. J. Z. Sadler, O. P. Wiggins, and M. A. Schwartz), ch. 9. Baltimore: Johns Hopkins University Press.

Fulford, K. W. M. (1995). Introduction: Just getting started, pp. 1–3. In: *Philosophy, Psychology, and Psychiatry* (ed. A. Phillips Griffiths). Cambridge: Cambridge University Press, for the Royal Institute of Philosophy.

Fulford, K. W. M. (1998). Mental illness, pp. 213–33. In: *Encyclopedia of Applied Ethic* (ed. R. Chadwick). San Diego, CA: Academic Press.

Fulford, K. W. M. (2000*a*). Philosophy meets psychiatry in the twentieth century — four looks back and a brief look forward. In: *Philosophy Meets Medicine* (ed. P. Louhiala and S. Stenman), pp. 116–34. Helsinki: Helsinki University Press.

Fulford, K. W. M. (2000*b*). Disordered minds, diseased brains and real people, ch. 4, pp. 33–47. In: *Philosophy, Psychiatry and Psychopathy: Personal Identity in Mental Disorder* (ed. C. Heginbotham). Avebury Series in Philosophy in association with the Society for Applied Philosophy. Aldershot, UK: Ashgate Publishing.

Fulford, K. W. M. (2000*c*). Teleology without tears: naturalism, neo-naturalism and evaluationism in the analysis of function statements in biology (and a bet on the twenty-first century). *Philosophy, Psychiatry, and Psychology*, **7**(1): 77–94.

Fulford, K. W. M. (2001). Philosophy into practice: the case for ordinary language philosophy, pp. 171–208. In: *Health, Science, and Ordinary Language* (ed. L. Nordenfelt), ch. 2. Amsterdam: Rodopi.

Fulford, K. W. M. and Hope, R. A. (1993). Psychiatric ethics: a bioethical ugly duckling? pp. 681–95. In: *Principles of Health Care Ethics* (ed. R. Gillon and A. Lloyd), ch. 58. Chichester, UK: John Wiley.

Fulford, K. W. M., Murray, T. H., and Dickenson, D. (eds) (2002). Many voices pp. 1–19. In: *Healthcare Ethics and Human Values: An Introductory Text with Readings and Case Studies*. Oxford: Blackwell.

Fulford, K. W. M., Woodbridge, K., and Williamson, T. (2002). Values-Added Practice. *Mental Health Today*, October, 25–7.

Garber, D. (1992). *Descartes' Metaphysical Physics*. Chicago: University of Chicago Press.

Gardner S. (1993). *Irrationality and the Philosophy of Psychoanalysis*. Cambridge: Cambridge University Press.

Garety, P. A. and Freeman, D. (1999). Cognitive approaches to delusions: a critical review of theories and evidence. *British Journal of Clinical Psychology*, **38**: 113–54.

Gillett, G. (1999). *The Mind and its Discontents*. Oxford: Oxford University Press.

Glover, J. (1970). *Responsibility*. London: Routledge and Kegan Paul.

Glover, J. (1988). *I: The Philosophy and Psychology of Personal Identity*. London: Penguin.

Gould, R. A., Mueser, K. T., Bolton, E., Mays, V., and Goff, D. (2001). Cognitive therapy for psychosis: an effect size analysis. *Schizophrenia Research*, **48**: 335–42.

Graham, G. and Stephens, G. L. (1994). Eds. *Philosophical Psychopathology*. Cambridge, Mass: MIT Press.

Hare, R. M. (1952). *The Language of Morals*. Oxford: Oxford University Press.

Harré, R. (1997). Pathological autobiographies. *Philosophy, Psychiatry, and Psychology*, **4**(2): 99–110.

Harré, R. and Gillett, G. (1994). *The Discursive Mind*. London: Sage.

Hawton, K., Salkovskis, P. M., Kirk, J., and Clark, D. M. (1989). *Cognitive Behaviour Therapy for Psychiatric Problems: A Practical Guide*. Oxford: Oxford University Press.

Heidegger, M. (1962). *Being and Time*. New York: Harper Row.

Hempel, C. G. (1961). Introduction to problems of taxonomy. In: *Field Studies in the Mental Disorders* (ed. J. Zubin), pp. 3–22. New York: Grune and Stratton. (Reproduced in Sadler, J. Z., Wiggins, O. P., and Schwartz, M. A. (1994). *Philosophical Perspectives on Psychiatric Diagnostic Classification*, pp. 315–31. Baltimore, MD: The Johns Hopkins University Press.)

Hemsley, D. R. and Garety, P. A. (1986). The formation and maintenance of delusions: a bayesian analysis. *British Journal of Psychiatry*, **149**: 51–6.

Hinshelwood, R. D. (1995). The social relocation of personal identity as shown by psychoanalytic observations of splitting, projection and introjection. *Philosophy, Psychiatry, and Psychology*, **2**: 185–204.

Hinshelwood, R. D. (1997). Primitive mental processes: psychoanalysis and the ethics of integration. *Philosophy, Psychiatry, and Psychology*, **4**(2): 121–44.

Hobson, R. P. (1991). Against the 'theory of mind'. *British Journal of Developmental Psychology*, **9**: 33–51.

Hobson, R. P. (2002). *The Cradle of Thought*. London: Macmillan, Pan Books.

Human Rights Watch/Geneva Initiative on Psychiatry (2002). *Dangerous Minds: Political Psychiatry in China Today and its Origins in the Mao Era*. New York: Human Rights Watch.

Hundert, E. M. (1989). *Philosophy, Psychiatry and Neuroscience*. Oxford: Clarendon Press.

Husserl, E. (1970). *The Crisis of the European Sciences and Transcendental Phenomenology*. Evanston: Northwestern University Press.

Jackson, M. and Fulford, K. W. M. (1997). Spiritual experience and psychopathology. *Philosophy, Psychiatry, and Psychology*, **4**(1): 41–66.

Jaspers, K. (1912). *Allgemeine Psychopathologie*. Berlin: Springer (trans. in Hoenig, J. and Hamilton, M. W. (1963). *General Psychopathology*. Manchester: Manchester University Press; new paperback edition (1997), with foreword by P. R. McHugh, from Johns Hopkins University Press, Baltimore, MD).

Jaspers, K. (1913*a*). Causal and meaningful connexions between life history and psychosis. Published as Chapter 5 in Hirsch, S. R. and Shepherd, M. (eds) (1974). *Themes and Variations in European Psychiatry*. Bristol: John Wright.

Jaspers, K. (1913*b*). The phenomenological approach in psychopathology. *Zeitschrift fur die Gesamte Neurologie und Psychiatrie*, **9**: 391–408. Published in translation (on the initiative of J. N. Curran) as *British Journal of Psychiatry*, 1968; **114**: 1313–23.

Judd, Lewis, L. (1990). The decade of the brain. Prospects and challenges for the NIMH. *Neuropsychopharmacology*, **3**(5–6): 309–10.

Kendell, R. E. (1975*a*). The concept of disease and its implications for psychiatry. *British Journal of Psychiatry*, **127**: 305–15.

Kendell, R. E. (1975*b*). *The Role of Diagnosis in Psychiatry*. Oxford: Blackwell Scientific.

Kenny, A. J. P. (1969). Mental health in Plato's Republic. *Proceedings of the British Academy*, **5**: 229–53.

Kuhn, T. S. (1970). *The structure of scientific revolutions*. Chicago: University of Chicago Press.

Lakatos, I. (1974). Falsification and the methodology of scientific research programmes. In: *Criticism and the Growth of Knowledge*, 3rd edn (ed. I. Lakatos and A. Musgrave), pp. 91–196). Cambridge: Cambridge University Press (first published 1969).

Megone, C. (1998). Aristotle's function argument and the concept of mental illness. *Philosophy, Psychiatry, and Psychology*, **5**(3): 187–202.

Midgley, M. (1996). *Utopias, Dolphins and Computers: Problems of Philosophical Plumbing*. London: Routledge.

Monk R. (1990). *Ludwig Wittgenstein: The Duty of Genius*. London, Jonathan Cape.

Moore, M. S. (1984). *Law and Psychiatry: Rethinking the Relationship*. Cambridge: Cambridge University Press.

Morrison, A. (ed.) (2001). *A Casebook of Cognitive Therapy for Psychoses*. Cambridge: Cambridge University Press.

Mundt, C. H. (1992). The history of psychiatry in Heidelberg, pp. 16–31. In: *Phenomenology, Language and Schizophrenia* (ed. M. Spitzer, F. Uehlein, M. A. Schwartz, and C. H. Mundt). New York: Springer.

Nagel, T. (1986). *The View from Nowhere*. Oxford: Oxford University Press.

Nordenfelt, L. (1997). The stoic conception of mental disorder: the case of Cicero. *Philosophy, Psychiatry, and Psychology*, **4**(4): 285–92.

Parnas, J. and Zahavi, D. (2000). The link: philosophy–psychopathology–phenomenology, pp. 1–16. In: *Exploring The Self* (ed. D. Zahavi). Amsterdam: Benjamins.

Petitot, J., Varela, F., Pachoud, B., and Roy, J.-M. (2000). *Naturalizing Phenomenology: Issues in Contemporary Phenomenology and Cognitive Science*. Cambridge: Cambridge University Press.

Phillips Griffith, A. (1994). *Philosophy, Psychology and Psychiatry*. Cambridge: Cambridge University Press.

Philpott, M. J. (1998). A phenomenology of dyslexia: the lived-body, ambiguity, and the breakdown of expression. *Philosophy, Psychiatry, and Psychology*, **5**(1): 1–20.

Ralph, R. O. (2000). Recovery. *Psychiatric Rehabilitation Skills*, **4**(3): 480–517.

Reznek, L. (1991). *The Philosophical Defence of Psychiatry*. London: Routledge.

Ricoeur, P. (1970). *Freud and Philosophy* (trans. D. Savage). London: Yale University Press.

Roberts, G. (1991). Delusional belief systems and meaning in life: a preferred reality? *British Journal of Psychiatry*, **159**(Suppl. 14): 19–28.

Robinson, D. (1996). *Wild Beasts and Idle Humours*. Cambridge, MA: Harvard University Press.

Rossi Monti, M. and Stanghellini, G. (1996). Psychopathology. An edgeless razor? *Comprehensive Psychiatry*, **37**(3): 196–204.

Sabat, S. R. (2001). *The Experience of Alzheimer's Disease: Life Through a Tangled Veil*. Oxford: Blackwell.

Sabat, S. R. and Harré, R. (1997). The Alzheimer's disease sufferer as semiotic subject. *Philosophy, Psychiatry, and Psychology*, **4**(2): 145–60.

Sadler, J. Z. (1992). Eidetic and empirical research: a hermeneutic complementarity, pp. 103–14. In: *Phenomenology, Language and Schizophrenia* (ed. M. Spitzer, F. Uehlein, M. A. Schwartz, and C. H. Mundt). New York: Springer.

Sadler, J. Z., Wiggins, O. P., and Schwartz, M. A. (1994). Eds. *Philosophical Perspectives on Psychiatric Diagnostic Classification*. Baltimore, MD: The Johns Hopkins University Press.

Schneider, K. (1980). *Clinical Psychopathology*, 4th edn. Stuttgart and New York: Thieme.

Spitzer, M. and Maher, B. (1990). *Philosophy and Psychopathology*. Heidelberg: Springer.

Spitzer, M., Uehlein, F. A., and Oepen, G. (1988). *Psychopathology and Philosophy*. Berlin: Springer.

Spitzer, M., Uehlein, F., Schwartz, M. A., and Mundt, Ch. (1992). *Phenomenology, Language and Schizophrenia*. New York: Springer.

Stanghellini, G. (1997). For an anthropology of vulnerability. *Psychopathology*, **30**: 1–11.

Stanghellini, G. (2000a). *Anger and Fury, Philosophy and Psychopathology*. Basel: Karger.

Stanghellini, G. (2000b). The doublets of anger (editorial). *Psychopathology*, **33**(4): 155–8.

Stanghellini, G. and Mundt, Ch. (1997). Personality and endogenous/major depression: an empirical approach to typus melancholicus. 1. Theoretical issues. *Psychopathology*, **30**: 119–29.

Stengel, E. (1959). Classification of mental disorders. *Bulletin of the World Health Organization*, **21**: 601–63.

Stephens, G. L. and Graham, G. (2000). *When Self-Consciousness Breaks: Alien Voices and Inserted Thoughts*. Cambridge, MA: MIT Press.

Szasz, T. S. (1960). The myth of mental illness. *American Psychologist*, **15**: 113–18.

Szasz T. S. (1976). *Schizophrenia: The Sacred Symbol of Psychiatry*. New York: Basic Books.

Thornton, T. (1997). Reasons and causes in philosophy and psychopathology. *Philosophy, Psychiatry, and Psychology*, **4**(4): 307–18.

Thornton, T. (1998). *Wittgenstein on Language and Thought*. Edinburgh: Edinburgh University Press.

Tyrer, P. and Steinberg, D. (1993). *Models for Mental Disorder: Conceptual Models in Psychiatry*, 2nd edn. Chichester, UK: John Wiley.

Walker, C. (1994*a*). Karl Jaspers and Edmund Husserl — I: The perceived convergence. *Philosophy, Psychiatry, and Psychology*, **1**(2): 117–34.

Walker, C. (1994*b*). Karl Jaspers and Edmund Husserl — II: The divergence. *Philosophy, Psychiatry, and Psychology*, **1**(4): 245–66.

Walker, C. (1995*a*). Karl Jaspers and Edmund Husserl — III: Jaspers as a Kantian phenomenologist. *Philosophy, Psychiatry, and Psychology*, **2**(1): 65–82.

Walker, C. (1995*b*). Karl Jaspers and Husserl — IV: Phenomenology and empathic understanding. *Philosophy, Psychiatry, and Psychology*, **2**(3): 247–66.

Wiggins, O. P. and Schwartz, M. A. (1995). Chris Walker's interpretation of Karl Jaspers' phenomenology: a critique. *Philosophy, Psychiatry, and Psychology*, **2**(4): 319–44.

Wilkes, K. V. (1988). *Real People: Personal Identity Without Thought Experiments*. Oxford: Clarendon Press.

Williams, B. (1985). *Ethics and the limits of philosophy*. London: Fontana.

Wing, J. K., Cooper, J. E., and Sartorius, N. (1974). *Measurement and Classification of Psychiatric Symptoms*. Cambridge: Cambridge University Press.

World Health Organisation (1967). *Mannual of the international statistical classification of diseases, injuries and causes of death* (ICD-8). Geneva: WHO.

World Health Organisation (1978). *Mental disorders: glossary and guide to their classification in accordance with the ninth revision of the International classification of diseases*. Geneva: WHO.

World Health Organisation (1992). *The ICD-10 Classification of Mental and Behavioural Disorders: Clinical Descriptions and Diagnostic Guidelines*. Geneva: World Health Organisation.

Yuasa, Y. (1987). *The Body. Toward an Eastern Mind–Body Theory*. New York: State University of New York Press.

Yamaguchi, I. (1997). *Ki also leibhaftige Vernunft, Beitrag zur interkulturellen Phànomenologie de Leiblichkeit*. Munich: Fink.

Zahavi, D. (2000). *Exploring the Self*. Amsterdam: Benjamins.

Section 1 Recycling History?

2 Towards a psyche for psychiatry

Russell Meares

Origins

The origins of dynamic psychiatry, as is well known, centred on Salpêtrière in Paris. The ideas that were being developed at that time were resonant with a particular mood, or state, of Western culture. Indeed, it can be said that the form of a particular culture is manifest, indirectly, in the expressions of those individuals who have created the culture. Although each one believes that he or she is making an expression that is purely personal, there is, underlying, the powerful influence of the world in which those people live. The writers, painters, architects, psychologists, politicians, and scientists of a particular age show in their own unique way something of the mind, if we can use that term, of that particular age.

The age in which dynamic psychiatry began was one in which the notion of personal existence, the immediacy of going on being, was a dominant theme. It is shown most clearly in the works of impressionist painters. Here is expressed the pleasure of ordinary life (Clark 1984, p. 3). What is depicted, however, is not merely people lunching, or boating, or going to bars and having picnics, but something also of that experience of well-being, of the movements of consciousness that are expressed in William James' term 'the stream of consciousness'. The rippling, dappled light of Renoir's work shows, as much as the actual subjects, the feeling of life going on.

In philosophy, the dominant voice was that of Henri Bergson, who was pre-occupied by the notion of personal existence, of the nature of the present moment (Bergson 1911), and with the idea that our experiences make up a reality that is different to the reality of Newtonian science. Neither zone of reality contradicts or cancels out the other. The statement that the sun sets in the west is true in one reality; that it does not set in the west is true in another. 'No philosophical doctrine,' he wrote, 'denies that the same images can enter at the same time into these two distinct systems' (Bergson 1911, pp. 13–14).

The philosophy of Henri Bergson was paralleled by the psychology of William James. The core of his great work of 1890 is an examination of the fundamentals of the experience of personal existence. He corresponded and conversed with Bergson. Both men developed a conception of the human time experience that differed from scientific time. Both men also described two forms of memory.

'The first records, in the form of memory-images, all the events of our daily life as they occur in time' (Bergson 1911, p. 92). The second kind of memory involves no such awareness of an event or episode from the past, but only the fact or movement that was learnt at that time (James 1890, pp. 648–650).

In psychiatry, the star of Paris was Pierre Janet. He had been to the same school as Bergson and continued his relationship with him into adult life. Janet was working towards a model of mind as the basic background to mental illness. The essential feature of this model was a hierarchy of mental functions. At the highest level was the function of présentification (Ellenberger 1970, p. 376), the creation of the present moment, a concept that resembled Bergson's 'attention to present life' (Bergson 1911, p. 226).

Janet's studies of people suffering from a disorder then called 'hysteria' became a principal basis of a kind of psychiatric practice in which the psychiatrist tries to understand the patient's illness in psychological terms. Jung wrote in 1908, when he was still a strong supporter and ally of Freud: 'The theoretical presuppositions on which Freud bases his investigations are to be found in the experiments of Pierre Janet' (Jung 1961, p. 10). William James considered that Janet's *Mental State of Hystericals* (Janet 1893) was worth 'all exact laboratory measures put together' (Myers 1986, p. 374).

In literature, the novel that is now seen as the great work of the era, that of Proust, was being written. Its focus was memory, in particular that kind of memory in which an event is recalled as if in 'the mind's eye'. Underlying Proust's quest seemed to be the implicit idea that the 'aliveness' of personal existence depended upon this faculty (Meares 2000, p. 93). It seems peculiarly appropriate that a cousin of Proust married Bergson.

1913

The value given to the sense of personal existence, expressed in many different fields, was lost quite spectacularly and suddenly. The change in consciousness is displayed in artwork.

The watershed year can be seen as 1913, the year in which Watson announced his behaviourist manifesto, when Freud and Jung exchanged their last letters, and when Henry Ford started his assembly line, in which the human functioned as part of a machine (Smith 1993).

The movement towards 1913 is shown by the changes in the work of Marcel Duchamp. At the first part of the twentieth century he was painting like an impressionist. Soon, however, he began to paint small machines. This culminated in his famous picture displayed at the Armory Show of 1913, one of the most influential art exhibitions of the twentieth century in the United States. Duchamp was one of the stars of the show. His 'Nude descending a staircase' was a sensation. It shows a human being depicted as a kinetic mechanism, person as machine.

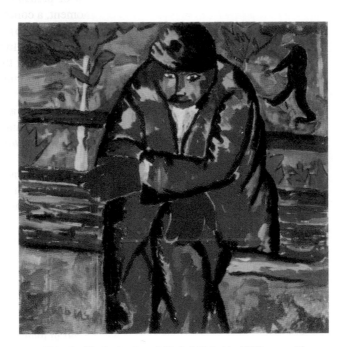

Plate 1 'On the boulevard' (Kazimir Malevich, 1911), see p. 44

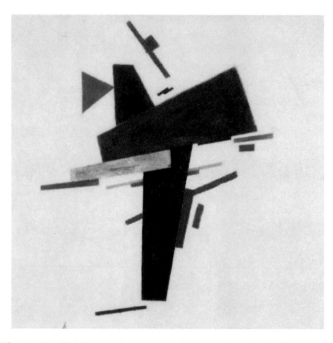

Plate 2 'Untitled (suprematist composition)' (Kazimir Malevich, 1916), see p. 45.

Another star of the show was Francis Picabia. He too began to paint in the style of the impressionist. There was a rapid change in his work, with the turning point around 1913 with his painting at the Armory Show, which was of a mechanical kind. Soon after this Picabia was portraying the human as a mechanism. Sadness is a screw-like machine; his girlfriend, Marie Laurencin, is an aircraft engine.

This sudden change in which the human was portrayed as a machine was evident across Europe. In England there were the Vorticists, headed by Wyndham Lewis. In Italy the futurists made a worship of the machine. The change in representation, shown so dramatically by Duchamp and Picabia, was demonstrated equally dramatically by Malevich in Russia. In 1911 and 1912, Malevich was portraying peasants in a simple, rustic style (Fig. 2.1). A picture entitled 'The scissors grinder', displayed in 1913, shows something quite different. In it the man and the machine have become one. Soon after this, Malevich abandoned the representation of the human, and his art became geometric, consisting of patterns (Fig. 2.2).

This new mode of artistic expression was epitomised by Mondrian, who became a new hero of the art world. His patterning form of expression was based on a philosophy in which that which was human was devalued. The ordinary world of living, both human and non-human, was excluded in order to attain to something that was seen as purer and 'higher'. Such was his rejection of the natural world that on one occasion, while lunching in the country with a fellow artist, he asked to sit with his back to the window so that he would not have to observe the green landscape (Holtzmann and James 1993, p. 7).

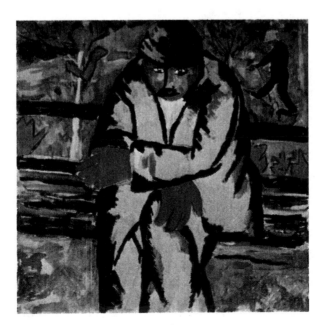

Fig. 2.1 'On the boulevard' (Kazimir Malevich, 1911).

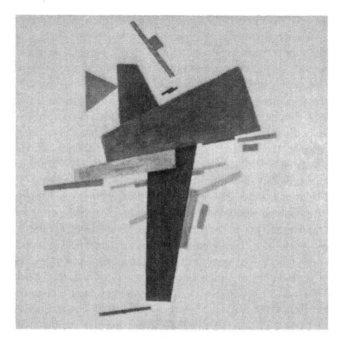

Fig. 2.2 'Untitled (suprematist composition)' (Kazimir Malevich, 1916).

Devaluation of personal being

The form of expression advocated by Mondrian persisted in the West. By the 1950s and 1960s it was a dominant mode in New York, where painters such as Frank Stella, Barnett Newman, and Kenneth Noland enjoyed a vogue.

In architecture, the first building of the new order appeared in 1914, designed by Gropius, founder of the Bauhaus (Pevsner 1957, p. 201). In this new world of architecture, a house was a machine for living, as Le Corbusier famously put it. Memory was abolished. A room of Le Corbusier is swept clean of a past, a scene of exhilarating purity. In contrast, a room of the bourgeoisie in the late part of the nineteenth century was full of memorabilia, of objects that reminded the occupants of their family, of stories from their past. There were gifts, portraits, souvenirs, and pieces of old furniture. The Le Corbusier room is purged of all this. It was an age when Henry Ford could announce: 'History is more or less bunk' (Ford 1919).

Just as memory was swept away in the world of architecture, so it was in the field of psychology and philosophy. I am speaking now of that peculiarly human form of memory in which an episode of the past is suddenly recovered and, as it were, 'viewed', as if in 'inner space'. This kind of memory was not only central to the writing of Proust but was also investigated from the philosophical and psychological points of view by Bergson and James. After the

First World War, both Bergson and James lost influence. In the new world of positivism and behaviourism, memory was only something that could be measured.

In psychology, the notion of self, because it is not directly measurable, was considered to be beyond the pale of respectable scientific inquiry and was banished in what has been called 'a radical behaviourist purge' (Harter 1983, p. 226). The same thing happened in philosophy. In England, the dominant philosophies of Russell, A. J. Ayer, and Ryle prevailed. Their ideology was most clearly expressed by Gilbert Ryle (1949) in his *Concept of Mind*, a hugely influential work in which his aim, as he himself admitted, was to deride the notion of an interior life and the metaphor of 'the mind's eye'.

From this temporal vantage point, the success of Ryle's polemic seems extraordinary. His argument, reduced to its fundamental form, depends on assertion. The principal assertion was that there is no such thing as inner experience because, in his view, those images that are a prominent part of this experience have no correlative physiology of the kind that is produced by external stimuli. 'The opinion' that 'imaging is a piece of near-sentience' is, he concluded, 'completely false' (Ryle 1949, p. 251).

Ryle's opinion that this 'opinion is completely false' is, of course, itself, completely false. Even the imaging of the congenitally blind shows activation of the visual cortex (Sadato *et al.* 1996). That Ryle was so respectfully received suggests that his viewpoint was consistent with, and mirrored, an age of ideological brutalism, in which the ordinary verities of living could be trampled on and denied (Arendt 1968, p. 167).

Similar viewpoints to those of Ryle persisted, like that of Mondrian, and became manifest not only in certain philosophies but also in a new genre of literature. Baudrillard described the characteristics of the 'new novel'. He wrote: 'The project is already there to empty out the real, extirpate all psychology, to move the real back to pure objectivity' (Baudrillard 1983, p. 142–3).

The conception of the human as a machine, a system in which the personal world of feelings and imagination is ignored or devalued, was clearly expressed in scientific circles. For example, W. Ross Ashby, who, with Norbert Wiener, was the originator of cybernetics, wrote in *Design for a Brain* (Ashby 1960, cited by Fischer 1963, p. 200):

> Throughout the book, consciousness and its related subjective elements are not used, for the simple reason that at no point have I found their introduction necessary . . . Vivid though consciousness may be to its possessor, there is as yet no method known by which he can demonstrate his experience to another.

Psychiatry and psychoanalysis could not resist these cultural influences. In psychoanalysis the change towards mechanism, and the conception of human as machine, was evident when the world of 'self', embodied in the figure of Jung, was cast out into an oblivion in which both he and his ideas were 'shunned as though they did not exist' (Kirsner 2001, p. 247).

In the new psychoanalysis, Freud's first model of mind was revised. 'Ego' became the dominant theory, particularly in the United States. 'Ego' began to be talked about as a machine — 'the psychic apparatus', it was called. Critics recognized that this theory left no room for the self (Rycroft 1972, p. 149). The language typically used to describe the mechanism of ego was as laborious and clanking, as removed from ordinary experience, as the contraption itself.

Psychiatry abandoned Janet, who by the 1950s and 1960s had become merely a footnote in many Anglo-American textbooks. His idea of basing psychiatry on a sophisticated model of a hierarchy of mental function was given up. The attempt to understand mental illness, to see it as a manifestation of a disruption of a dynamism, was largely rejected by mainstream psychiatry. In 1980, the syndrome upon which Janet had developed his postulates was formally jettisoned by the *Diagnostic and Statistical Manual* (DSM) and split up into its main constituent parts, as if they were unrelated (Meares *et al.* 1999*a*).

A faltering revival

The hegemony of the positivist–behaviourist ideology began to fail around 1970. Ellenberger's great book renewed the reputation of Janet (Ellenberger 1970). In 1972, the neuropsychologist Endel Tulving brought back into the discipline of psychology the notion of memory, which had been described within their different disciplines by James, Bergson, and Proust. He called it 'episodic memory' and distinguished it, as James had done, from another kind of memory system that involves fact and knowledge of the world. This latter memory function does not involve the double experience of an episode from the past that is linked to knowledge of a particular fact, such as the values of coins, the names of birds, and so forth.

In psychoanalysis, Winnicott's *Playing and Reality*, published in 1971, was covertly and unobtrusively revolutionary. Implicitly, he placed the experience of 'going on being' as the central issue that confronts us in our work. In the same year, Heinz Kohut, in the United States, overtly declared a revolution with his *The Analysis of the Self*. In psychology, the notion of self returned quite suddenly and James reappeared. Also quite suddenly, studies of mother–infant interaction began as if somewhere within this interaction the child's 'self' was emerging. Coincidentally with these changes was the emergence of a non-linear mathematics of living things, and a new kind of architecture began in which there was an escape from the rigidity of straight lines and box-like structures in favour of the curves and symmetry of the natural world. Utzon's Sydney Opera House is an example.

This shift in consciousness included a return to some of the basic ideas that had preceded the shift of 1913. However, the new manner of thinking faltered. It seemed that in psychiatry it had very little effect.

It can be suggested that the faltering was a consequence of the success of the totalizing positivist–behaviourist era, which had destroyed an intellectual world by neglect and derision. Kohut, for example, could not define 'self' (Kohut 1977, p. 310–11). There was no intellectual background against which he could work. Such a failure to find a suitable foundation stone upon which to build the psychology of 'self' is clearly a massive impediment to the development of the theory. It is necessary to develop a theory, which has a scientific value, of what might be called 'personal being'. This is so not only in order to develop logically based treatments for personality disorder, upon which Kohut focused, but also to approach the whole range of mental illness. All mental illnesses involve disturbances of 'personal being' or 'self'. This is a complex experience, involving multiple dimensions such as affect state, body feeling, cohesion, continuity, temporality, spatiality, privacy (boundedness), the feeling that it is one's own, and the sense that we have control of its movements. It seems possible that each form of mental illness is underpinned by disruptions of particular dimensions of 'personal being'. For example, certain kinds of anxiety states might depend upon a diminished sense of ownership (Meares 1986), obsessive compulsive disorder may be related to a deficiency in boundedness (Meares 1994, 2001), borderline personality disorder to a failure of integration and the reflective function (Meares *et al.* 1999*a*), and eating disorders to a very limited sense of control of inner life (Russell and Meares 1997).

Psychiatric care is concerned with the vicissitudes of our ordinary sense of personal existence, with the variations in the 'myself' who appears in the following statement: 'I was not myself when you saw me last'. If psychiatry is to move forward as a science' we must develop a model of this central experience in order to understand the manner of its disruptions. The way in which such a model might be built is illustrated in the work of Hughlings Jackson (1835–1911), the first person to use the word 'self' in the medical literature (Jackson 1931–2, vol. 2, p. 96).

The Jacksonian self

Jackson has been called the father of English neurology. A large part of his opus, however, is devoted to the concept of mind and to a theory of mental illness. These theories influenced James, who corresponded with Jackson and quoted him in his main work. Jackson also influenced Janet in his attempt to build a hierarchy of mental function. Jackson's ideas anticipate, to a remarkable extent, ideas that are current at the moment.

Jackson's approach was logical and methodical. He saw the study of mental illness as, at bottom, an experimental investigation of mind, or self. Accordingly, the first step must be to identify and define this experience. He conceived it as double, consisting of subject and object, or as he put it, 'subject consciousness', symbolized by 'I, and 'object consciousness'. He acknowledged that this distinction is an abstraction, remarking: 'Each by itself is nothing, [each] is only half itself' (Jackson 1931–2, vol. 2, p. 93). In essence, self depends upon the emergence of what he called 'the introspection of consciousness', but it is not equivalent to it (Jackson 1931–2, vol. 2, p. 96).

Jackson's concept of a duplex self was echoed by both Janet (1803, p. 34–5) and James. James made the necessary experiential elaboration of the concept with his description of 'the stream of consciousness'. I am taking this experience as implicit in Jackson's model.

The next task was to understand how this experience arises. Jackson argued that it had its basis in a particular kind of brain function. He warned, however, against the confusion of psychical states with brain states. Rather, there is a 'concomitant parallelism' between brain and mind (Jackson 1931–2, vol. 2, pp. 42, 85).

Jackson's idea about the kind of brain function that underpins the experience of self was based in evolutionary theory. He considered that the organization of the brain was decreed by evolutionary history. He built his theory about what he understood to be the basic units of central nervous system function. These are reflexive — the smallest elements of sensorimotor function. Each of these units he considered to be a representing system. In organisms at an early evolutionary stage, these simple representations are relatively uncoordinated. At a later period of evolution, when the brain is larger, rather than new representations being recorded, there is re-representation and greater coordination (Jackson 1931–2, vol. 2, p. 42). At a higher stage still, there is a re-re-representation and a still further and more complex coordination. This idea must have seemed exotic, even outlandish, in Jackson's time. In our era, however, his supposition has been confirmed. In the visual cortex, for example, it has been shown that there are multiple representations of the visual field rather than a single neural map (Allman 1987, p. 636).

The appearance of self, Jackson suggested, is a manifestation of the most recent evolutionary changes, and so emerges late in human development. The evolution and development of 'self' is a reflection of a more complex coordination than encountered at early phases of evolution and development. Self, seen in this way, is not a structure, or a series of representations, but a process, as James was to later maintain.

Jackson rejected the idea that mind or self requires a special new form of neural function to be built into the human brain. He wrote: 'There is no autocratic mind at the top to receive sensations as a sort of raw material, out of which to manufacture ideas, etc. and then to associate these ideas' (Jackson 1931–2, vol. 2, p. 98). Nevertheless, self is dependent on the evolution of anatomically new structures. Jackson suggested that the evolutionary development of the prefrontal cortex is necessary to the emergence of self (Jackson 1931–2, vol. 2, p. 399). However, this is not to say that self resides in the prefrontal cortex. Rather, the new structure allows a more complex coordination of the fundamental units of the central nervous system.

Jackson's model is resonant with current work on the development of a neural model of 'self', of the kind undertaken by, for example, Damasio (1994). It also anticipates mathematical models of mind based on the emergent mathematics of chaos and complexity.

A testable model

The idea that the brain–mind system is, in essence, a machine is not, in itself, objectionable. The principal objection to the mechanical conceptions of human existence developed during the positivist–behaviourist era is that they exclude fundamental aspects of this experience, and that the conceptions are based not on how the brain–mind system works but on how a particular machine, such as a computer, operates. Jackson himself was proposing a machine. He called the brain–mind system 'a sensori-motor mechanism, a co-ordinating system, from top to bottom' (Jackson 1931–2, vol. 2, p. 41). His hypothetical machine, however, was built in the opposite way. Instead of working from machine to mind, he argued from mind to machine. He began with personal experience, with what seemed to be the central experience of self. The next step, based on meticulous observation of neurological patients, led him to imagine a machine that underpins this form of consciousness. It resembles modern conceptions of a self-organizing system (Capra 1996, pp. 264–85).

Jackson's main hypothesis was that assaults on the brain–mind system cause a retreat down the hierarchy of mental function laid down in evolutionary history. He called this process 'dissolution'. Those functions that appeared last in evolutionary history and emerged late in human development are the most fragile, the most easily overthrown. This hypothesis is testable and provides a means of understanding certain pathological states. Examples include dissociation (Meares 1999) and borderline personality disorder (Meares *et al.* 1999*a*).

Jackson's pioneering model of mind is, of course, limited and preliminary. It lacks, for example, the developmental perspective and the effect of environment. Nevertheless, this perspective is implied. Those functions, which include what Jackson was calling 'self', and which appeared last in evolutionary development, are, he pointed out, 'incomplete', relative to earlier functions. Maturation must depend upon environmental factors.

The complexity of maturation is evident when we reconsider the implications of the statement: 'I was not myself when you saw me last'. The speaker here uses three words, 'I', 'me', and 'myself', that point to different aspects of personhood. Do they all emerge together? Because the experience of personal being is unified, the common sense answer is yes. However, the statement itself suggests something different. The speaker implies a certain stability for 'I' and 'me' but a variability for 'myself' — a potential fragility. The Jacksonian 'dissolution' hypothesis predicts that 'myself' develops considerably later than 'I' and 'me'. Developmental studies support this prediction.

The 'I', a system of awareness and response, is present in early form at birth (Bower 1974). The 'me' is evident at about 18 months when the child can point to his or her image in a mirror or photo and say, 'That's me' (Amsterdam 1972; Lewis and Brooks-Gunn 1979). However, such has been the scientific neglect of the sense of personal being, the self of Jackson and James, that the next major step in this maturation, the appearance of the third term, was not known until quite recently, when it was shown that the development of the concept of 'inner' experience is attained at about 4 years of age (Meares and Orlay 1988). The dating of this milestone is consistent with the findings of Flavell *et al.* (1993), suggesting the child discovers the 'stream of consciousness' at age 4, 5, or 6 years, and also with inferences from so-called 'theory of mind' experiments (Astington *et al.* 1988; Gopnik and Astington 1988; Hobson 1991; Perner 1990; Wellman 1990). The establishment of this milestone provides the starting point for the construction of a plausible schema for the development of the experience of 'myself' (Meares 2000). This schema suggests that it arises and is manifest in conversation (Hobson 1985; Meares 1993, 1998, 2000), the idea that underpins what Hobson called 'the Conversational Model'.

This idea offers a means of overcoming, at least to an extent, a major obstacle in the way of treating self as an object of scientific enquiry, which is that 'self' cannot be observed. However, the notion that the Jamesian self is manifest linguistically leads to the possibility of its fluctuations being charted by words, used in the natural manner, in conversation. Seen in this way, the structure of language reflects a state of self. Linguistic analyses conducted in the author's department in association with the linguistics department of Macquarie University, Sydney, are being employed to study the process and progress of therapy in an ongoing programme for patients with borderline personality disorder (Meares *et al.* 1999*b*; Stevenson and Meares 1992). The analyses used include studies of cohesion (Samir 2001), of transitivity (Henderson-Brooks 2000), and of the complexity of the time–space domain (Garbutt 1997). A principal underlying idea is that human conversation is made up of a mingling of two main forms of language, one related to the environment and the other to self (Meares 1993, 1998, 2000; Meares and Sullivan 2002).

Phenomena to theory

Science moves forward in a way that is represented in the progression from Linnaeus, who classified us and gave us the name of *Homo sapiens*, to Darwin, who proposed a theory of our origins. Both approaches are necessary: one does not supersede the other. An open pathway must remain between the two systems, so that there is a continuing interplay between them, as intimated by Schiller (1801) in his essay on the main themes of 'matter' and 'form'.

Hughlings Jackson used the methods of both Linnaeus and Darwin in his attempt to develop a theory that provided a basis for understanding certain mental illnesses. He began with a precise observation of phenomena, both psychic and neurological. These gave him the ground out of which a theory could grow.

Janet's approach was similar in confronting a condition that other observers had maintained was too protean in its manifestations to bring 'together under one and the same formula'. He searched for the 'rigorous laws' (Janet 1893, p. 484) that underlay and determined these phenomena. In particular, his aim was to go beyond Briquet (1859).

Briquet had worked at Salpêtrière in the 1850s. In the manner of an epidemiologist, he simply catalogued all the most salient clinical and biographical details of 430 people given the diagnosis of hysteria at that hospital. Such a method is useful as a 'starting point', as Janet acknowledged (p. 487), but it offers no means of understanding the condition, no theoretical framework to guide the direction of treatment.

It is of interest that Briquet's catalogue became the basis for DSM-III's 'somatization disorder', when the word 'hysteria' was officially removed from the psychiatric lexicon. This diagnosis was based on a checklist that failed to include essential features of the syndrome identified by Janet, most notably conversion and personality disorder. Although there have been rectifications in DSM-IV, the diagnosis of 'somatization disorder' is emblematic of the deficiencies of the DSM.

The DSM does not reflect a proper empiricism in the manner of Linnaeus, in which phenomena are observed without preconception. Although the tradition of Linnaeus is maintained — a physician, he devised an early psychiatric classification — it is muddied by the interpenetration of various traditions, ideologies, and viewpoints. One ideology and tradition that appears to be particularly influential is that which dominated Western thought in the years after 1913, and in which the phenomena of consciousness are devalued. The diagnostic criteria of 'somatization disorder', in a manual of mental disorders, include not one mention of psychic life. Janet's careful observations of the disturbed consciousness of his patients remain disregarded, as is his view that 'retraction of the field of consciousness', characteristic of the condition (Janet 1893, pp. 496–507), is related to a disturbance of cerebral function (pp. 507–8). No state of consciousness is an isolated phenomenon. It arises as a consequence of the brain's interplay with the sensory environment. The possibility that the unusual life history of pain exhibited by those with so-called 'somatization disorder' is related to deficiencies in sensory processing, as demonstrated in a number of studies (Horvarth et al. 1980; James et al. 1989, 1990), is not contemplated in the DSM-IV narrative concerning diagnostic category 300.81. The approach is firmly behavioural, locked in the mode of thought epitomized in the expressions of Watson and Ryle. It is a diminished form of psychiatric practice that is based in such limited conceptualizations.

To develop a psychiatric practice based on adequate theory, we need to acquire the data out of which to create such a theory or theories. The phenomena of consciousness that were once the main subject of philosophy and psychiatry are no longer studied in any systematic way. In order to go beyond our present level of conceptualization and practice in psychiatry, we must employ the modes of thinking exemplified by Jackson, James, and Janet, and return the psyche to psychiatry.

Karl Jaspers wrote: 'All life reveals itself as a continuous interchange between an inner and an outer world' (Jaspers 1962, p. 12). Out of this interchange arises the third thing, the experience of 'myself'. Unless psychiatric institutions of teaching and research restore to the experiences of 'inner' life the value given to them before the shift in Western consciousness that occurred round 1913, we are in danger of developing and propagating a discipline that is, in a fundamental way, lifeless.

References

Allman, J. M. (1987). Evolution of the brain in primates. In *The Oxford Companion to the Mind* (ed. R. L. Gregory). pp. 633–9. Oxford: Oxford University Press.

Amsterdam, B. (1972). Mirror self image reactions before age two. *Developmental Psychology*, **26**: 738–44.

Arendt, H. (1968). *Totalitarianism*. New York: Harvest, Harcourt, Brace and Jovanovich.

Ashby, W. R. (1960). *Design for a Brain*. London: Chapman and Hall.

Astington, J. W., Harris, P. L., and Olson, D. R. (1988). *Developing Theories of Mind*. Cambridge: Cambridge University Press.

Baudrillard, J. (1983). '*Simulations* (trans. P. Foss, P. Patton, and P. Beitchman). New York: Semiotext (e).

Bergson, H. (1911). *Matter and Memory*. London: Allen and Unwin.

Bower, T. (1974). *Development in Infancy*. San Francisco: Freeman.

Briquet, P. (1859). *Traité de Clinique et Thérapeutique a l'Hystérie*. Paris: Baillière.

Capra, F. (1996). *The Web of Life: a new scientific understanding of living systems*. New York: Anchor, Doubleday.

Clark, T. J. (1984). *Farewell to an Idea*. New Haven: Yale University Press.

Damasio, A. (1994). *Descartes' Error*. New York: Grosset, Putnam.

Ellenberger, H. F. (1970). *The Discovery of the Unconscious*. London: Allen Lane Press.

Fischer, E. (1963). *The Necessity of Art* (trans. A. Bostick). Harmondsworth, UK: Penguin.

Flavell, J., Green, F., and Flavell, E. (1993). Children's understanding of the stream of consciousness. *Child Development*, **64**: 387–96.

Ford, H. (1919). *New York Times*, May 20.

Garbutt, M. (1997). *Figure Talk: Reported Speech and Thought in the Discourse of Psychotherapy*. PhD thesis, Macquarie University, Sydney.

Gopnik, A. and Astington, J. (1988). Children's understanding of representational change and its relation to the understanding of false belief and the appearance-reality distinction. *Child Development*, **59**: 26–37.

Harter, S. (1983). Developmental perspectives on the self system. In *Handbook of Child Psychology*, vol. 4 (ed. P. Mussen). New York: Wiley.

Henderson-Brooks, C. (2000). An investigation of the language of a person with borderline personality disorder during psychotherapy. BA (hons) thesis, Macquarie University, Sydney.

Hobson, R. F. (1985). *Forms of Feeling: The Heart of Psychotherapy*. London: Tavistock.

Hobson, R. P. (1991). Against the theory of 'theory of mind'. *British Journal of Developmental Psychology*, **9**: 33–51.

Holtzmann, H. and James, M (ed. and trans.) (1993). *The New Art — New Life: The Collected Writings of Piet Mondrian*. New York: Da Capo Press.

Horvarth, T., Friedman, J., and Meares, R. (1980). Attention in hysteria: a study of Janet's hypothesis by means of habituation and arousal measures. *American Journal of Psychiatry*, **137**: 217–20.

Jackson, J. H. (1931–2). *Selected Writings of John Hughlings Jackson*, vols 1 and 2 (ed. J. Taylor). London: Hodder.

James, L., Gordon, E., Kraiuhin, C., and Meares, R. (1989) Selective attention and auditory event related potentials in somatization disorder. *Comprehensive Psychiatry*, **30**: 84–9.

James, L., Gordon, E., Kraiuhin, C., Howson, A., and Meares, R. (1990). Augmentation of auditory evoked potentials in somatization disorder. *Journal of Psychiatric Research*, **24**: 155–63.

James, W. (1890). *Principles of Psychology*, vols I and II. New York: Holt.

James, W. (1892). *Psychology: Briefer Course*. London: Macmillan.

Janet, P. (1893). *The Mental State of Hystericals* (trans. C. R. Corson). New York: Putnam, 1901.

Jaspers, K. (1962). *General Psychopathology*. Manchester: Manchester University Press.

Jung, C. G. (1961). Freud and psychoanalysis. In *C. G. Jung: The Collected Works*, vol. 4 (trans. R. F. C. Hull). London: Routledge and Kegan Paul.

Kirsner, D. (2001). Off the radar screen. *Psychoanalytic Studies*, **3**: 247–54.

Kohut, H. (1971). *The Analysis of the Self*. New York: International Universities Press.

Kohut, H. (1977). *The Restoration of the Self*. New York: International Universities Press.

Lewis, M. and Brooks-Gunn, J. (1979). *Social Cognition and the Acquisition of Self*. New York: Plenum.

Meares, R. (1986). On the ownership of thought: an approach to the origins of separation anxiety. *Psychiatry*, **21**: 549–59.

Meares, R. (1993). *The Metaphor of Play: Disruption and Restoration in the Borderline Experience*. Northvale, NJ: Jason Aronson.

Meares, R. (1994). A pathology of privacy: towards a new theoretical approach to obsessive-compulsive disorder. *Contemporary Psychoanalysis*, **30**(1): 83–100.

Meares, R. (1998). The self in conversation: on narratives, chronicles and scripts. *Psychoanalytic Dialogues*, **8**(6): 875–91.

Meares, R. (1999). Hughlings Jackson's contribution to an understanding of dissociation. *American Journal of Psychiatry*, **156**(12): 1850–5.

Meares, R. (2000). *Intimacy and Alienation: Memory, Trauma and Personal Being*. London: Routledge.

Meares, R. (2001). A specific developmental deficit in obsessive-compulsive disorder: the example of the Wolf Man. *Psychoanalytic Inquiry*, **21**: 289–319.

Meares, R. and Orlay, W. (1988). On self boundary: a study of the development of the concept of secrecy. *British Journal of Medical Psychology*, **1**: 305–16.

Meares, R. and Sullivan, G. (2002). *Two Forms of Human Language*. In *Language Development: Functional Perspective in Evolution and Autogenesis* (ed. G. Williams and A. Lukin). London: Continuum. (in press)

Meares, R., Stevenson, J., and Gordon, E. (1999*a*). A Jacksonian and biopsychosocial hypothesis concerning borderline and related phenomena. *Australian and New Zealand Journal of Psychiatry*, **33**(6): 831–40.

Meares, R., Stevenson, J., and Comerford, A. (1999*b*). Psychotherapy with borderline patients. Part I: A comparison between treated and untreated cohorts. *Australian and New Zealand Journal of Psychiatry*, **33**(3): 467–72.

Myers, G. (1986). *William James: His Life and Thoughts*. New Haven: Yale University Press.

Perner, J. (1990). *Understanding the Representational Mind*. Cambridge, MA: MIT/Bradford.

Pevsner, N. (1957). *An Outline of European Architecture*. Harmondsworth, UK: Penguin.

Russell, J. and Meares, R. (1997). Paradox, persecution and the double game: psychotherapy in anorexia nervosa. *Australian and New Zealand Journal of Psychiatry*, **31**(5): 691–9.

Rycroft, C. (1972). *A Critical Dictionary of Psychoanalysis*. Harmondsworth, UK: Penguin.

Ryle, G. (1949). *The Concept of Mind*, London: Hutchinson. Harmondsworth: Penguin. (The 1963 edition is cited here.)

Sadato, N., Pascual-Leone, A., Grafman, J., Ibanez, V., Deiber, M. P., Dold, G., *et al.* (1996). Activation of the primary visual cortex by Braille reading in blind subjects. *Nature*, **380**: 526–8.

Samir, H. (2001). *Resonance in Therapeutic Conversation and the Emergence of Self.* Master of Medicine (Psychotherapy) thesis, University of Sydney.

Schiller, F. (1801). *On the Aesthetic Education of Man* (ed. and trans. E. Wilkinson and L. Willoughby). Oxford: Oxford University Press, 1967.

Smith, T. (1993). *Making the Modern, Art, and Design in America*. Chicago: University of Chicago Press.

Stevenson, J. and Meares, R. (1992). An outcome study of psychotherapy in borderline personality disorder. *American Journal of Psychiatry*, **149**: 358–62.

Tulving, E. (1972). Episodic and sematic memory. pp. 382–404. In *Organization of Memory* (ed. E. Tulving and W. Donaldson). New York: Academic Press.

Wellman, H. (1990). *The Child's Theory of Mind*. Cambridge, MA: MIT Press, Bradford Books.

Winnicott, D. (1971). *Playing and Reality*. London: Tavistock.

Section 2   A New Kind of Philosophy

3 Wittgenstein's method and psychoanalysis

Gordon Baker

It is known that Wittgenstein conceived of philosophy primarily as a kind of therapy. He offered therapies for particular philosophical problems (Wittgenstein 1953, §§133, 255).[1] Evidently his procedure is rational discussion; he offers a 'talk cure'. But what is treated? What are the illnesses? What precisely is the nature of the treatment? What are its goals? There seems to be room for diversity in giving answers to these questions.

Even in the case of medicine, we are faced with a choice between different models of therapy. At a minimum there are contrasts between preventive and curative medicine, between the practice of a general practitioner and the conduct of public health campaigns. The targets of these activities are correspondingly different: obesity or lack of aerobic exercise, cancer or smallpox, burns and broken limbs. What is the intended analogy? Which one makes best sense of an activity? This seems an important question to consider, even if any answer is conjectural.

The concept of a disorder has a range of applications to non-medical conditions and, correlatively, the concept of therapy extends far beyond the practice of medicine. There are behavioural, affective, sensory, social, and intellectual disorders of individuals, and there are all kinds of suggested therapies: drugs, behavioural therapy, 'cognitive therapy', etc. Do any of these practices provide an analogy that illuminates Wittgenstein's philosophical investigations?

Some fix on his particular conception of therapy can be derived from his suggestions that there are some similarities between his philosophical investigations and psychoanalysis. This is a muted, but recurrent, theme. Wittgenstein also made definite, though sparing, use of some of Freud's terminology in the course of his investigations: 'the unconscious', 'acknowledgement', 'sublimation', 'censorship', and 'resistance'.

It is, of course, debatable just what similarities he saw and what dissimilarities, and also how much importance is to be attached to comparisons of his philosophical activities with psychoanalysis. 'Not much' seems to be the

---

[1] The abbreviation 'BT' in the text refers to the 'Big Typescript' TS 213 in von Wright (1982). References are to section numbers when prefixed with the sign '§', otherwise to page numbers.

prevalent view,[2] but it can scarcely be denied that there is evidence for a contrary assessment. Some of this is internal:[3]

> We can only convict another person of a mistake . . . if he (really) **acknowledges** this expression as the correct expression of his feeling.

> For only if he **acknowledges** it as such, *is* it the correct expression. (**Psychoanalysis**.) (BT, p. 410)

> Difficulty of philosophy, not the intellectual difficulty of the sciences, but the difficulty of a change of attitude. **Resistances** of the will to be overcome. (**BT**, p. 406)

Other evidence is external:

> W. had himself talked about philosophy as in certain ways like psychoanalysis . . . When he became a professor at Cambridge he submitted a typescript to the committee. . . . Of 140 pages, 72 were devoted to the idea that philosophy is like psychoanalysis.[4]

Full clarification of this comparison and resolving the dispute about its importance would be an enormous undertaking even if one could avoid disputes about alternative interpretations of Freud. At a minimum, it would require investigation of the extent of Wittgenstein's knowledge of Freud, especially of how he understood the methods of psychoanalysis and what he thought to be of interest and value in this practice. It would require thorough investigation of his conception of philosophical problems. Ideally, it would involve a comprehensive survey and detailed analysis of the problems he addressed and the therapeutic methods that he exhibited in his writings, dictations, and lectures. And it might even require considering why many analytical philosophers exhibit strong resistance to acknowledging analogies between psychoanalysis and his diverse philosophical investigations.

My goal in this chapter is more limited: to study in some detail the conceptual investigations that are the immediate context of one remark making an explicit comparison with psychoanalysis. This material occurs in the 'Diktat für Schlick'[5], a text dictated to Friedrich Waismann, most probably in

---

[2]P. M. S. Hacker (*Wittgenstein: Meaning and Mind*, pp. 90–92) lists a number of respects in which the analogy is illuminating.

[3]In all quotations, *italics* are used to mark the author's own emphasis, and bold to mark emphases that the author has added. Translations are the author's own; occasionally they modify published ones.

[4]This is part of a reported conversation in August 1949 (Bouwsma 1986, p. 36). The typescript referred to here is the pre-war version of *Philosophical Investigations* (TS 220 in von Wright (1982)).

[5]This is TS 302 in von Wright (1982).

December 1932. Since the whole text has remained hitherto unpublished and little studied, careful investigation of the remarks in Diktat für Schlick (pp. 28–30) offers the possibility of throwing some fresh light on Wittgenstein's therapeutic methods.[6]

Let's begin with the methodological remark itself:

> Our method resembles psychoanalysis in a certain sense. To use its way of putting things, we could say that a simile operating in the unconscious can be made harmless by being articulated. And the comparison with psychoanalysis can be developed even further. (And this analogy is certainly no coincidence.) [7]

Six things are immediately noteworthy. First, it is 'our method' (not philosophy in general) that is said to bear some resemblance with psychoanalysis. Second, the resemblance is claimed to hold only *in a certain sense* (not in all respects).[8] Third, the ostensible topic is the explicit articulation of *a simile*, which is working *unconsciously* in somebody's thinking (cf. BT, p. 410). Fourth, it is suggested that a simile may be *damaging* as long as it is unconscious, whereas it can be rendered *harmless* by *articulating* it and acknowledging it *as a simile*. (This is a specific application of the general therapeutic technique that is characteristic of psychoanalysis.) Fifth, the analogy of 'our method' with psychoanalysis holds, too, *in some other (unspecified) respects*. Finally, the analogy itself is *not accidental*, but rather *essential* to 'our method'; hence grasping certain respects in which Wittgenstein's practice resembles psychotherapy is necessary for understanding what he is trying to do.

This remark is interpolated into an otherwise uninterrupted discussion. Its placement suggests that the purpose of the remark is to clarify the strategy being pursued in the surrounding text. So, the immediate question is how exactly that discussion makes clear that Wittgenstein's method does indeed resemble psychoanalysis *in a certain sense*.

The immediate topic of discussion is broached a few sentences earlier:

> If we want to deal with a proposition such as 'The nothing noths' or the question 'Which is prior, nothing or negation?', then in order to do it justice

---

[6] The original German text together with a translation into English is to appear in Waismann (2002).

[7] Original text: 'Unsere Methode ähnelt in gewissem Sinn der Psychoanalyse. In ihrer Ausdrucksweise könnte man sagen, dass im Unbewusstsein wirkende Gleichnis wird unschädlich, wenn es ausgesprochen wird. Und dieser Vergleich mit der Analyse lässt sich noch weithin fortsetzen. (Und diese Analogie ist gewiss kein Zufall.)'

[8] What are the respects in which the analogy does *not* hold? This important question is not investigated here.

we ask ourselves 'What did the author have in mind with this proposition?'
[or] 'Where did he get this proposition from?'[9]

The topic is the treatment of a pair of paradigms of *philosophical* utterances taken from Heidegger.[10] The first is notorious. And the second one frames a quintessentially philosophical question by making use of the concept of priority. (Other such questions are 'How is it *possible* that . . . ?', 'What are the *real* properties of . . . ?', 'Of what things can one be *absolutely certain*?', etc.)

Given the widespread impression that Wittgenstein's general business is to frog-march words back from their metaphysical to their everyday use (Wittgenstein 1953, §116; BT, p. 412), one might expect him to lodge strenuous objections to this pair of propositions. Should not he condemn Heidegger for uttering nonsense?[11] Objections spring immediately to mind. The expression 'das Nichts' ('the nothing') is ill formed: like 'everything', 'nothing' cannot be combined with the definite article. There is no such verb as 'nichten' ('to noth'). What could it possibly mean to compare 'nothing' with 'something' in respect of priority? Can 'negation' be called some *thing*? Could a logical operation (negation) occur prior to anything other than another logical operation? And so forth.

Less pedantically, one might make fun of what Heidegger said:

> When it comes to noth-ing, is it only the nothing that can noth? Or could something noth? Unless something *can* noth, can there be any such thing as noth-ing? So if the nothing really noths, must the nothing be something? Otherwise there could be no noth-ing. So how then could it be true of the nothing that it noths?

But these are not Wittgenstein's procedures. Instead, in order to *do justice* to such a proposition (*um ihm gerecht zu werden*)[12], we must ask what *the author* had in mind in framing them, what he might have meant by them, or from what source he took them. These philosophical utterances are *patently* nonsensical; to the extent that the author is aware of this, it would be pointless to produce an argument in support of that claim. (Heidegger could scarcely have failed to notice this 'defect'.[13]) What we need to clarify

---

[9]Original text: 'Wenn wir einen Satz wie den "das Nichts nichtet" oder die Frage "was ist früher, das Nichts oder die Verneinung?" behandeln wollen, so fragen wir uns, um ihm gerecht zu werden: was hat dem Autor bei diesem Satz vorgeschwebt? Woher hat er diesen Satz genommen?'

[10]Both occur in his inaugural lecture 'What is metaphysics?' given in Freiburg in 1929.

[11]This is precisely what Rudolf Carnap did in some detail in the paper 'Überwindung der Metaphysik durch logische Analyse der Sprache' (Carnap 1932).

[12]This purpose is prominent in the 'Big Typescript': 'Our sole task is to be just [*gerecht zu sein*]' (BT 420); 'The goal . . . justice [*Gerechtigkeit*]' (BT 414). Later he indicated the need to avoid injustice [*Ungerechtigkeit*] in his assertions (Wittgenstein 1953, §131).

[13]In fact, as Carnap noted, Heidegger turns this 'logical' absurdity into a condemnation of the sovereignty of 'logic'.

is what *motivates* a particular individual to say obviously puzzling things.[14] We might do this by getting her to remind herself of how she herself uses words in everyday life — for the specific purpose of encouraging her to reflect on precisely how her philosophical utterances deviate from that pattern. We try to get her to direct her attention to her own motivation. She needs to work out *why* she feels *driven* to say what she does. What is pathological in her thinking is not the deviance of her philosophical utterances from everyday speech patterns, but the unconscious *motives* that give rise to her behaviour.

This strategy is pursued in a distinctive form of investigation — seeking for an unconscious analogy or picture, an unconscious conception or a way of seeing things. Wittgenstein's diagnosis of a philosophical problem (disquiet) is that a philosopher thinks that to convey an important insight he is compelled to say something that seems, *even to himself*, empty, self-contradictory or meaningless. He experiences an internal tension or conflict. What needs clarification are the motives that occasion such a conflict.

> When . . . we disapprove of these expressions of ordinary language (which are after all performing their office), we have got a picture in our heads which conflicts with the picture of our ordinary way of speaking. Whereas we are tempted to say that our way of speaking does not describe the facts as they really are . . . As if the form of expression were saying something false when the proposition *faute de mieux* asserted something true. (Wittgenstein 1953, §402)

The suggestion of an unconscious picture as the root of someone's intellectual trouble clearly requires to be confirmed by this individual's own acknowledgment. To put this strategy into practice is, in a certain sense, to treat a person seriously and with respect, i.e. to try to make sense of her saying something despite its apparently making no sense at all.

Aren't there parallels with Freud? The psychoanalyst's task is to uncover the *unconscious motives* for a patient's manifestly *absurd* ideas or behaviour, and to get the patient to *acknowledge* his motives. This is a difficult and delicate task. In particular, it may require helping the patient to overcome his own *resistance*.

---

[14]This strategy is pursued in Wittgenstein (1953, §§38–9). It is noted that '*strange to say*, the word "this" has been called the only genuine name'. (This seems a clear allusion to Russell.) Reasons are listed why the use of 'this' does not fall within the gamut of word-uses that are characterized by the term 'name' (§38c). 'But *why* does it occur to one to *want* to make precisely this word into a name, when it *evidently* is not a name? — This is just the reason. For one is tempted to make an *objection* against what is ordinarily called a name' (§39). A suggestion is then made: 'a name really ought to signify a simple'. But this will be a correct diagnosis of the motivation only if it is acknowledged by the imagined interlocutor. The emphasis of this whole passage is not on showing that the philosophical statement is mistaken, but on clarifying an individual's motivation for making such a patently strange claim.

This pattern of investigation dominates the subsequent stretch of 'Diktat für Schlick'. This explores *why* (for what *reasons*) Heidegger expresses himself in an extraordinary way, *why* he feels driven to run up against the limits of language (Wittgenstein 1953, §119). It looks for a picture that *unconsciously* shapes his thinking and it seeks to clarify the *sources* of this picture or the *materials* from which it has been derived. (Hence this investigation into motives has some general affinity with Freud's procedure of tracing the origins of neuroses in an individual's childhood experience.)

Wittgenstein first suggests the diagnosis that someone who is tempted to speak as Heidegger does is operating unconsciously with a particular simile. In this case, being or existence is pictured as an island in a sea of nothingness, and this sea is imagined as restlessly eating away at the solid land, and dissolving it away. In endlessly throwing up waves and causing erosion, the sea manifests an *activity*, and that is what Heidegger meant to signify by the verb 'nichten' ('to noth'). (This might be a paradigm of 'a simile that has been absorbed into the forms of our language' (Wittgenstein 1953, §112).[15])

What is the status of this suggestion? How could it be *demonstrated* that Heidegger must have been influenced by just this picture? It cannot be *shown* to be correct. (*Man kann es garnicht zeigen.*) Presumably *the individual* to whom this suggestion is made must *acknowledge* the simile as something that *did* influence her thinking. *Only* in this case is the diagnosis correct (BT, p. 410; Ambrose 1979, pp. 27, 40). Only then is *her* problem brought to light. Only then have we articulated something that *was* working *unconsciously* in *her* thinking.

Her acknowledgment need not be grounded in any memories of actual episodes of reasoning things out; indeed, if the simile was working unconsciously (*im Unbewussten*), this *could not* be her ground. Here, there seems to be a problem about validation of a statement that has the form of a memory-claim about an individual's past unconscious motives. (There is a parallel conceptual problem in psychoanalysis.) Does this make Wittgenstein's diagnosis pointless? Is the suggestion empty?

Arguably, what underpins my acknowledgment that this simile *has been* working unconsciously in my thinking is the recognition that reflecting on it now has the power to eradicate the drive or temptation for my making these particular philosophical pronouncements. I am now inclined to say both 'That's exactly the way I *meant* it' (*'ja, genau so habe ich es gemeint'*) and 'That is completely absurd' (cf. BT, p. 410). (Here, the manifest absurdity of thinking of non-existence as an activity is indicated by the ironic remark: 'In this sense of "activity" even resting (*das Ruhen*) would signify an activity'.) Philosophical

---

[15]Analogues might be the picture of the sequence of events as logs floating downstream in a river and passing under a bridge (Wittgenstein 1958, 107–8); the simile of immediate experience as the image cast on a screen by a film strip passing through a projector (BT 428); or the conception of measurement as juxtaposition of two things (Wittgenstein 1958, 26; Waismann 1965, 42).

theses and questions may be the manifestations of confusion (*Verwirrung*). If my particular confusion is now dissolved by reflecting on the simile that Wittgenstein proposes, then this discussion has achieved the sole desideratum (*das, was wir tun wollten*) of a philosophical clarification of concepts, namely eliminating a particular philosophical problem, i.e. a particular individual's disquiet, unrest, or torment, an individual's tormenting question (*quälende Frage*). We could imagine Heidegger simply dropping the assertion 'Das Nichts nichtet' because it has now lost all its interest or importance for him.

This is a very different criterion of success from proving that a question *cannot* be framed or that a statement *cannot* be made because it transgresses the bounds of sense.[16] In particular, success is strictly person-relative. The problem is *somebody's* mental *disturbance*. Hence philosophical problems, in contrast to all others, can be *completely* dissolved (BT, p. 421; cf. p. 431): the *individual's specific* disturbance may vanish completely. 'The problems are dissolved in the literal sense [*im eigentlichen Sinne*] — like a lump of sugar in water' (BT, p. 421). In this sense, conceptual analysis is essentially terminable, but *other people* may develop or continue to have the very same problems — or new ones. For these reasons, the general task of philosophical therapy is, in another sense, essentially endless (cf. Wittgenstein 1967, §447).

What seems crucial here is winning someone's acknowledgement of other possibilities. Pluralism is built into the very idea of a simile or picture: explicitly to regard something as a picture is to recognize that there are alternative conceptions of what is depicted. (This is arguably why articulating an unconscious simile gets rid of its damaging power and renders it harmless. It can no longer exercise tyranny if one acknowledges it as a simile.) If Heidegger were to acknowledge the proposed *simile* as the root of his thinking, and if he were really uneasy (*ungemütlich*) about saying 'Das Nichts nichtet', then he has available a way out of his difficulty, viz. dropping this picture. (This is perhaps easiest to achieve if he sees how to replace the first picture by another picture no less well 'justified' by what he says and thinks.) He would then lose the *drive* to make this philosophical statement. It gave expression to a disquiet that has now vanished away.

In what sense does this amount to treatment of a philosophical problem? Understanding why Wittgenstein thinks that a discussion of a picture with an individual is relevant to philosophical investigation depends on clarifying his distinctive conception of philosophical problems. This is exactly what he now proceeds to sketch.

'It might strike us as strange by what as it were trivial means [*durch welche gleichsam trivialen Mittel*] we can be freed from deep philosophical disquiets

---

[16]Carnap's explicit purpose is to show how Heidegger's questions and assertions violate logical syntax; in a logically adequate language, they could not be expressed. If his argument is cogent, its conclusion is impersonal, a theorem about the 'geometry' of language.

[*Beunruhiggungen*].' This does indeed seem remarkable. One might exclaim: 'How can discarding a mere picture eliminate a *conceptual* difficulty?' One might think that more impressive resources must be necessary, something comparable to inventing the theory of types or Russell's analysis of definite descriptions. It seems that *deep* problems must require non-trivial solutions. (This idea is expressed in the French proverb: Aux grands maux les *grands* remèdes.) But 'against this stands **our** conception that there is no such thing as a *big* problem in the intellectual sense' [*im Sinne der Wissenschaft*] (BT, p. 407).

Wittgenstein tackles this wonder as a sign of confusion. It must be equally astonishing that disquiets may also be eliminated by mere changes in notation.[17] In both cases the confusion is to suppose that these means of dissolving difficulties are really trivial. They are only '*as it were* trivial'! We are strongly inclined to speak of '*mere* pictures' and '*mere* changes in notation'. But these dismissive turns of phrase are misconceived — in respect of many philosophical problems.

He discusses two cases of dissolving worries by changes of notation. The first is 'the problem of identity in diversity' (von Wright 1982, TS 200, §99). We say: 'This rose is red'. Company this to the statement, 'Two plus two is four', we may suppose that the first statement claims that this rose is *identical with* the colour red. Or we might arrive at the more sophisticated idea of its really being true that the rose is red requires the *partial* identity of the rose and the colour red. (Even that has obviously paradoxical implications.) Here the problem can be dissolved by introducing two distinct logical symbols, 'ϵ' and '$=$', to distinguish two senses of 'is'. The first is used to translate 'This rose is red': this statement has the form '$a\epsilon A$' and says that this rose is a member of the set of red things. The second is used to translate 'Two plus two is four': this can be written in arithmetical notation as '$2 + 2 = 4$'. This change of notation frees us from the troubling question: 'To what extent is this rose the very same thing as the colour red?'. Or, more precisely, our puzzlement is removed provided that we *acknowledge* that 'ϵ' expresses what we meant by 'is' in 'This rose is red' (Waismann 1965, pp. 35–6).[18] 'It is characteristic of [*a certain kind of philosophical problem*] . . . that the questioner is *freed* from the problem through a certain change in his mode of expression'.[19]

---

[17]It is sometimes asserted that he holds the opposite view, as if, in describing our conceptual landscape, he endorsed the objection: 'What you want is only a new notation, and by a new notation no facts of geography are changed' (Wittgenstein 1958, p. 57).

[18]cf. Waismann 1965, 148: The rule that a speaker is now following might be one to which he *assents* when we *suggest* it to him. In this case it is a revocable *decision* which validates our taking this to be the rule that he is following (cf. Wittgenstein 1953, §82).

F 34: Die Zeichenregel ist dann die Regel, zu der der Sprechende sich *bekennt*.

Dieses Sich-zu-einer-Regel-bekennen ist auch das **Ende** einer philosophischen Untersuchung. Wenn man z. B. die Skrupeln über das Wort 'ist' dadurch weggeräumt hat, dass man den Menschen 2 oder 3 verschiedene Zeichen statt des einen zur Verfügung stellt, so hinge nun alles davon ab, dass er sich zu dieser Regel bekennt, ϵ sei durch $=$ nicht zu ersetzen.

[19]von Wright 1982, Band XI (MS 115) 36.

The second case is the 'Law of Identity'. The formula 'A = A' seems to be a fundamental proposition of logic; it has often been taken to be a logical axiom. But what does it mean? This question seems deep and in a certain sense mysterious. At the same time, 'A = A' seems to be utterly stupid and useless (cf. Diamond 1976, pp. 282–3). Compare this formula with 'A = B'; that may be construed as a licence to substitute 'A' for 'B' in any logical formula. But what point could there be in setting up a rule to license substituting 'A' for itself? It is remarkable that we can free ourselves from this disturbing question simply by introducing a notation that excludes the possibility of the formula 'A = A' (Wittgenstein 1961, 5.53, 5.533). Strange as it may sound, what seemed to us deep, fundamental, *a priori* about this formula we recognize again in its exclusion from our language by adoption of a new system of signs.[20] 'The deep problem lay, so to speak, simply in the fact that we felt uncomfortable [*ungemütlich*] in the old notation . . . ' On this conception, there is nothing in the least astonishing in the observation that a change in notation may eliminate someone's deep discomforts.

What these considerations bring out is Wittgenstein's distinctive conception of philosophical problems. These are not regarded as abstract puzzles that stand in need of solutions, like chess problems or riddles. They are not conceptual problems that have the accidental property of perplexing and troubling some thinkers. Equally, they are not discomforts that are caused or brought about by conceptual problems.[21] Rather they are individuals' *troubled states of mind*, which have as their intentional *objects* particular conceptual confusions, tensions, paradoxes, or puzzles. A philosophical problem *is* an individual's internal conflict: 'But *this* isn't how it is!', we say. 'Yet *this* is how it has to *be*!' (Wittgenstein 1953, §112).[22] There are many examples. Frege had the conviction that numbers must be objects if there is any possibility of knowledge in arithmetic, and yet he could see no coherent way to frame logical definitions of numbers as objects. Someone may be disturbed by the impression of disorder in his own concepts (BT, p. 421: *ein Bewusstsein der Unordnung in unsern Begriffen*) or by an apparent absence of systematicity in rules of inference (Waismann 2002: *die Regellosigkeit*). A person may be

---

[20]This thought might be generalized. If *essence* is expressed by grammar (Wittgenstein 1953, §372), and if every rule of grammar can be made to disappear by adopting a suitable notation (McGuinness 1967, 239–41), then what makes any proposition the expression of something fundamental and *a priori* is the possibility of eliminating it completely from language.

[21]For this reason, they are wholly unlike headaches. (That comparison is frequently drawn in order to make fun of the idea that Wittgenstein's therapy is directed at troubled *individuals*. It seems to inform Ryle's often quoted remark that Wittgenstein did not have 'a soothing bedside manner'.)

[22]It is common to confuse the objects of emotions with their causes, and thereby to take the relation of an emotion to its object to be external or hypothetical. Wittgenstein emphasized the importance of keeping this distinction clearly in focus.

seriously irritated at her apparent inability to describe fully her own immediate experience; e.g. her inability to say how many stars or raindrops she now *sees* (Waismann 2002: *'Phänomenale Sprache'*). She may feel frustrated or exasperated at becoming entangled in her own explanations of word-meanings or at feeling left in the lurch by them (e.g. in trying to explain what 'A = A' means). And so on.

This point is subtle but crucial. On Wittgenstein's conception, philosophical problems *are* deep disquiets (Wittgenstein 1953, §111), feelings of discomfort, torments, irritations, conflicts, etc. He targets 'philosophical problems, i.e. the particular disquiets of individuals which we call "philosophical problems"' (von Wright 1982, Band XI.35). 'Our method' is aimed at getting philosophical problems to disappear completely — *in this sense of 'problem'*. 'As I conduct philosophy, its **entire task** consists in shaping expressions so that certain **disquiets** [*Beunruhigungen*] . . . disappear' (BT, p. 421). Certain questions give rise to a peculiar mental disquiet, and activity that is philosophy might be characterized as 'the allaying of this disquiet'.[23]

This conception of philosophical problems is clear in 'Diktat für Schlick', even though it is only partially explained there. I have exploited roughly contemporaneous texts to bring it into sharper focus.

It is a corollary of this conception of a philosophical problem that philosophical investigation (or the clarification of concepts) *must* take the form of a discussion with an *individual* (actual or imaginary). Every problem is *someone's* problem, and another's problem is *another* problem (cf. Frege 1959, §27). Hence therapy for confusions is *essentially* person-relative.

It is equally clear that philosophical discussions *cannot* be adversarial. Suggestions are made, but the interlocutor must acknowledge a picture if it is to be root of his problem (BT, p. 410). Likewise, he must accept and make use of a notation that gets rid of his worry. Everything depends on his *free* acknowledgment (Waismann 1965, p. 36; cf. p. 148; Waismann 1956, pp. 18–21). This might leave one wondering how anything is achieved if nothing is *proven* — or at least why the achievement belongs to *philosophy*.

It is an essential feature of Wittgenstein's discussions that the interlocutor is free to reject any suggestions made. Someone who makes a philosophical utterance is offered a picture that may inform her thinking, or she is made aware of an alternative way of expressing things. She may be advised to put aside the question, 'What is meaning?', and to focus instead on the question, 'What's an explanation of meaning?' (Wittgenstein 1958, p. 1). Why not reject these suggestions? They might seem like evasions. She could object that they are not analyses of concepts. The answer indicated here is that the proposals are felt to relieve the problem-troubled individual of her disquiet or torment. *Her suffering* is the motive-force for her accepting a *possible* escape route when its

---

[23]'Philosophie ist die Stillung dieser Unruhe' (F. Waismann in the introduction to Schlick (1936)).

availability is clear to *her*.[24] (Here is another respect of analogy with psychoanalysis.) She feels: 'Thanks be to God! I now see how to drop that burden' (cf. BT, p. 416). She realizes the possibility of adopting a way of thinking or a notation that no longer leaves her feeling deeply ill at ease (*ungemütlich*). If I see the possibility of discarding the simile that drives me into saying 'Das Nichts nichtet', or if I see the possibility of replacing that simile by another that doesn't depict a kind of struggle between being and non-being, then I have found a good reason for laying aside this metaphysical proposition as something without further interest to me. What earlier seemed to me to be gold when I was, as it were, in the magic castle, now in the light of day strikes me as nothing but a piece of rusty metal (cf. Wittgenstein 1980, p. 11).[25]

One might describe this enterprise as dissolving 'the metaphysical aura' around certain expressions (Waismann 1965, p. 81).[26] 'One can't step twice into the same river.' 'Che sera sera'. 'What is done cannot be undone.' 'Everything is what it is and not another thing.' 'Another's idea is another idea.' 'One can never be certain what another thinks or feels.' 'There is only one number 0.' The temptation to say such things can be eliminated only by clarifying the *motives* that lead highly intelligent people into making these useless statements.

Suggesting to another person a simile or picture that may have unconsciously guided his thinking is a rather hit-or-miss method of diagnosis. It may be highly effective in some cases; it seems to be a compelling diagnosis of the source of Augustine's problem of how to measure time (Waismann 1965, p. 42). But it calls for imagination and empathy from the philosopher-therapist and for sensitivity and lack or resistance from the problem-tormented 'patient'. (It may fall far short of our ideal of a diagnostic *method*.[27]) What else can be done?

Wittgenstein now suggests applying his own distinctive method of investigation (*unsere Betrachtungsweise*). This is to clarify how the individual who formulates a philosophical proposition such as 'Das Nichts nichtet' means to *make use* of it. We should ask her: 'What inferences can you draw from it? What evidence do you take to support it? What kind of a proposition is it meant to be? Does it have the status of a scientific explanation? Is it a foundation-stone on which other propositions rest? . . . '. Wittgenstein declares that he will tolerate any answers whatever to these questions; he will take exception to no honest answer, including the negative answers that the proposition has no implications, no grounds, no explanatory status, etc. (*Ich erkläre mich mit **allem** einverstanden . . . Ich habe **nichts dagegen** . . .*), but

---

[24]This point is neglected in Ryle's ironic question: 'Why should the fly take the way out of the fly-bottle when it is pointed out to him?'.

[25]This is an application of this simile opposite to the self-effacing one that Wittgenstein made, but it seems no less apposite.

[26]One might add that it is *in this sense* that what *we* do is to bring words back from their *metaphysical* to their everyday use (Wittgenstein 1953, §116).

[27]That ideal may itself call for therapeutic treatment (cf. Wittgenstein 1953, §§100–8).

he insists on knowing precisely what role the proposition has or whether it is an idle wheel in the other's system of thinking (*ob er leer läuft*). The questions asked are genuine questions calling for sincere answers, and the interrogation is open-ended and exploratory. (Here is yet another parallel with psychoanalysis; the analyst may need to press the patient to answer questions and to cut off evasions, but he should not pass any judgements on the answers given.)

The next paragraph envisages the case in which the philosophical proposition turns out to have no real function. It proves to be something similar to a polite formula (*Höflichkeitsformel*), say an old-fashioned locution for closing business letters ('I remain, Sir, your most humble and obedient servant'). Propositions of this kind may be found in logical, mathematical, and scientific treatises (e.g. the Law of Identity). Here Wittgenstein mentions citations of the law of causality in books on mechanics; this may be included in the preface as the foundation of physics, and yet no further mention is made of it in the body of the work and no consequences are drawn from it. Frege commented on similar propositions included as 'definitions' in mathematics texts, and he described them as 'stucco ornaments' in contrast to load-bearing members in an intellectual aedifice (Frege 1979, p. 212).

The final paragraph of this discussion in 'Diktat für Schlick' further investigates the *motivation* driving authors to incorporate such *empty* propositions into formal, rigorous expositions of their ideas. Thinkers are prey to the illusion (*aufgetäuscht*) that these propositions say things of fundamental importance. They imagine that these principles constitute the foundations (*Grundsteine*) of their intellectual constructions. The Law of Identity has often been taken to be a basic law of logic.[28] Similarly the Principle of Induction or the Uniformity of Nature is often claimed to be the presupposition of all natural science. How can such a radical misconception come about?

Wittgenstein offers two very different explanations. The first characterizes philosophical pseudo-propositions as the products of a kind of displacement behaviour. (This explanation builds on an idea that Wittgenstein took from Heinrich Hertz.[29]) Here the matter is explained by a simile. Suppose that a person usually never eats his fill, i.e. that he rarely fully satisfies his appetite for food. He may then be inclined to take any sensation in his gut to be a form of hunger and to respond to it by eating something, even when the sensation arises in an exceptional case from indigestion occasioned by his having overeaten. In this case his responding by eating serves no purpose — or may even be dysfunctional. We are, Wittgenstein suggests, educated to respond to intellectual discomfort by searching for more fundamental principles. We respond to any felt difficulty by asking

---

[28]Leibniz called identities (e.g. 'Whatever is, is'; 'Each thing is what it is'; 'A is A'; etc.) the primary truths of reason, and he showed how to demonstrate the inferences of logic by means of identity (*New Essays*, 361–3, 366).

[29]The 1938 version of *Philosophical Investigations* had a motto from Hertz's *Die Prinzipien der Mechanik* (1910) that gave powerful expression to this idea.

for or providing an explanation.[30] This habitual response may then occur even when the difficulty is one that cannot be met in this way. That might happen if what bothers us is the apparent absence of any pattern or system (*Regellosigkeit*) in what we call 'rules of inference'[31] or 'propositions' or 'languages'. In such cases we ask: 'What is a rule of inference?' or 'What is the general form of the proposition?'.[32] What we are then likely to produce or accept is something that has the form of an explanation even though it has no real function at all.

This way of thinking may culminate in the desire to begin philosophy with something that is the foundation for all the sciences. 'Here we fall into a similar confusion as the one that could arise from designating as the foundation of a house, at one time the lowest course of bricks, at another time solidity itself.' According to this explanation, somebody producing philosophical pseudo-propositions is something detrimental to her intellectual welfare, i.e. a kind of disease. It prevents her effectively dealing with the sources of her intellectual discomfort. The immediate discomfort in a particular case may be eliminated by reshaping her forms of expression (BT, p. 421). In this way certain vexing questions may disappear completely from her intellectual agenda — because she ceases to *want* to ask them.[33] Therapy for this kind of intellectual dysfunctionality would require teaching another how to differentiate among his various difficulties and how to satisfy his real needs from case to case.

The second explanation recognizes the possibility of there being some positive value in philosophers' nonsense. (This explanation is said to build on architectural ideas expressed by Adolf Loos.[34]) Stucco ornaments may serve an aesthetic purpose even if not a structural one. They may be requirements of style. Tautologies have this role in structuring arguments; the law of excluded middle may be prefixed to a complicated argument having the form of a constructive dilemma in order to make this pattern conspicuous. In the same way, propositions without any explanatory content may be used to give a particular shape to a body of thought — a shape that is for some reason especially satisfying. There is appeal, for instance, in the idea that the whole world is supported by a tortoise, that it is held up by Atlas, or that it was created in six

---

[30]von Wright 1982, MS 219.8: *What* is disastrous in the scientific way of thinking (which today rules the whole world) is that it wants to respond to every discomfort by giving an explanation.
[31]This problem is discussed in the dictation 'Rechtfertigung der Grammatik' (Waismann 2002).
[32]Contemporary philosophers ask obsessively: 'What is consciousness?'.
[33]This is precisely the message of the motto from Hertz. Even a physicist may ask 'What is force?' or 'What is electricity?', or may state that the nature of force is a mystery. In doing so, the physicist seems to be expressing some kind of dissatisfaction or bewilderment in respect of the complexity of the scientific knowledge that he or she has. 'When these painful contradictions are removed, the question as to the nature [of force] will not have been answered; but our minds, **no longer vexed**, will **cease to ask** illegitimate questions.' (Hertz) In this sense, one might say, 'offenbar irrt die Frage in Bezug auf die Antwort, welche sie erwartet' [evidently the question is mistaken in respect to the answer which it invites] (Wittgenstein 1958, 169). To that extent the question is illegitimate [*unberechtigte*].
[34]Loos occurs in listings of the thinkers who have most influenced his own thinking (Wittgenstein 1980, 19).

days by God; in form, if not in fact, this closes off the disquieting spectre of an infinite regress. A mere ornament (say a cornice on a house or a wardrobe) has the power to emphasize the limits of what is bounded — and conversely a different pattern of decoration may serve to disguise these limits from view. Either role may yield a deep kind of satisfaction (or dissatisfaction). In this way even a philosophical pseudo-proposition may have an important positive role in somebody's system of thought. Arguably this was precisely the role of the nonsensical metaphysical propositions of the *Tractatus*: not to give any kind of justification, but simply to make perspicuous and satisfying the activity of analysis there advocated as the proper activity of philosophizing.

What is the upshot of this whole discussion? In particular, what have we learned from his practice about Wittgenstein's *methods* for dissolving philosophical problems?[35] Three things stand out.

First, there is the suggestion that some philosophical utterances can be traced back to similes or pictures that unconsciously shape an author's thinking. (This might destroy the appearance that these propositions express 'something deep in the nature of things . . . foundation stones that human thinking can overstep but never displace' (Frege 1959, p. xvi).)

Second, there is the suggestion that many philosophical propositions are idle wheels that engage with nothing in the mechanism of thought; they do no real work. (This is a mechanical metaphor that crops up frequently in Wittgenstein's writings.) They say little or nothing (e.g. Wittgenstein 1953, §13), yet, despite their vacuity, they impose demands and generate dissatisfaction and confusion. We may feel that we must call the utterance 'I have toothache' a description and then agonize over the question of what it describes. In this way, philosophical problems arise when language goes on holiday (*freiert*), not when we are guided by practical purposes in framing propositions (BT, p. 427).

Third, Wittgenstein suggests that philosophical propositions are a kind of displacement behaviour; they attempt to deal with all intellectual disquiets by constructing intellectual explanations (on the model of mathematics or physics), whereas what is needed are alternative pictures to make our own linguistic practices surveyable (*übersichtlich*) — on the model of depicting intensity of conviction by speech intonation (Diktat für Schlick, p. 21). He urges the importance of acknowledging other possibilities for the purpose of breaking the grip of specific *prejudices*.

All three of these activities are evidently meant to be 'clarifications of concepts' or 'descriptions of the grammar of our language'. But this activity takes a very distinctive and unexpected form. Wittgenstein engages in sympathetic, open-ended discussion that demands the interlocutor's active participation. There is no attempt to assemble a dossier of grammatical facts, and no attempt to frame adversarial, coercive arguments. Discussion is strictly person-relative,

---

[35]His methods might have fruitful application to resolving other kinds of problems such as entrenched disagreements about matters moral, aethetic, or political. Cora Diamond has made some intruiging suggestions along these lines, but such wider possibilities are not explored here.

and there is scrupulous respect for the interlocutor's freedom. The goal is to change her ways of thinking — with her consent (cf. Waismann 1956, pp. 20–1). In these respects, the practice of 'our method' is very far removed from the paradigms of 'conceptual analysis' to be found in Carnap[36] and Ryle.[37]

Let us now go back to the beginning. What are the resemblances of 'our method' with psychoanalysis? There is one quite general one: the purpose of providing therapy for individuals' troubled states of mind (*Beunruhigungen*), but there are also resemblances in certain specific respects. Three are evident in 'Diktat für Schlick'. Arguably all three of them are to be regarded as *essential* to the practice of 'our method'; i.e. they are constitutive of the identity of this distinctive practice of philosophizing.

First, the primary concern is helping individuals to bring to consciousness their own motivations and desires. Philosophical utterances, which are often patently absurd, are taken to manifest unconscious cravings, drives, prejudices, and pictures. It is these things that are the targets of Wittgenstein's therapeutic activities, not the utterances generated by them. An individual needs to acknowledge a picture that holds him captive (Wittgenstein 1953, §115) or prevents his seeing clearly his own use of words (Wittgenstein 1953, §§5, 110). He needs to become aware of his own cravings (Wittgenstein 1958, pp. 17–18), his urges to misunderstand the workings of language (Wittgenstein 1953, §109)[38], or his strong desires to see things in particular ways (BT, pp. 406–7). Wittgenstein's purpose is to win acknowledgment from suffering individuals of what unconsciously influences them. Proof and refutation are just as alien to his investigations as they are to Freud's practice of psychoanalysis.

Second, Wittgenstein's writings resemble Freud's in respect of teaching a *method* by means of detailed case studies. 'Demonstrating a method by means of examples, and the series of examples can be broken off' (Wittgenstein 1953, §133). The only product of the teaching is imparting a skill. (Results are of limited interest. Heidegger's confusions are unlikely ever to be repeated exactly.) Case studies are of interest in respect of the methods exhibited in the treatment of absolutely specific individual difficulties: what is demonstrated are procedures for untying the particular knots that someone has tied in her own thinking (Wittgenstein 1975, p. 52; BT, p. 422) or for putting a derailed wagon back precisely on the rails so that it can roll (BT, p. 410). The importance of the methods is independent of the generality of the difficulties. It is in precisely this respect that 'our conception [*is*] that there is no such thing as *big*, essential problem in the sense in which such problems arise in intellectual disciplines' (BT, p. 407).

---

[36]This contrast is particularly striking in respect of their treatments of Heidegger's metaphysical uses of words.

[37]The differences are often thought to be mostly stylistic, the similarities profound. Cf. Kenny 1989.

[38]These might be what is flagged by the phrase 'grammatical illusions' (Wittgenstein 1953, §110), and the results may be what is called 'grammatical fictions' (§307).

Third, 'our method' is intended to be therapeutic in a strong sense: the over-arching concern of *therapy* is with enhancing *human welfare*. Intellectual tor-ment signals intellectual disease (confusion, prejudice). Like pain or neurotic discomfort, it is a form of ill-fare; hence it calls for treatment (cf. Wittgenstein 1953, §599). The programme is to make the unconscious conscious in order to break its thrall and render it harmless (*unschädlich*); it is to break the grip of prejudices or superstitions. The target is not opinions (or mistakes), but ways of thinking. The aim of Wittgenstein's therapy is to increase freedom — just as psychoanalysis aims to set patients free from neurotic behaviour cycles. We *cannot* engage in critical investigations of aspects of our own thinking of which we are *unaware* (cf. Wittgenstein 1953, §129). We may be held captive by pictures (§115). We may get stuck in pointless repetition: 'But *this* is how it is . . . ', I say to myself over and over again (§113). The goal is to eliminate neurotic confusion, as it were; but not ordinary confusion resulting from lazi-ness, inattention, ambiguity, vagueness, fallacious inferences, etc.[39]

Accepting Wittgenstein's methods of therapy as a form of *philosophical* inves-tigation presupposes reconceptualizing the boundary between logic and psychol-ogy.[40] On his view, dealing with compulsions, obsessions, prejudices, torments, and so on is the *proper business* of philosophy. So, too, is facilitating or effecting changes in ways of thinking about things. Discussion is less a matter of con-structing rigorous arguments from secure premises than of making propaganda for alternative points of view. It is subversive in aiming to shake up entrenched habits of thought (*Denkgewohnheiten*) (BT, p. 423), including prejudices about the nature of philosophical argument and philosophical problems. Hence the method that Wittgenstein sought to demonstrate clearly in his practice is likely to encounter yet further severe *resistance* among analytical philosophers![41]

What Wittgenstein offers us is a distinctive conception of the method and purpose of concept clarification.[42] His discussion of Heidegger in 'Diktat für Schlick' shows precisely how 'our method is, in a certain sense, similar to psychoanalysis' (p. 28). We need to *do justice* to this statement by clarifying what he had in mind.[43]

---

[39]So too, Freud treats neurotic distress, not everyday unhappiness.

[40]It might be better to recognize the variety of boundaries drawn by philosophers between logic and psychology. For example, Frege denied that modality is relevant to discriminating logical forms of judgement or inference, whereas TLP is built on the principle that every significant proposition must be contingent, so that any 'necessary truth' must be logically unlike any contin-gent proposition, and any inference in logic or in mathematics must be completely different from inferences relating significant propositions (Wittgenstein 1961, 6.1263).

[41]It has some real affinities with the methods exhibited in the work of Nietzsche and Merleau-Ponty.

[42]Waismann (1956) expounded a somewhat similar conception in his article 'How I See Philosophy'. Much of the description of method (but not the particular examples considered for treatment) is closely based on material that Wittgenstein dictated to him in the early 1930s. However, Waismann says nothing about this pedigree, nor does he claim that the method there advocated is (or was) Wittgenstein's.

[43]It would be a moral defect in us to make fun of this statement along the lines that Carnap makes fun of Heidegger.

Arguably, this particular conception of therapy — the essence of 'our method' — runs through and unifies all of his later philosophy, although making a thorough case for that ambitious claim would need book-length treatment.

References

Ambrose, A., ed. (1979). *Wittgenstein's Lectures: Cambridge 1932–5, from the notes of Alice Ambrose and Margaret MacDonald*. Oxford: Blackwell.

Bouwsma, O. K. (1986). *Wittgenstein: Conversations 1949–1951*. Indianapolis: Hackett.

Carnap, R. (1932). Überwindung der Metaphysik durch logische Analyse der Sprache. *Erkenntnis II*.

Diamond, C., ed. (1976). *Wittgenstien's Lectures on the Foundations of Mathematics*. Sussex: Harvester.

Frege, G. (1893). Preface. *Die Grundgesetze der Arithmetik*.

Frege, G. (1959). *Foundations of Arithmetic*. Ed. 2. Tr. J. L. Austin. Oxford: Blackwell.

Frege, G. (1979). *Posthumous Writings*. Edd. H. Hermes, F. Kambartel, and F. Kaulbach. Trs. P. Long and R. White. Oxford: Blackwell.

Hacker, P. M. S. (1990). *Wittgenstein: Meaning and Mind*, pp. 90–2. Oxford: Blackwell.

Hertz (1910). *Die Prinzipien der Mechanik*.

Kenny, A. (1989). *The Metaphysics of Mind*. Oxford: Clarendon.

McGuinness, B. F., ed. (1967). *Ludwig Wittgenstein und der Wiener Kreis*, shorthand notes recorded by F. Waismann. Oxford: Blackwell.

von Wright, G. H. (1982). *Wittgenstein*. Oxford: Blackwell.

Waismann, F. (1936). Introduction. In: Schlick, M. (1936). *Gesammelte Aufsätze*. Vienna: Gerholt.

Waismann, F. (1956). *How I See Philosophy*. Ed. Harré, London: Macmillan.

Waismann, F. (2002). *Voices of Wittgenstein: Preliminaries to the Vienna Circle Project* (ed. G. Baker). London: Routledge.

Waismann, F. (1965). *The Principles of Linguistic Philosophy*. London: Macmillan.

Wittgenstein, L. (1953). *Philosophical Investigations* (ed. G. E. M. Anscombe and R. Rhees, trans. G. E. M. Anscombe). Oxford: Blackwell.

Wittgenstein, L. (1958). *The Blue and Brown Books*. Oxford: Blackwell.

Wittgenstein, L. (1961). *Tractatus Logico-Philosophicus*. Trs. D. F. Pears and B. F. McGuiness. London: Routledge & Kegan Paul.

Wittgenstein, L. (1967). *Zettel*. Edd. G. E. M. Anscombe and G. H. von Wright. Oxford: Blackwell.

Wittgenstein, L. (1975). *Philosophical Remarks*. Ed. R. Rhees. Trs. R. Hargreaves and R. White. Oxford: Blackwell.

Wittgenstein, L. (1980). *Culture and Value*. Ed. G. H. von Wright in collaboration with H. Nyman, Tr. P. Winch. Oxford: Blackwell.

4   How can a mind be sick?

Eric Matthews

How can a mind be sick?

It is largely taken for granted in modern culture that psychiatry is a branch of medicine: that being a doctor of the soul is more or less the same kind of professional activity as being a doctor of the kidneys or the heart. I say it is 'largely' taken for granted: this is not the same as saying it is universally accepted. There is a persistent current of thought that is suspicious of the whole notion of mental disorder as an illness in the medical sense, and this suspicion does not seem to be entirely perverse. Mental disorder (as opposed to mental handicap) does not seem to be characterized by a breakdown in function, in the way that, say, kidney disorders or heart disorders are. In the latter cases, the disorder is normally taken to consist of the failure of the organ in question to perform its normal biological function, or to perform it with reasonable efficiency, where efficiency is judged by biological criteria such as survival to a normal lifespan, ability to carry out species-specific bodily activities, and so on. But the 'mind' is surely not an organ at all, and even if we can say it has biological functions (for instance, learning from experience with a view to providing better for our biological needs), then it is not a breakdown in these that is the chief feature of most of the disorders listed in the standard psychiatric classifications. For example, the delusions from which mentally disturbed people may suffer are not the result of non-functioning of their thought-processes, but of their functioning in a humanly undesirable way: someone who has the delusion of being pursued by agents of a foreign power is not incapable of deriving conclusions from evidence, but derives conclusions from evidence that does not justify them by normal standards of human rationality.

Dementia, with its consequence of decline in memory, may be seen as a breakdown in one key area of mental functioning in this sense; but is that really the central feature of, say, schizophrenia, depression, or the phobias? Any of these conditions is, of course, liable to reduce biological efficiency and so increase the risk of death: but these are indirect consequences of the condition, not a direct outcome as in the case of kidney or heart failure. What makes these conditions 'disorders' seems to be rather that they affect our human, rather than our biological, functioning: that is, that they affect our behaviour in a broad sense, including our thoughts and feelings, towards ourselves and others in a human or social context. We do not think, or feel, or act in a 'normal' way: our condition is described as disordered in relation to social or human norms of how we should relate to one another, and of what constitutes a desirable human life, rather than in relation to biological norms of how our bodies should operate if we are to continue living and acting in the ways characteristic of our species. One illustration of this is the difficulty often experienced in translating the terms used in psychiatric diagnosis into different languages, belonging to different cultures. For example, I understand that in Chinese the same word is used for 'anxiety', 'tension', and 'worrying', which refer to different symptoms in English psychiatric diagnoses.

One way in which this is relevant is that we think of illness in the medical sense as something that happens to people, rather than something they choose; something they suffer from (they are 'patients'). Because of this, it is inappropriate to blame someone for being ill (except in the sense that some of their voluntary behaviour, such as smoking or overeating, may have made them more vulnerable to illness — but even then the illness itself is something that overtakes them, not something they have chosen). But we normally think of behaviour as something that is within our power to choose, so that, if mental disorder is a disorder of behaviour, it looks as though it is something that, to some degree at least, we can choose to have or not have. This is reflected in the popular usage of 'sick' in relation to minds, with its overtones of condemnation rather than sympathy. Actually, saying that someone has a 'sick mind' or is 'sick in the head' curiously combines the idea that they are to be disapproved of with the idea that, in some way or other, the behaviour resulting from their mental condition is not a matter of fully deliberate choice, but somehow an expression of the kind of person they are. Being 'sick in mind' seems to be thought of as a description of what we are, rather than of a condition into which we happen to fall. This seems to be a manifestation of the same way of thinking that condemns cats, for instance, because they seem to enjoy playing with the mice they kill: somehow this is taken both as a manifestation of the cat's ineluctable nature and as something to be condemned.

Anthony Kenny (1969), in a well known paper, claims that the concept of 'mental health' (and hence 'mental illness') was 'invented' by Plato, in the *Gorgias* and the *Republic*, when he developed the long-standing metaphor of a 'healthy mind' in such detail as effectively to turn it into something more than a metaphor. But, as I have said in a previous paper (Matthews 1999), what strikes me about Plato's account is that he treats mental health as a matter to be dealt with by judges and legislators, rather than by doctors: as something that consists in a morally good state, rather than the kind of well-being that we think of in the case of bodily health. (A further complication, of course, is that Plato, as commonly in Greek thought, gives moral overtones even to the notion of physical health.) Here again, we see evidence of a long tradition of thinking of mental 'disorder' as a different kind of human malaise than bodily 'illness'. But to think of mental disorder in this way seems to lead to a conclusion that, whether justified or not, is alien to the way in which most of us nowadays think about people with mental disorders. It is the conclusion that, to some degree at least, those with such disorders are liable to moral judgement for being in that condition. This seems to most of us both inhumane and unscientific.

A way of avoiding this conclusion that has attracted many people, especially psychiatrists, is to say simply that so-called 'mental disorders' are in fact a subset of bodily disorders, namely, disorders of the brain and central nervous system. To take this line has a robust feeling of scientific materialism about it: many seem to think that only a Cartesian dualist could think of psychiatric illness as anything other than brain malfunction. Furthermore, it seems to fit in well with the obvious success of drug and other 'physical' treatments in alleviating the distress of psychiatric patients, and with the increasing evidence of correlations between brain abnormalities and mental disorders. Finally, it would, if it was accepted, make it clear that mental disorder could, like any other illness, be the result of causes beyond the disordered person's control: we know that brain functioning, as much as liver functioning, can be affected by injury or disease. So it would confirm the generally held view, referred to at the beginning, that mental disorder is (or can be) 'illness' in exactly the same sense as liver failure or bronchitis, a subject for compassion rather than condemnation. *If* it was accepted — but can it be? One doesn't, surely, need to be a Cartesian dualist, treating thought, emotion, and will as processes occurring in some kind of mental substance that is totally unlike anything else in the universe, in order to deny that mental disorder is brain malfunction. Nor does one need to deny the importance of brain functioning in mental disorder, including the possibility of reducing the distress of mental disorder by acting directly on the brain's operations. For the moment, these will have to remain simple affirmations, without justifying argument, which I hope to be able to supply later.

We seem, therefore, to be in something of an *impasse*. Either we say that mental disorders (with some exceptions such as dementia) are deviations from human norms, in which case we seem to be committed to treating them as, in effect, moral disorders, freely chosen, and so not really 'illness' in anything except a purely metaphorical sense. Or we say that they are types of brain disorder (as in the old-fashioned usage 'nervous diseases' — cf. the 'institution for the very, very nervous' in Mel Brooks' film 'High Anxiety'), and so are genuine illnesses; but then it seems difficult to account for some of the distinctive features of our concept of psychiatric disorder. However, is the situation really as bad as all that? Is it not possible to develop a conception of 'sickness of the mind' that can do justice to the peculiar features of psychiatric disorder? I believe it is, if we begin by challenging some of the assumptions that give rise to the apparent *impasse* in the first place — assumptions about the nature of the distinction between the 'mental' and the 'physical', and consequent assumptions about the nature of the distinction between 'mental disorder' and 'physical illness'.

The root of the problem

At the root of the problem is something profoundly philosophical, namely, the troublesome concept of 'mind' itself. As Gilbert Ryle pointed out 50 years ago, the fact that 'mind' is a noun leads us to attribute it to the category of 'things' or 'substances'. Then we either, like Descartes, conclude that, since it does not seem like any ordinary tangible or visible ('material') thing, it must be some special kind of intangible thing. Or else, like traditional materialists, we conclude that, because we cannot accept the existence of intangible things, it must be an ordinary material thing — the most promising candidate being the brain. Neither of these conclusions seems entirely satisfactory, so perhaps, Ryle concluded, we ought to go back to our starting point and re-examine it. Perhaps we were wrong to jump to the conclusion that, because 'mind' is a noun, it must name some thing called a 'mind'. Perhaps in a sense there is no such thing as a 'mind'. But that does not imply the unreality of human mental life. Human beings plainly do go in for what Ryle liked to call 'mental operations' — they think, feel, wish, desire, formulate purposes, and so on. Some of the things people do, equally, can be called 'purely physical'; for instance, they breathe, and digest, and get hot and cold. These 'operations' are not normally such as to involve 'mental' activity at all: they go on, we hope, without our having to think about them. But there are many other human 'operations' that seem neither 'purely physical' nor 'purely mental'. Human beings walk and talk and play football and paint pictures and form relationships with other human beings, and join political parties and churches, and so on and so on. Although they involve bodily movements, these operations also involve thoughts, feelings, etc. We decide to go for a walk, we join a political party or church because we share its values and beliefs; our relationships with other human beings involve emotions, common purposes, ideas about life, and so on. None of this suggests a picture of human beings as made up of two distinct parts, each responsible for one kind of activity. Human beings do not 'have' bodies and minds, they live their lives in ways that involve thought, feeling, purpose, will and bodily movements of various kinds, all integrated together.

So, Ryle concluded, we should not think of a human being as a 'ghost' attached to a 'machine', but simply as a human being, a member of the species *Homo sapiens*, who thinks, feels, wishes, desires, breathes, digests, goes for walks, votes, falls in love, etc. — a startlingly radical conclusion indeed! The French phenomenologist Maurice Merleau-Ponty, expressed much the same idea when he said that we should think of human beings as 'body-subjects', essentially embodied creatures who are 'in-the-world' both in the ways in which all objects are and in a special way of their own that involves subjectivity – thoughts and feelings and intentions relating to the objects about them. And it is the same idea that lies behind the contention of a later British philosopher, Peter Strawson: what is primary is not the concept of a 'body' or a 'mind', but of a 'person', who has both 'bodily' and 'mental' attributes. However obvious this conclusion is to common sense, it is something that needs to be affirmed; as Wittgenstein said, things often escape our attention when we are in philosophical mode precisely because they are so obvious. It is not only Cartesian dualists who have failed to notice the obvious truth that saying that people think and feel as well as breathe and digest does not entail that they have some special organ which 'does the thinking'. Classical materialists make the same mistake, only substituting 'brain' for 'mind' or 'soul' as the entity that thinks and feels. But it is not either the mind or the brain that thinks and feels: *people* think or feel, using their brains (as we now know) to do so.

This thus offers a much more sensible framework for thinking about the distinction between the 'mental' and the 'physical' in general, as different sorts of human activities rather than as the activities of different sorts of things. We do not need to deny, for example, that we could not think without a brain, and that the character of our thinking may well be affected by the nature and structure of our brains. But we equally do not need to draw the conclusion from that that our thinking is a brain process, or that certain kinds of thinking are nothing more than certain kinds of brain process. Given that we are biological creatures, all human activity, from thinking about philosophy to digesting our dinner via going for a walk, necessarily involves certain things going on in our brains and central nervous systems, but there are nevertheless important distinctions to be made between different kinds of human activity. For example, thinking about philosophy necessarily requires that one has a concept of philosophy, which is a concept that has a meaning in a particular culture, so that to say someone is thinking about philosophy is not only to talk about what is going on in their head but also about their membership of a particular culture. (The same applies to 'going for a walk', 'falling in love', and so on.) Digesting one's dinner, on the other hand, does not necessarily require any concept of dinner, or any concept at all: mice digest their dinners in exactly the same sense that human beings do. So, talking about someone as digesting their dinner is talking only about what is going on in their stomachs and other parts of their bodies.

This has a bearing on our present topic. If we can't talk about 'bodies' and 'minds' as separate entities, then it clearly follows that we can't distinguish 'bodily' from 'mental' illness on the basis of the entities that they affect. Once again, we had better say that it is human beings who are 'well' or 'ill', not 'bodies' or 'minds'. And to be 'ill' will then clearly mean being in an undesirable state of some kind, however that state has been produced and by whatever standards its undesirability is measured. Thinking of 'illness' in that way will make it plain that, even if there may be pragmatic reasons (perhaps of several different kinds) for making distinctions between 'bodily' and 'mental' illness, there is no metaphysical reason for making such a distinction. This is important, if only because pragmatic distinctions are unlikely to be absolute, in the way that a metaphysical distinction is; in particular, they do not rule out the possibility that some ways in which things can go wrong for people may not be readily classifiable either as clearly 'bodily' or clearly 'mental'. Or again, some conditions that count as 'bodily' by one pragmatic criterion might count as 'mental' by another. One distinction between bodily and mental illness that has been tacitly taken as metaphysical up till now could be seen as pragmatic: namely, that bodily disorders consist of the breakdown of functioning of particular bodily systems or organs (as, for example, heart disease consists of the failure of the heart to perform its biological functions, or to perform them efficiently), whereas mental illness consists of deviation from some human norm of socially desirable functioning, as depression consists, amongst other things, of a psychological inability to maintain a socially normal level of activity such as getting out of bed in the morning. This is a 'pragmatic' basis for distinction, in that it is founded on the ways in which we try to help those suffering: in heart disease we try to restore normal biological functioning to the heart, in depression to help the patient live a socially normal life.

A related pragmatic distinction is this: bodily illnesses are those we can understand causally — we look for what has caused the bodily organ or system in question to go wrong in this way (injury, a virus or bacterium, malnutrition, or whatever) — whereas mental disorders are those we can understand in terms of reasons — we ask why (for what reason) this person has deviated from certain social norms (for instance, what life crisis has induced our patient to lose his or her normal human engagement with the world, to regard the world as 'meaningless'?). This is a pragmatic basis, again, in that it has to do with how we relate professionally to the two kinds of patients: do we seek to treat them by manipulating the cause of their distress, or by understanding them as fellow human beings responding to a difficult situation, and helping them to find a solution to their problems? Neither this nor the preceding criterion provides a basis for an absolute or metaphysical distinction. For instance, obesity may well be considered a bodily disorder, in that it consists of a breakdown of biologically desirable functioning, but may nevertheless be understood as a response to difficult emotional and personal situations, and so treated as a mental disorder; conversely, dementia may be considered a mental disorder in that it consists of an inability to maintain ordinary social relationships, but a bodily disorder in that it can be causally explained by disease of the brain.

The problem of choice

Talking of mental disorder as something that can be understood in terms of reasons seems again to raise the problem of choice. After all, to say of someone that she has acted for particular reasons normally implies that she has acted freely, out of choice. However, it was said to be a characteristic feature of our concept of illness that illness is not chosen, but suffered. This is not merely arbitrary, because we think of illness, as said earlier, as something deserving compassion and help rather than moral condemnation. (We think of people who tell those with depression to 'pull themselves together!' as unenlightened.) So, saying that at least some kinds of thing we call 'mental illnesses' can be understood in terms of the person's reasons seems to imply that they are not really 'illnesses' at all, but moral failings. Perhaps, however, we need to question this assumption about the connection between acting for reasons and 'choice', or (what amounts to the same thing) to question the excessively narrow conception of 'choice' that is involved in this way of thinking. This is a conception of choice as necessarily and always involving conscious deliberation and weighing of alternatives, as when I have to decide a moral issue such as whether I should invest in companies with a bad environmental record. What I choose in such a case is (or ought to be) based on moral principles, such as the principle of providing for my family by savings, the principle of not fostering practices that harm the environment, and so on. Only if it is based on such explicit and personally held principles, as opposed to gut reactions, is it truly a moral decision. However, a decision based on gut reactions, without much thought, is still a decision, still a free choice. Gut reactions are still reasons for acting: I act according to those gut feelings that seem most important to me. And someone whose reasons for acting were formed, for instance, by the circumstances of her upbringing, rather than by reflection on general principles, could both act for reasons and still not deserve moral condemnation — just as someone who hadn't had much of a mathematical education might arrive at certain mathematical conclusions by reasoning (would not be a mere automaton that arrived at the conclusion because of the workings of its inner mechanism), but still not deserve moral condemnation for getting them wrong.

In the same kind of way, we might suggest that those sorts of mental illness that we can understand as based on reasons might still be genuinely deserving of compassion rather than moral condemnation. To say, for example, that someone might become depressed as a natural human reaction to desperate life circumstances (bereavement, traumatic experiences such as participation in a brutal war, betrayal by someone one loves, extreme poverty, or whatever) is to say that they have reasons for being in a depressive state, but that clearly does not entail that they should be morally condemned for their depression: the only appropriate reaction is human sympathy for their distress and for their reasons for being distressed. Nothing in what I have said implies that depression is always a reasoned response in that sense, rather than, say, a result of serotonin levels in the brain. That is an empirical question that I do not, as a mere philosopher, presume to answer. However, it is worth saying that there is some empirical evidence that such life circumstances do sometimes play a part in the development of depression, for example in the apparent success of cognitive therapy in treating many depressives (admittedly, helped along by medication). All I do want to say (and this *is* a philosophical question) is that there is no logical incompatibility between seeing depression (or any other condition) as based on reasons and treating it as an illness.

So what is the upshot of all this? The view I want to defend is a permissive or pluralistic one: that there are several ways in which 'minds' can be regarded as 'sick', or rather, as I should prefer to say, in which people can be regarded as sick in their minds. Some of these may indeed be considered as forms of brain disease: they consist of the failure of the brain to perform certain functions typical of the human brain, either at all or in a biologically effective way, a failure that results directly from biological or biochemical damage to the mechanisms by which those functions are normally performed. If anything can help someone with this kind of sickness, it is neurosurgery, or medication, or some other purely bodily treatment; sickness of the brain, in this sense, is part of ordinary medicine, like sickness of the heart or the kidneys. Other kinds of sickness of the mind may be purely 'mental', in the sense that they represent human attempts to solve difficult life problems of one kind or another; they come within the purview of therapy, rather than that of the simple giving of advice, because the attempts do not involve explicit conscious deliberation to any significant degree (that is what differentiates them from Thomas Szasz's 'problems in living'). However, they can still be understood in terms of reasons, rather than causally explained. This kind of mental sickness is the appropriate domain for psychotherapy in its various forms. And there is probably a third, intermediate, type of mental sickness, which consists of unfortunate solutions to life problems which are themselves (the solutions, that is) adopted, at least in part, under the influence of biological or biochemical damage to the brain or related systems, or because of such things as genetic predispositions to favour certain sorts of solutions over others. This, perhaps, is the field of operation of the psychiatrist, as distinct from either the neurologist or the psychotherapist.

I will make one or two closing remarks in an attempt to fend off some misunderstandings of what I have been trying to say. First, in any given case, any one of the conditions listed in the standard psychiatric classifications such as the DSM may fall within any of the three types: for instance, depression may sometimes be of the first type, sometimes of the second type, and sometimes of the third type (this is not an empirical statement, but one of logical possibility). Second, in any given case, a particular person's condition may belong to two different types simultaneously, or even to all three. Someone may be anorexic, for example, both for reasons that can be understood and as a result of biochemical causes: both will then need treatment if the person is to be helped. Third, and consequently, psychiatry seems to be the basic discipline for helping people who are sick in their minds, and psychiatry is simultaneously a branch of medicine like any other and something very different from other branches of medicine, in that human understanding of patients is not merely a useful therapeutic aid (like a good 'bedside manner') but an integral part of what the therapy consists of. And, finally, I am certainly *not* defending Szasz's thesis that mental illness is a 'myth': to say that it is is to fall victim to precisely the unexamined assumptions about 'body', 'mind', and 'illness' that I have tried to undermine. Being sick in the mind, whatever it means, is at least as serious a form of human suffering as being sick in the body, and deserves to be treated with as much respect and compassion.

Consciousness in the world: the phenomenology of Maurice Merleau-Ponty

The problems about the concept of 'mental illness', I have suggested, arise largely from unexamined assumptions about the concepts of 'mind' and 'body'. In what remains of this chapter, I want to develop a view of the mind which I believe can avoid many of these problems. The key notion which we have to examine is that of 'consciousness'.

When scientists and philosophers consider the nature of consciousness, they generally take it for granted that they know what they mean by 'consciousness', but perhaps they are wrong to do so — certainly, the lack of real progress on these questions would suggest so. In talking of 'what they [or we] mean by "consciousness" ', I am not talking primarily of what the word 'consciousness' means in English, or what cognate terms mean in other languages. That would be settled by an examination of the way the word is used in common situations, and the answer to the question would probably be that it has several different meanings, perhaps related by a family resemblance. But this would not be any help in itself with the scientific and philosophical questions I mentioned: it would still need to be determined which, if any, of these ordinary-language senses corresponded to the one the scientists and philosophers were interested in (or is it *all* of them together?). And, even more important, it would remain to be clarified what exactly we are talking about when we use the word 'consciousness' in the preferred sense(s). To use a mode of expression that has not exactly been in favour in recent analytical philosophy, it is not the meaning of the *word* 'consciousness' that is at issue, so much as the meaning of the 'thing' consciousness.

That mode of expression is potentially misleading, although I can think of no way of avoiding it in English. It is misleading because it suggests that consciousness is something or other — something locatable somewhere, whether in the brain or somewhere else. It could be a 'something or other' in the sense in which, say, a brain or a neuron or a kidney is: a substantial entity that clearly is located somewhere. Or it could be a 'something' in a less substantial sense, such as a process or an activity, which is locatable in the sense that it goes on somewhere or other, or perhaps in the sense that a place is — the sense in which, for example, a clearing in a forest is something, even though it has no substance. But it is precisely part of the point of the question that I am wanting to ask ('What do we mean by consciousness?') to decide whether or not consciousness is a something in any of these senses or whether what we mean by it cannot be thought of in this way. Many of the ways in which the word 'consciousness' is used in ordinary language do indeed suggest that consciousness is something in one of the senses mentioned. The very fact that 'consciousness' is a noun suggests a view of it as a substantial thing (this is part of Ryle's point in *Concept of Mind* (Ryle 1949)). Talk of 'recovering consciousness' suggests an idea of consciousness as something that we can lose and then regain. William James famously talked about consciousness as like a 'stream', implying that consciousness was something that flowed through (through where? — the brain, presumably). Ordinary language, not to mention Freudian talk of 'thoughts coming into consciousness', implies that consciousness is a place, like a clearing in a forest. The identification by some scientists and philosophers of consciousness with cognitive activities, for which we can hope to discover the 'neurological basis', implies a view that it is 'something' in the sense of a set of activities of a certain kind, which are located in the brain and central nervous system.

Once we get into the habit of thinking of consciousness as a 'something', then it seems obvious that we can avoid Cartesian dualism and make our account of consciousness fit with all that we increasingly know about neurophysiology only by locating consciousness in the brain. For Descartes, too, thought of consciousness as a 'something'; in his case it was a substantial something, namely, an immaterial substance. The problem with this is that, by Descartes's own account, 'immaterial' meant 'non-spatial', so that there are obvious difficulties about saying where exactly this 'something' is located. Furthermore, if we take science seriously, we have to accept that, as we know more about the connections between brain processes and mental life, it becomes increasingly clear that a living and active brain is at least a necessary condition for consciousness. This is difficult (although not impossible) to combine with a view that consciousness is a substance entirely independent in its existence and nature from anything material. The pressure to some form of materialism is therefore obvious. But the influence of Descartes retains its force even in the reaction against him, in that materialists treat consciousness also as a thing, only a material rather than an immaterial thing.

My primary aim in this chapter is not to question (or to defend) materialism or Cartesian dualism, but to examine critically this common assumption: that 'consciousness' is the name of something or other, whether a substance (or substances), or an activity, process, or property (or set of activities, processes, or properties). The method I shall adopt will be based on Maurice Merleau-Ponty's version of phenomenology, at least as I understand it. I choose Merleau-Ponty's version rather than any other (Husserl's, for instance) both because I am more familiar with it and because Merleau-Ponty is more engaged with the kinds of questions about consciousness that I want to address here. What phenomenology seeks to do, according to Merleau-Ponty (1989, p. vii), is 'to give a direct description of our experience as it is, without taking account of its psychological origin and the causal explanations which the scientist, the historian or the sociologist may be able to provide'. Thus, in this case, a phenomenology of consciousness would aim to describe our actual experience of being conscious, without bringing in any presuppositions derived from scientific or philosophical theories about, say, the causal conditions for being conscious. The purpose of doing this is precisely to answer the sorts of question about consciousness that I mentioned earlier, namely, what do we mean by 'consciousness'? Answering such questions is not, Merleau-Ponty argues, a matter of 'analysing concepts', if that is taken to be a special kind of activity that can be undertaken without any reference to the world in which our concepts are anchored. Concepts cannot be analysed without relating them to the experiences that give them their meaning, just as (to use one of Merleau-Ponty's own images) we cannot understand what the symbols on maps mean if we do not know how to find our way round the countryside to which maps refer.

Nowhere is this more obvious than in the case of the key concept of consciousness itself. Before we even begin to do science or philosophy, and to develop technical terms such as 'consciousness' to enable us to do so, we all already have the experience from which that term derives its technical meaning. Consciousness is 'identifiable with what we are' (Merleau-Ponty 1989, p. xv). To find what consciousness means, therefore, we have to reflect on what we are, not what science can tell us about human beings, nor what we can conclude from a philosophical analysis of the concept of experience or subjectivity, but the way in which we actually experience the world. And here, even in those very words, we see the beginnings of what a phenomenological reflection on consciousness can reveal. 'Experience' is always experience of the world; consciousness is always consciousness of some object or other. That is, consciousness, as we know from our own case, is not an introspectible object, as Cartesian dualism would suggest, nor identifiable with a physical object such as the brain, or with the operations or some subset of the operations that take place within that object, as standard versions of materialism imply. Consciousness is not an object at all, neither material nor immaterial; rather, to say that we are conscious is to say that we stand in a certain relation to the world, or to objects.

Being-in-the-world

The focus of attention thus shifts from 'consciousness' to 'ourselves as conscious', from 'subjectivity' to 'ourselves as subjects'. A phenomenological investigation of consciousness is not an inquiry into the nature of any kind of object, but reflection on the way in which we are in the world by virtue of being conscious subjects. Merleau-Ponty, like Sartre, takes over from Heidegger the notion that human being is 'being-in-the-world', as a way of marking that shift in focus. It might be said that *all* being of anything at all is being-in-the-world, because what it means to 'be' is to be part of a world. But Merleau-Ponty uses the expression 'being-in-the-world' precisely to mark the additional feature that distinguishes the way in which human beings are from the way in which mere objects are. Human beings are, of course, a species of objects, which, like other objects, have a spatial location in the world and are causally affected by other objects. But, unlike mere objects (such as chairs, trees, or computers), human beings also relate to the world in another way than spatially or causally. Human beings relate to the world *as subjects* or *intentionally*; when, for instance, I am conscious of a lecture-room and the people in it, this is not just a matter of being located in the room and spatially related to the people, nor of being causally affected by the room and people (light being reflected from them and affecting my retina and optic nerve in certain ways). It is also a matter of my seeing all this *as* a room with people in it — moreover as a room in which I am giving a paper and people who are the audience for this paper. In this sense, the relation of consciousness to objects is one that attributes meaning to objects, by virtue of their relation to the person whose consciousness it is.

'Being-in-the-world', in the sense of having a subjective or intentional relation to the world, of course presupposes that one is in the world in the causal and spatial sense. I can be aware of the lecture-room as the place in which I am giving a paper only because my senses are causally affected by it and because of the way in which they are affected. If what was coming in through my eyes was a representation of a busy railway platform, then I could not (literally) regard this place as the location for my paper. (I could, of course, imaginatively pretend that the railway station was a lecture room; or, if I was mentally disturbed, delude myself into thinking that it was, but both of those are different sorts of experience, and have different sorts of intentional relations to what I am seeing.) Our experience of the world is always an experience of it from a certain point of view, defined by our bodies and their presence in the world, both in the sense of a literal point of view, defined by our body's present spatial location and spatial relations to the objects experienced, and in a more metaphorical sense, defined by the peculiarities of our body's modes of experiencing objects (as, for instance, a blind person's experience of this room will be different from that of a sighted person). Hence, Merleau-Ponty says that we are 'body-subjects', that our subjectivity is essentially embodied. The 'meaning' that we find in the objects of our experience is thus inseparable from our bodily dealings with them, the ways in which someone with a body such as ours must be in the world. To take a simple example, we see an apple as tasty because beings with our sorts of bodies have to eat and to evaluate objects in part in terms of their goodness to eat.

However, saying that our subjectivity is essentially embodied is not the same as identifying our subjectivity with our bodies, or with any part of them, such as our brains. That would be to treat our subjectivity as a certain kind of object, rather than as a way of referring to the peculiar kind of relationship we have with the world. Nor is it even identifying our subjectivity with certain kinds of processes going on in our bodies or brains (such as cognitive processes), because that would be again to treat subjectivity as an object that must be located somewhere. The whole point of the talk of 'being-in-the-world' is that consciousness or subjectivity is not any kind of object, and so does not have to be located anywhere, either inside us or outside us. It might indeed be better to cease talking about 'consciousness' at all, and to speak instead about human beings and their peculiar way of relating to the world. Then we might avoid some of the misleading ways of talking and thinking that we are otherwise led into.

People are only too fond, for instance, of such locutions as 'The brain organizes incoming sensory data to form a unified picture of the world', when the brain is strictly incapable of doing anything of the sort. In order to 'organize sensory data' in this way, the brain, an electrochemical system, would have to be able to recognize sensory data as such, to see them as disorganized, and to have the aim of imposing organization on them, but to have that ability the brain would have to be able to form concepts (of sense data, of an organized picture of the world), and that would require it to be a person in its own right, capable of participating in communication with other persons in which such concepts could be given meaning. How could a brain so participate, independently from the rest of the body, which enables actual persons to engage in communicative activity with other persons (for example by speaking to them using a shared language)? It would be better to say that *people* organize what they see to form a coherent and meaningful picture of the world; this organization certainly involves considerable brain activity, and would not be possible without it, but that is far from saying that the brain itself does the organizing.

In short, the phenomenological view, as presented by Merleau-Ponty, is that talk of consciousness is talk of the peculiar way in which human beings relate to the world — meaning-giving, as well as causal and spatial. But how does that connect with the pressure on any one who respects science, and in particular the achievements of neurophysiology, to adopt some form of materialism? Is it compatible? Clearly it is not compatible, for instance, with 'central state materialism' or the 'mind-brain identity thesis'; for to say that mind (consciousness) is identical with the brain is to treat consciousness as an object in exactly the same sense that the brain is, and that is inconsistent with the view that consciousness is not an object at all. Nor is it compatible (although this may not seem so obvious) with the form of the identity thesis that speaks of identity, not between 'brain' and 'mind', but between 'brain processes' and 'mental operations (such as thoughts)'. For brain processes are still objects in the sense of needing to be located somewhere — in some set of neurons. However, thoughts are not located anywhere; my present thoughts, for example, are not anywhere — not in my head, nor in my 'mind' (whatever that might mean), nor in my behaviour, facial expressions, spoken utterances, or whatever. To speak of my thoughts is to speak of a particular way in which I relate to the world, which certainly involves my brain processes, my behaviour, my facial expressions and spoken utterances, but cannot be identified with any of these on their own. To say that I am thinking a particular thought is not to identify any particular process going on anywhere, but to talk about a particular relation in which I stand to objects, one mediated by concepts that belong to a language I share with others.

On the other hand, the view of consciousness I have been describing does provide a basis for a form of materialism, at least in a negative sense, for it gives no reason to postulate anything non-material, any mental substance in which to locate thoughts, emotions, sensations, or whatever. If my thoughts are not in my head, they are (and for the same reason) not in my 'mind' either. Since the desire to find a home for such mental operations as thoughts is one of the principal motives for belief in an immaterial as well as a material substance, this at least strengthens the position that all there really is in a human being is material. When we talk about human consciousness, on this view, we are simply talking about the way in which a certain kind of material object, namely a human being (a biological organism), is in the world.

Even if we do not need to locate thoughts and other conscious operations, do we not need to explain their possibility? Materialism, it might be said, is the view that neurophysiology provides a complete explanation of this possibility, or at least would do if we knew enough about it. Immaterialism is then the view that neurophysiology cannot, even in principle, provide such an explanation, and that we need therefore to invoke something non-material to do so. However, given the account of consciousness developed here, it seems that both materialism and immaterialism must be wrong, although they are wrong for different reasons, and materialism is less wrong than immaterialism. Take a particular example of a conscious operation, say, someone's intention to go for a walk. In order for this person to have this intention, certain preconditions are necessary: first, the person must, as far as we know in the present state of science, have a functioning brain, since being able to think seems to require the possibility of certain processes taking place in the brain; second, the person must have the concept of 'going for a walk', which implies belonging to a society and culture in which that concept is given meaning.

It is because the second condition is necessary that neurophysiology cannot provide a complete explanation of the possibility of this thought (a thought, as has been said earlier, is not simply something that takes place in the brain — one could not open up the brain and discover the thoughts within it). In this sense, materialism in the sense described earlier is mistaken. However, this explanation certainly does not invoke the existence of anything non-material: belonging to a culture does not require the existence of any non-material thing within oneself, only that one stands in certain kinds of relations to other human beings, in particular communicative relations. If someone says that such communicative relations require the existence of non-material minds, because communication is possible only between beings who can understand the meaning of each other's utterances, then the answer is that understanding each other's utterances is itself a matter of relating to each other in certain ways — responding appropriately in context to what the other person says, for example. The meaning of an expression is not, as most philosophers would now accept, an 'idea' in someone's 'mind', but what is given by the way the expression in question is used in particular contexts.

In this sense, materialism, although mistaken, is at least less mistaken than immaterialism, because it does not require the postulation of anything non-material in order to explain the possibility of consciousness. It is not my primary aim in this chapter, as I said earlier, to defend or attack either materialism or dualism, but what does concern me is to show that the phenomenological view of consciousness is perfectly compatible with a recognition of the scientific facts of neurophysiology as we know them — the recognition that provides one of the prime motives for materialism. This view agrees with the materialist at least in so far as the proper functioning of certain neurophysiological processes is certainly a necessary condition of the possibility of having consciousness, and differs only in denying that it is a sufficient condition, and still more that having consciousness and being in certain neurophysiological states are identical. (The dualist is not logically required to accept even that neurophysiological functioning is necessary to consciousness.) That brain functioning, and other body functioning, is necessary to consciousness is implicit in the whole way in which human being-in-the-world has been described, in the idea of the necessary embodiment of subjectivity above all.

Biology and the mind

If neurophysiological processes of certain kinds are necessary conditions of the possibility of being conscious, then it follows that the kinds of ways in which it is possible for human beings to be conscious depend on the nature of human neurophysiology. What desires we can have, to take a simple instance, depend essentially on the nature of our brains and nervous system: we can have desires for food and sex, for example, because 'that is the way we are made'. Of course, many of the more sophisticated desires we have are not directly dependent on our biological constitution in this way. A desire to do philosophy, for instance, does not depend on any different biological structures than a desire to think about English literature. Whether a particular individual becomes a philosopher or a literary scholar depends not on their biology, but more likely on various cultural and social factors. Have they ever been introduced to philosophy? Were their teachers of literature more attractive people than their teachers of philosophy? Have they developed in the course of their lives more of a bent for reflecting on very general problems of human knowledge and values or more of an interest in the uses of the imagination in storytelling and poetry? And so on. But it does not follow that their interest is entirely independent of neurophysiology: unless certain processes functioned effectively, they could not have an interest in either philosophy or literature.

Again, even the basic biological desires such as hunger and sex can, of course, be influenced in their expression by cultural and social factors. What kinds of food we find good to eat, and what kinds of people we find sexually attractive, can differ even in people whose basic biological structures are identical. Here we might say that social and cultural development builds on, and perhaps to a certain extent transforms, our biological inheritance. But this is clearly not to say that we do not have a biological inheritance, or that this inheritance is not fundamental to understanding human consciousness. One way in which this may become clear is when something 'goes wrong' in human behaviour (a subject about which Merleau-Ponty has a good deal to say) — when, for instance, someone loses the desire to eat or to have sexual relations, or when these desires are directed towards objects that are deemed to be inappropriate in a particular society (as when someone in our society desires to eat human flesh or to have sex with small children). Then, depending on the case, we may say that this abnormality is caused either by neurological changes or by sociocultural factors, or perhaps by both.

In conclusion, I want to consider another significant feature of Merleau-Ponty's view of consciousness that is closely connected to the issues I have just been discussing. If to be conscious is to be-in-the-world in a certain way, a way that essentially involves one's body, then we do not need to identify consciousness with *explicit* consciousness alone. This sounds peculiar to us, in part again because of the continuing influence of Descartes, who effectively defined 'consciousness' as equivalent to 'explicit consciousness', in that to be conscious is to be conscious of being conscious: if I am having a certain desire, then I know that I have it. From this, of course, spring all of the alleged philosophical difficulties with notions of unconscious thoughts, desires, purposes, etc., but one can surely be-in-the-world in a certain way without knowing that one is — without being immediately and without further reflection able to formulate explicitly how one is in the world. I may, for instance, have the purpose of passing the ball to my team-mate on the opposite side of the football field even though no explicit thought to that effect ever 'passes through my mind'; it is still a purposive action, not a mere automatic reflex, a purely physiological response over which I have no control. Similarly, the action of someone who rapidly adds up the change she receives at the supermarket till and checks that it is correct is different from the purely mechanical operation of the calculator in the till itself; the shopper, unlike the calculator, is 'doing mental arithmetic', even though she never says to herself that that is what she is doing, and may even do it from force of habit.

That consciousness (i.e. purposiveness, thoughtfulness, intentionality) is not coextensive with explicit consciousness is connected with the fact that subjectivity is not disembodied but necessarily embodied. If the fundamental intentions that I can have towards the world depend essentially on the structure of my body, then conversely my bodily structures themselves have a certain intentionality, a directedness that does not necessarily require explicit formulation. For example, to feel hunger is to stand in a certain purposive relation to the world, whether or not I am explicitly aware of that purpose (in this case of my desire to eat something). My bodily reactions towards objects have a directedness to them. Merleau-Ponty argues that many of the reactions to their environment even of organisms as primitive as a dung beetle have to be understood in intentionalistic or purposive terms rather than causally explained in a mechanistic fashion. The animal's response varies according to the nature of the external situation and its relation to the animal's own internal needs. In this sense, the organism itself 'chooses the stimuli in the physical world to which it will be sensitive' (Merleau-Ponty 1965, p. 13). This view does not imply any mystical vitalism, but it does imply a certain conception of the body, namely, that it cannot be understood in a purely mechanistic fashion, but only by using such concepts as 'need', 'the good of the animal', 'adaptation', and the like. One significant difference between the mechanistic conception and the alternative is that mechanism treats the body simply as a collection of externally related processes, each of which can be causally explained on its own in terms of the laws of physics and chemistry, whereas Merleau-Ponty's alternative view treats the living body as an organized whole, which has needs as a whole — needs that must be satisfied if the whole is to survive as such. This is not mystical vitalism because it is not a view about ontology, the postulation of an additional entity or domain of reality (the 'life-force' or *élan vital*), but a phenomenological description of what we actually find: we experience bodies, our own and those of other organisms, as wholes rather than as collections of parts. What is mystical is to deny the distinctiveness of our experience of living organisms, to reduce them to elaborate machines.

Being embodied also allows us to retain memories of the past, not only in the form of explicit recollections, but also in the form of habits of behaviour and response. It is this retention of the past that Merleau-Ponty refers to as 'sedimentation'. These sedimented habits also enter into our present conception of the world and its meaning for us, but, once again, they do so not as part of our explicit awareness but as an 'unconscious' framework of our present experience. To say all this is not, of course, to deny that human beings, unlike dung beetles and perhaps unlike more complex animals such as chimpanzees, are capable also of explicit consciousness. The difference in the human case is that much of our behaviour is symbolic; it involves the use of signs, both linguistic and other, that allow 'a possibility of varied expressions of the same theme' (Merleau-Ponty 1965, p. 122). Language-using animals such as ourselves can describe objects in different and individual ways, and these descriptions can have a truth-value: our conduct is therefore 'open to truth and to the proper value of things' (p. 122). When that stage is reached, behaviour has become fully meaningful, and intentional explanation is even more clearly the only satisfactory way of understanding it. It is nevertheless important, in Merleau-Ponty's view, to see intentionality as extending all the way down into the most primitive forms of organic reaction, including our own less sophisticated reactions.

It is not my contention that a phenomenological approach of this kind can resolve all the problems about the nature of consciousness, but it does seem to me to go a considerable way to illuminating those problems more clearly than most other approaches.

References

Kenny, A. (1969). Mental health in Plato's *Republic*. *Proceedings of the British Academy*, **5**: 229–53.

Matthews, E. (1999). Moral vision and the idea of mental illness. *PPP: Philosophy, Psychiatry, Psychology*, **6**(4): 299–310.

Merleau-Ponty, M. (1989). *Phenomenology of Perception* (trans. C. Smith, with revisions by F. Williams and D. Gurrière). London: Routledge.

Merleau-Ponty, M. (1965). *The Structure of Behaviour* (trans. A. L. Fisher). London: Methuen.

Ryle, G. (1949). *The Concept of Mind*. London: Hutchinson.

Section 3   A New Kind of Ethics

5   Psychiatry and law

Daniel N. Robinson

Introduction

This brief chapter is intended to draw attention to certain issues of moral and political significance arising from the very purposes of psychiatry and of law, and of the more subtle influences each may have on the other. Lest there be any misapprehension regarding the perspective in which these remarks are grounded, three major points need to be made clear: First, I do not regard mental illness as a 'myth', nor do I accept the thesis that the very concept of illness is correctly applied only to physiological processes. It is in the very phenomenology of mental illness that the findings from neurology or neurochemistry would be relevant, and surely not vice versa. Thus, although there is much to recommend in Thomas Szasz's critique of psychiatry, his controversial conclusion, featured as the title of his best-known work (Szasz 1961), is not accepted here.[1] Further, and quite obviously, I do not confuse what for many years was rightly condemned as 'Soviet psychiatry' with the aims of worthy governments seeking to provide necessary psychiatric assistance to those in need. Finally, I do not take the unavoidable controversies and shifting perspectives within psychiatry as evidence that all is 'relative'. Put another way, I do not regard mental illness as a merely social 'construct', contingent on what are no more than local customs and hardened prejudices.[2] As for the diversity of perspectives, science at large has featured the same and, during stages of the greatest progress, has hosted controversies great enough to pose a threat to life and limb. In short, then, although profound conceptual and philosophical issues suffuse psychiatric theory and practice, the concerns addressed here are somewhat external to this, rooted instead in

---

[1]For the same reason there is little to recommend in Stephen Stitch's *From Folk Psychology to Cognitive Science* (Stitch 1983). In whatever sense mental disturbances might be 'supervenient' on events in the brain, it is the resources of 'folk psychology' that must be counted on even to express the problem. In this connection, see Chapter 3 of Strawson (1983).

[2]So-called 'social constructionism' is now advanced in such widely differing ways and applied in so willy-nilly a manner as to be largely useless for purposes of scholarly criticism. Here it is sufficient to say that 'social constructionism' is a poor account of, for example, the efficacy of neurosurgery in eliminating antisocial behaviour in those suffering from temporal lobe focal epilepsy.

the realities of complex societies striving to achieve and preserve states of robust but ordered liberty.

It is also important at the outset to put to rest certain commonplaces that would, if true, immunize psychiatry against the very matters at the centre of this essay. To be clear on this point as well, I would urge upon readers the essentially civic and theoretical frameworks within which the psychiatric mission must be located if it is to be even intelligible. On this point the targets of criticism must be those who would claim for psychiatry some sort of moral and political aloofness as regards any developed axiology or system of justice; those who would affirm so radical a version of eclecticism as to resist any general propositions regarding the nature of human nature and the conditions that favour its flourishing; those so metaphysically opposed to any form of essentialism as to have no stable ground on which to establish a nosology; those who think of the consulting room as defined more by contractual and social bonds than by covenantal terms. If 'social constructionism' is a useful code-term for all this, its influences have not gone unnoticed within clinical psychology. One experienced clinician, recognizing the consequences of these tendencies, reaches this conclusion (Woolfolk 2001, p. 288):

> As we begin this new millennium, humanistic perspectives in mental health professions have been all but washed away by the objectivist tide. Sadly, one of the most vigorous countertrends to scientism in psychotherapy is the relativistic and ultimately nihilistic set of views that derives from social constructionism.

Against this I would call attention to those theoretical and civic presuppositions on which the practice — the very idea — of psychiatry depends. Two illustrations will help to make the point. Consider first the public health officer sent to a village in response to reports of some general malaise. Among other tests, she measures the core temperature of the entire population and discovers that two members of the community have temperatures of 98.6 °F, with the remaining 200 members of the community giving readings of 104 °. Clearly, the examiner will not conclude cheerfully that there are only two seriously deviant cases! Instead, the news will be that some sort of epidemic has broken out with only two citizens apparently spared. Owing to the possession of a developed and tested theory of normal physiological function, the health officer is able to ignore mere statistical trends. She is thus able to recognize that nearly everyone in the community is in a pathological state. In the absence of such a developed theory of normal function, the diagnostic tests would simply have no place to go. They would have no tale to tell. They would not even be 'findings' in any informed sense of the term.

Consider a second illustration, fully intended to be grotesque. Here we find the commandant of a concentration camp visiting the camp's psychiatrist and complaining of reduced efficiency. He finds that, of late, he seems to have lost some interest in maintaining high rates of extermination and asks whether there is something in the pharmacy that might help him reach former levels of performance. I offer this as a reminder that it is not every complaint that warrants solicitude. The Nazi executioner, who finds himself plagued by his mission and unable to pursue it with zest, is not one needing help, but one who is rather 'on the mend'. Thus, not every complaint is the sign of a disorder, whereas there are some forms of 'success' that may signal pathologies of the worst sort.

What should be clear from these admittedly overdrawn examples is that forms of psychological therapy cannot plausibly be chosen in either a theoretically or a morally neutral manner. If only implicitly, the therapist has embraced a conception of human nature that cannot be stripped of moral features, and a conception of the sort of world, both local and wider, in which any decent person and any worthy life will be inclined to make adjustments and accommodations — the sort of world in which both doctor and patient have a reason to maintain membership.

If there is an implicit theory of human nature at the core of psychiatric practice, there is also — and dependently — a recognition of the essentially *civic* aims served by successful therapy (see also Robinson 1997). The most tragic figure presented in the *Iliad* is one Homer refers to as the 'heartless, lawless, stateless man'.[3] Severe forms of psychopathology have this much in common: They are marked by a departure from the world as given, and thus the abandonment of that very setting in which one's identity, purposes, attachments, and achievements find expression and nurturance. Therapy is not extended to isolates, but to those intended and intending to return to places populated by others; by spouses and children, by colleagues and neighbours, each with a set of expectations, each holding out the promise of some meaningful contribution to one's life. Moreover, this essentially civic dimension of therapy is displayed just as vividly when the therapist recognizes that the client must be removed from a destructive environment as it is when the aim is to restore the client to a decent one.

It cannot escape notice that the aims of psychotherapy, achieved in different — sometimes medical and scientific — ways, have much in common with the aims of law, at least where law is part of a larger political context respectful of the dignity of the person. Therapy and law both seek to enhance life by enlarging the possibilities for what is finally the good in life. Both are intended to be 'liberating', where liberation includes freedom from what is otherwise destructive of life's higher purposes. Both, then, rest on certain assumptions about the goods of life — assumptions that arise from a conception of human

---

[3]The description is given by wise Nestor in Book IX of Iliad at [**63**]. The words *aphrEtOr* ('clanless), *athemistos* (lawless) and *anestios* (heartless) are repeated by Aristotle (1972) in his *Politics* [**1253ª5–7**].

nature as this conception has been tested and refined over the course of millennia. In these respects, the data of human history are vastly more richly and relevantly informing than anything concocted in the Orwellian simplicity of the 'psych lab'. On such matters, neither psychiatrist nor legislator must stand by until the 'analysis of variance' has yielded the requisite levels of significance!

In referring to political regimes respectful of human dignity, however, one must have in mind not merely homage paid to the genre but respect for each individual of which the genre is constituted. Moral progress in the political world is measured by the degree to which the individual person is valued, even at the expense of the wishes of the collective, just as long as this person poses no threat to the fundamental interests of the collective. Stated in more familiar terms, moral progress includes the recognition that no one is to be regarded merely as the tool of another.

In the very nature of things in an imperfect world, noble aspirations are no bar to conflict and failure. Just where a respect for the moral standing of one citizen is to be suspended on behalf of the respect owed to another cannot be settled by computers or galvanometers, but must be subjected to what we are pleased to call judgement. The institutionalization of such judgement then appears as the settled law of the community or polis, the *rule of law*. As there is many a slip between the cup and the lip, so there is much room for mischief between the stated aims of law and its actual administration. There is more than one cynically named 'People's Republic' in which the law neither defends the people nor secures a republic. There is, then, a test that can be applied to determine whether the rhetoric so respectful of the dignity of the person predicts the actual fate of its intended beneficiaries. The test, I suggest, is in the form of counting certain barriers and measuring their height and thickness. Which barriers? The barriers that are just those legal protections available to the individual as the otherwise unopposable power of the State — the otherwise unopposable power of large majorities or insolent kings or well-armed police — would revoke or significantly constrain the liberty of that same individual.

Clarity on this point is especially important. As Aristotle instructed, a given goal can be attained by various means. There is no inflexible 'model government' on offer here as the only expression of genuine respect for the dignity of the person. A government that is non-intrusive as the population becomes addicted to drugs, as its children acquire and proceed to use weapons, as its armies engage in rape and pillage, is a government with no claim to the fidelity of moral beings. That government, too, must lose support when it finds in the eccentric and even perverse desires of the individual a sufficient reason to disregard the decent expectations of an entire community. A strident *individualism*, indifferent or even hostile to the interests and wishes of others has lost any right to expect others to defend individualism itself. Again, there must be a tested and therefore realistic conception of human nature as a guide in the matter of just where the exploits of the person are to be blocked so that the authentic interests of others may be respected.[4]

I would also not wish to be heard as a defender of 'rights' in the sense in which that word has come to be understood. I have argued elsewhere that rights, if they match up with anything in the world of really existing entities — that is to say, if they amount to anything other than words on a page — match up with a certain class of *vulnerabilities* and, as such, should be extended well beyond the realm of the exclusively human (Robinson and Harré). To have a 'right' in this sense is to be vulnerable to what others might do by way of defeating one's significant interests. And note that one may have an interest even while being unable to take an interest. As this has been treated at some length elsewhere, I need only sketch the contours of a political regime worthy of the support and esteem of rational purposive beings. However, I am most assuredly not sketching the contours of a self-indulgent collective addicted to 'rights' as the best way to avoid duties.

Respect for the person under the rule of law inevitably raises the question of the grounds on which to justify *coercion*. If, in a regime of justice, each person is of value, then the regime must accept as valuable what each person prizes, including not only one's possessions but also one's activities, associations, deeply held beliefs, summoning aspirations, and even idle pleasures. Again, the momentous question has to do with the conditions necessary and sufficient to relieve the regime of what might be called the burden of respect for all this and more, the conditions that justify the application of coercive force against one who had previously enjoyed a life of liberty.

There are three grounds that have been advanced traditionally as justifying the constraint of liberty; first, where the exercise of liberty constitutes actual or likely *harm* to others; second, where the exercise of liberty causes great *offence* to others; and, third, where the exercise of liberty creates a public *nuisance*.[5] Instances of each are easily imagined, and no detailed justification of the use of coercive force would seem to be required. A brief rehearsal is sufficient. To wit: the police power of the State, fundamentally established to secure citizens in their lives and possessions, is surely justly applied in preventing harm to the innocent. Nor must an entire community confront what is grossly offensive each time the public byways are used. As for legions of solicitors proclaiming their religious beliefs in hotel lobbies and airport waiting rooms, although we are not harmed by their conduct and may not be at all offended, we agree that the State has a legitimate right to reduce the level of

---

[4]The literature here is vast and subtle. An influential contemporary statement of the strong rights thesis is given by Dworkin (1977). A critical appraisal of the thesis, within the framework of a perfectionist theory of morals, is found in George (1993). My own position is closely allied with the latter work.

[5]A full discussion of this grounding of coercion is found in Feinberg (1970). I discuss this within the context of therapies in Robinson (1974).

nuisance. There are, then, countless instances in which coercion is at least arguably permissible, even when there is no threat of actual physical harm or property damage or loss.

This much acknowledged, we recognize that regimes of justice — the ones that have any claim on our affection and allegiance — are, as noted, the ones that erect barriers both numerous and high, lest coercion replace reasoned discourse. The number and height of the barriers increase in proportion to the liberty that hangs in the balance. The number and height of the barriers are greatest where a citizen's life hangs in the balance, and only slightly lower where civic freedom itself is at risk. Thus does the State, at least the State in which justice is a real aspiration, if not an accomplished fact, give criminal defendants the widest assortment of protections against the State itself. Death and incarceration both put an end to civic life. Both — one finally and the other significantly — remove one from the polis, rendering one, as it were, 'heartless and stateless'. Before the State can succeed in effecting so great a transformation, the targeted citizen enjoys, first and most importantly, the presumption of innocence. Nor is there any duty to assist the State that seeks to confine him or her. The citizen need give no evidence that would incriminate. To be sure these protections are enjoyed fully; there is the right to counsel, the right to face and challenge one's accusers, the right to bail, the right of appeal, the right to a determinate sentence.

Specifically rejected, even as the State seeks to preserve the lives and possessions of all citizens, are justifications for coercion based on calculated probabilities or imagined possibilities. Prior restraint is still an incompletely tested juridical precept, although it has been soundly repudiated in the matter of freedom of the press in the United States. Surely, in time of war, the plan to publish material giving aid and comfort to an enemy might well result in prior restraint. But the precedent or principle that allows the State to confine citizens, merely on the expectation that they might do something unlawful, is fraught with danger and is defensible only where the State itself is imperiled.[6] This is the case even where the predictive efficiency of indicators is very high. Surely the best predictor of criminal behaviour is a history of such behaviour. None the less, once prisoners have completed their terms, they are free. That they fall into a category of likely offenders has no bearing whatever on this freedom. Justice is, in the relevant sense, 'blind' to the future. The social contract promises liberty to those who use it rightly and threatens its withdrawal where it has been misused. Punishment is none the less *after the fact as proven*, and never on a hypothesis.

To aim for a state of ordered liberty is noble. To expect to achieve it in its fullness is naive. In this connection, consider the theory of signal detection, which seems here to fit too well to be a metaphor. We expect the radar system

---

[6]The matter of quarantine fits readily under the *harm* principle. It is not a necessary feature of harm that it be intended in order for the State to protect potential victims.

to report if two planes are likely to collide. We expect that same system to say nothing when two sparrows fly past each other. If we seek perfection, however, our case becomes hopeless, for the only way the system will never fail to report an impending collision is by always treating the sparrows as aeroplanes! We do not want the innocent held hostage to the wayward intentions of the career criminal. We do not want to incarcerate a citizen merely on the likelihood of an offence. But the only way we can achieve the former aim flawlessly is by never releasing anyone from prison. And, of course, the only way we can be sure that no innocent person is ever constrained of liberty is by never convicting anyone.

If signal detection theory is more than a metaphor — if it is even something of a guide — then we know how to increase the number of correct decisions without a corresponding increase in mistaken ones. First, the system needs a good and accurate memory, for to know that no sparrow ever attains a speed of 600 miles per hour is already to make some progress in air traffic control. The system also must allow the manipulation of the *pay-off matrix*: the relative costs assigned to each of the two possible errors, and the relative benefits paid for each of the two correct decisions. In a regime of justice respectful of the dignity of the individual, the 'pay-off' is set in such a way that it is far more likely the guilty will go unpunished than that the innocent will lose their liberty. This is not one of the failures of the system, but a measure of the success of a system that can do no better than what reality actually affords.

To this point, I have ignored political aspirations and have considered only the central aspirations of *regimes of justice*. In fortunate times, the two go hand in hand. But political power has often been wielded at the expense of justice, even when the words on the page are lofty. In noting that the aims of psychiatry and of law are comparable, I have not suggested, therefore, that the aims of either are *political*, at least in the sense of a 'political agenda' or 'party politics'. Rather, both seek to enlarge the canvas of the authentically lived life; both seek to render us fit for friendship and other nourishing modes of association; both seek to promote what the record of history offers as a valid picture of human nature as it expresses itself under favourable conditions.[7] Both psychiatry and law are, then, theory driven in their points of origin and civic in their larger projections.

Politics and politicians, owing to the powers vested in office, stand at once as the guardians of and as potential threats to ordered liberty. This, too, is an unavoidable gift of reality: whatever power is necessary and sufficient to secure freedom is sufficient to curtail or even eliminate it. Again, law is the barrier to political abuse as it is the barrier to personal abuse. Consider once more harm, offence, and nuisance. It is a worthy and designated duty facing political leaders that citizens be protected in their lives and possessions, be

---

[7]On the political grounding of conditions favouring 'civic friendship', see Robinson (1999).

spared exposure to the grossly offensive, and be freed from the stultifying impositions of the public nuisance. Governments are derelict should they fail in these respects. However, to succeed they must constrain; to constrain they must use their police powers; and to use their police powers — in all but two spheres of civic life — they must successfully negotiate the formidable barriers to mere political oppression. These two spheres are occupied by legal infants and by those judged to be mentally ill. To reside in either of these spheres is to be judged as unfit for the rule of law. If it is to be protected from the punishments of law, it is also to be classified as something of a ward of the State. With the infant, this status is intended to protect the infant; with the mentally ill, to protect them as well as others.

What should the relationship be between and among the aims of law, the aims of psychiatry and the aims of governments? This is a vexed question, bound to embarrass neat and direct answers. In no defensible sense should psychiatry seek to be or be accepted as a *branch* of government. There is an implicit cooperative mission on which the healer and the law-giver serve, namely that of creating the conditions of authentic human flourishing. But politics *qua* politics is not to be a medical subspecialty. Nor would it be defensible for psychiatry to set itself up as a substitute for the law itself or as an ultimate arbiter on questions of justice. Rather, it should be a principal commitment of psychiatry to develop and express as generous a disposition toward the dignity of the person as is found in the law itself. It is this point that I would expand by way of conclusion.

Respecting the dignity of the person includes a respect for life's wider, if not wiser, possibilities and the need some have to sample offerings perhaps less visited by the many. There are, to be sure, limits to eccentricities, even those that result not always in harm to others but in offence, discomfort, fear. William Galston, a committed defender of cultural diversity, describes the limits in these terms (Galston 1991, pp. 38–9):

> We may argue interminably about distributional entitlements, but the violation
> if basic decency — of the rules that make human life possible and tolerable —
> is an undeniable affront. The victim's cry — it isn't right, it isn't fair — is not
> so much claiming a share as it is expressing fear, suffering and humiliation.

Respect for the person does not include respect for all the choices made by that person, only for the value of choice itself and the 'suffering and humiliation' that attends either the total denial of choice or the exercise of choices grossly demeaning of others.[8] At this juncture, however, there is a fundamental

---

[8]In saying 'the value', I would not want to be taken as defending a 'choice-above-all' thesis. Nor need one regard liberty as an absolute value in order to recognize its place among the higher values. Even for those for whom liberty is an instrumental value (e.g. George 1993), it is a great and abiding value.

distinction between psychiatry and law, and one that confers on psychiatry a range of options otherwise and correctly denied to the law itself. As noted earlier, the number and height of the barriers the State must hurdle are determined by the interests that might otherwise be utterly defeated by the actions of the State. But psychiatry — unless it finds itself in league with the State — has no such power. Its counsels and exhortations are those of the teacher or good friend; its medicines and therapies are for those who would choose to take them.

There is a moral world of difference between instruction and coercion. Recognizing the aims of just laws as compatible with the aims of wise counsel, psychiatry can find direction and refinement in the reasoning and the canons of developed law. It can be reminded of the value of diversity, the grim consequences of imposed homogeneity, and yet the ever-present need to preserve an ordered liberty if liberty itself is to have a beneficiary. Practically, what psychiatry can and must learn from developed law is that the barriers against the application of the State's police powers are the creation of whole ages and epochs, some marked by revolution and the shedding of blood. These are not to be conveniently set aside to make it easier for politicians to achieve short-term objectives or to implement some pet theory of civic life. As you would heal the distressed mind, so must you defend the citizen at risk. Indeed, it may well be that the healing of that mind begins in earnest when the client is recognized less as a patient and more as a citizen in waiting.

References

Aristotle (1972). *Politics*. (trans. H. Rackham). Cambridge, MA: Harvard University Press.

Dworkin, R. (1977). *Taking Rights Seriously*. Cambridge, MA: Harvard University Press.

Feinberg, J. (1970). *Doing and Deserving*. Princeton, NJ: Princeton University Press.

Galston, W. (1991). *Liberal Purposes: Goods, Virtues, and Diversity in the Liberal State*. Cambridge: Cambridge University Press.

George, R. (1993). *Making Men Moral*. Oxford: Oxford University Press.

Robinson, D. N. (1974). Harm, offense and nuisance: some first steps toward the establishment of an ethics of treatment. *American Psychologist*, **29**: 233–8.

Robinson, D. N. (1997). Therapy as theory and as civics. *Theory and Psychology*, **7**(5): 697–703.

Robinson, D. N. (1999). Fitness for the rule of law. *Review of Metaphysics*, **52**: 539–54.

Robinson, D. N. and Harré, R. (1995). On the primacy of duties. *Philosophy*, **70**: 513–32.

Stitch, S. (1983). *From Folk Psychology to Cognitive Science*. Cambridge, MA: MIT Press.

Strawson, P. (1983). *Skepticism and Naturalism: Some Varieties*. New York: Columbia University Press.

Szasz, T. (1961). *The Myth of Mental Illness*. New York: Harper & Row.

Woolfolk, R. (2001). 'Objectivity' in diagnosis and treatment. In: *Critical Issues in Psychotherapy* (ed. B. Slife, R. Williams, and S. Barlow). London: Sage Publications.

6 Understanding dementia: a hermeneutic perspective

Guy A. M. Widdershoven and Ineke Widdershoven-Heerding

Introduction

Persons with dementia may confront us with expressions or reactions that pass comprehension. A sudden outburst of anger may be embarrassing. How should one react to strange demands or unjustified reproaches? A common reaction to strange expressions accompanying dementia is to consider them as being caused by the underlying disease or disturbances in the brain. If this approach is taken, the utterances of the person with dementia are no longer considered as meaningful. They are regarded as the natural consequences of the illness, not as the individual expression of a human person.

Understanding dementia involves more than just a cognitive operation. A person's requests or demands call for specific actions or omissions. How to deal with unexpected likes or dislikes? What is to be done when a person with dementia resists an offer of care that seems appropriate? How to act on conflicting values? Should a person with dementia's refusals be respected, or may they be ignored? If one considers the person with dementia's utterances as caused by an underlying disease, the inherent claims may be overruled. Thus, a causal explanation results in disregarding the wishes of the patient and the values expressed in them.

A causal approach to dementia may be quite natural, given the strangeness of the behaviour of the person with dementia. Yet there are other ways of dealing with strangeness. From a hermeneutic perspective, strange phenomena do not have to be regarded as meaningless. A strange encounter may have meaning, in that it urges one to reconsider one's expectations and prejudices. Strange behaviour may confront us with a new perspective and make us aware of the limitations of our own perspective. It may induce a process of broadening one's view and of finding new ways of dealing with the situation.

In this chapter we will elaborate this hermeneutic approach to dementia. First we consider the question of how strange attitudes and behaviours, which are often characteristic of persons with dementia, can be understood. We distinguish a dialogical hermeneutic approach from an objective explanatory approach on the one hand, and an interpretative subjectivist approach on the other. Next, we explain how the hermeneutic approach leads to new ways of dealing with conflicts of values between persons with dementia and their caregivers. We will contend that declaring one party in the right, as both the explanatory and interpretive approaches require, does not solve such conflicts. The hermeneutic approach, by contrast, leads to a series of practical ways of acknowledging, and often reconciling, the values of both parties. Finally, we argue that the hermeneutic understanding of dementia is a matter of practical wisdom or *phronesis*.

Case

Mrs C is a patient on the psychogeriatric ward of a nursing home. She suffers from a moderate degree of dementia. She has lucid moments, during which she clearly indicates what she wishes. At other times she is difficult to address. Mrs C is a widow. Her children (one son and one daughter) visit weekly. She recognizes them most of the time and then she enjoys their company. On average Mrs C is a compliant patient.

One afternoon the daughter pays a visit to Mrs C. She notices that her dress is dirty. She has spilled food on it. The daughter asks the nurses why they have left her mother like this. This is not in accordance with her mother's concern for her appearance. The nurses explain that her mother, contrary to her normal compliant behaviour, showed resistance and refused to take off her dress. She accused them of mislaying her things. In view of her strong resistance, they could not think of any other solution than to let her be, at least for a while.

The daughter tries to explain to her mother that she had better change into a clean dress. Then Mrs C becomes angry. She blames her daughter for trying to arrange things behind her back — and she does not mean the dress alone. She says that she knows quite well that her daughter has spent all her money. Then the anger turns into grief over her daughter's treason. The daughter denies strongly having touched the money: her brother takes care of it. This doesn't solve much though, as their mother now claims that apparently they are both conspiring against her.

Understanding strange behaviour

Caregivers are sometimes confronted with strange behaviour from persons with dementia. An ordinary request or a simple suggestion may elicit an incongruous reaction. Mrs C's refusal to put on a clean dress is an example. Her refusal is odd. Normally, one would wish to replace the dirty dress.

Remaining dirty is not done. Moreover, Mrs C is known to be attached to neatness and cleanliness. Her resistance is a surprise to those around her (first the nurses, then her daughter). Stranger still is her motivation. She claims that the caregivers mislay her things. Such a reproach is not a common reaction to the question of whether to put on a clean dress. To the nurses, Mrs C's reaction is perplexing. Therefore, they let her be; she remains sitting in her dirty dress. Acting on her unaccountable utterances, there seemed to be no alternative. The experience of oddness is also apparent in the interaction between Mrs C and her daughter. Her suggestion to take off the dress is again followed by a refusal and reproaches. Continuing the argument is not helpful, as the mother's reactions become more and more forceful. It is increasingly difficult for the daughter to respond adequately to her mother. The end of the story is a situation of frustration and misunderstanding for all parties involved.

Situations like this, characterized by oddness and incomprehension, require explanation. How do we gain insight into Mrs C's behaviour? Where do her reactions stem from? One possible explanation is that Mrs C's behaviour is a consequence of her disease. Mrs C is forgetful and therefore she loses her things. Trying to explain this, she blames others for it. Her refusal and her reproaches are caused by her cognitive limitations. The oddness (the rejection, the anger) can be accounted for by knowledge of general psychological regularities and rules. This type of explanation may render Mrs C's behaviour understandable and acceptable to those around her. In this approach, a person with dementia's reaction is explained, but at the same time it implies an attitude of distance and superiority towards this person. Mrs C's reproaches are explained as a consequence of her disease, not as individual meaningful expressions.

Another approach, different from the above, is to regard the odd behaviour of a person with dementia as meaningful because it fits into this person's concept of the world. This is what we will call the interpretive approach. What appears odd at first sight may become intelligible when it is related to the person with dementia's view of the world. Understanding from within is what matters in this approach. One has to put oneself in the place of the person with dementia. To understand Mrs C's behaviour, we should interpret it as a consequence of her specific way of experiencing the world. To Mrs C, those around her are threatening. She feels that they wish to rob her of her belongings. From this point of view it is understandable that she wishes to hold on to her things and that she wants to keep her dress on. Her violent reaction towards the nurses and her daughter is born from her wish to keep a grip on her own life.

Whereas in the explanatory approach the odd behaviour is rendered comprehensible by understanding it as a consequence of an underlying process (the disease), the interpretative approach is directed to the meaning of this behaviour in relation with the person's point of view. In the first case an objective world functions as the standard against which the person with dementia's expressions are assessed. In the second case attention is focused on the subjective experience of the person with dementia, of which there can be no objective test. A consequence of the latter approach is that eventually all odd behaviour becomes meaningful, understandable, and even acceptable. It is always possible to fit it into *some* conception of the world. This leads, as in the explanatory approach, to a certain distance from what is happening — not because one possesses a better insight than the person involved, but because it does not really matter what he or she says or does. In the end all will become meaningful.

Next to the objectivist explanatory approach and the subjectivist interpretative approach, there is a third alternative: hermeneutic or dialogical understanding (Gadamer 1960). In this approach odd behaviour is seen first and foremost as a breach of our expectations, the most important effect of which is to bring out and make explicit our own presuppositions. Odd, unexpected experiences make us aware of the limitations of our ordinary world view. The incomprehensible expressions of a person with dementia, according to this hermeneutic approach, thus put to the test the presuppositions of the caregivers. They imply that a certain situation is not quite what the caregivers assumed. It shows 'dissimilarity in horizon' between the person with dementia and those around him or her. Both parties view the situation from a different perspective. In our case, Mrs C expresses her discontent towards the nurses and her children. She is dissatisfied with the way her personal things and possessions, including her financial matters, are taken care of. Her resistance is a mark or signal that the definition of good care is not shared by those concerned (the caregivers) and Mrs C (the relevant person).

The recognition that experiencing the unexpected opens our eyes to a broader horizon forms the core of the hermeneutic approach. Instead of waving away the perspective of the person with dementia as irrelevant (as happens in the explanatory approach), or of treating it as the only relevant point of view (as in the interpretative approach), the hermeneutic approach claims that the confrontation of perspectives may lead to a new and better (shared) perspective. Mrs C's dissatisfaction may bring the nurses to a redefinition of good care. What in her present situation is important to Mrs C? She likes to know where her things are when she needs them. She wants her possessions (her dresses, her money) to form a part of her own world, in which she feels confident. Her indignation shows that she does not regard the help her caregivers offer as helpful, but on the contrary as a hindrance. From a hermeneutic point of view the question arises whether the offered care, efficient as it may be, is adequate. Does it reach its aim, is it in accordance with the needs of the person involved, or can it be ameliorated. Is it possible to take care of Mrs C in such a manner that she keeps feeling supported and at home in her own world, including her own belongings?

How to deal with conflicting values?

Ethical aspects of care for people with dementia come to the fore specifically when a tension arises between the person with dementia's wishes and the caregiver's notion of good care. These situations can be labelled as conflicts of values. In our case, this conflict breaks out over the question whether or not to change her clothes. Mrs C does not want to take off her dress, whereas those around her — the caregivers, the nurses, her daughter — think it necessary. How to act in such a situation? The three above-mentioned approaches all offer a different solution.

From the explanatory perspective, the values of the person with dementia are not deemed essential. They are not relevant to the definition of good care. The person with dementia's perception of the situation is unsound. One may try to correct the person with dementia's opinion and try to establish a more accurate perception of the world. The adepts of *reality orientation therapy* advocate this approach (Folsom 1968). According to this method, fighting has to be avoided. This means, in Mrs C's case, that there is to be no argument, but the caregivers will keep stressing the fact that reality differs from what the person with dementia thinks. When they do not succeed in reforming this person's notions, it is legitimate to neglect them in the future. In Mrs C's case, her refusal and reproaches may be disregarded as irrelevant when a decision has to be made about what will happen in the future. As a result of her disease, Mrs C has no right of speech. She is, in technical terms, incompetent; other persons, who act in her best interest or according to her (former) character, are to take the decisions. It is to be expected that the decision will be to put on the clean dress. It is improbable that she would have refused a clean dress, had she been competent. And it is not in her interest to appear unkempt and undignified.

An interpretative approach proposes a totally different method to solve this conflict of values. The values of the person with dementia are of the utmost importance. These notions should not be ignored or corrected. On the contrary, according to the so-called *validation approach*, they should be acknowledged and confirmed, in order to make the person with dementia feel accepted (Feil 1984, 1989). In the case of Mrs C, this implies that the caregivers comply with her claim, that the nurses and her children wrong her. Isn't this what she experiences? To her, this is reality. And one can and should respond to her indignation with support and sympathy. This gives room for her fears and it creates a situation in which they may be lessened.

Such an interpretative perspective abstains from judgements about the adequacy of the person with dementia's perceptions. The only important thing is to respect his or her views. When Mrs C feels threatened, she should be comforted and appeased by joining her experience and helping her to express her wishes. This implies holding back from attempts to make her give up her resistance. When Mrs C does not want to take off her dress because she fears it will disappear, then she must be allowed to continue wearing the dress.

The interpretative approach thus offers, in the case of conflicting values, an unequivocal pattern of action that is the opposite of the actions proposed by the explanatory approach: respect the person with dementia's will and refrain from trying to break her resistance and from trying to make her change her mind.

The hermeneutic approach stresses that, in the definition of good care, the values of both parties — the person with dementia and the surrounding caregivers — are relevant. It claims a position beyond the objectivism of the explanatory approach and the relativism of the interpretative approach (Bernstein 1983). The person with dementia's notions should not be put aside because they are irrelevant, as in the explanatory approach, nor should they attain an infallible status, as in the interpretative approach. They should stimulate those involved to offer to the person with dementia a form of care that fits his or her needs best. Mrs C is not necessarily wrong or right when she suspects that others mislay her things or hide them. Her accusations make clear that the caregivers should pay more attention to her knowing where her possessions are. What matters is not whether Mrs C puts on a clean dress against her will or not, but how to structure the care given to her in such a manner that she knows what happens to the clothes she has taken off. The possibility for the person with dementia to identify him or herself with the situation is crucial (Agich 1993). The acceptance of the offered care is the culmination of a well-structured caring process (Tronto 1993).

There are three key characteristics of the hermeneutic position. The first is to pay close attention to the developing identity of the person with dementia as an ongoing historical process. From the explanatory perspective, the biography of the patient has only a factual importance as information. On the basis of this information conclusions may be drawn about the person with dementia's preferences, had he or she still been competent. In this case one looks back to the past. The interpretative approach on the other hand focuses on the actual experiences of the person with dementia. The current phase of life is, in principle, of equal importance as the former phases. As in historicism, all phases must be understood separately. The hermeneutic approach, however, places the actual experiences of the person with dementia in the broader perspective of his or her life history. Developing certain preferences and notions is part of a continuing process rooted in the past and influenced by relevant others (family, caregivers).

The second characteristic of the hermeneutic approach is the claim that conflicts of value are not necessarily solved by judging one of the parties to be in the right. A conflict of values, according to the hermeneutic approach, should serve rather as an inducement to search for new patterns of action that are better adjusted to the values of all those involved. For example, one might propose to Mrs C that she make her own choice of a dress from her wardrobe to replace the dress she is wearing. This would allow her to get a better grip on her possessions and she may well put on a clean dress as well. Similar suggestions can be made with regard to her financial matters, for instance asking her to sign her own cheques. All these actions are guided by the wish to make Mrs C a partner in the caring process. (We return to the practical implications of the hermeneutic approach below.)

The third characteristic of the hermeneutic approach is to stress that a person's values are never fixed. All adequate visions are temporary and prone to change. The notions embraced by caregivers and persons with dementia develop in a continuing process of communication, deliberation, and sometimes conflict (Emanuel and Emanuel 1992; Widdershoven 1999). This does not imply a total rejection of former values: it is a continual adaptation of the pattern of values. During this process, conflicting values are rephrased and modified. They are no longer incompatible. New notions arise that may supplement, and even enrich, the former situation.

From the hermeneutic point of view, in a case of conflicting values there is no requirement to put the values of the caregiver above those of the person with dementia or the other way around. What really matters is to find a solution that does justice to both parties, a solution in which both parties recognize themselves. Moody (1992) calls this *negotiated consent*. It implies the employment of several possible interventions by the caregiver to reach an agreement with the person with dementia. Moody's 'scale of interventions', as he calls it, includes:

1. *Advocacy* — adjustment of the surroundings to the person with dementia's wishes.
2. *Empowerment* — stimulating the person with dementia to overcome some resistance.
3. *Persuasion* — convincing the person with dementia.
4. *Substitution* — taking over the person with dementia's decision.

These interventions should be regarded as falling in a spectrum from less to more intrusive interventions. One has to bear in mind that it is best to intervene to the minimal possible degree. The suggestion to make Mrs C a partner in the process of choosing a dress, or signing cheques, may be regarded as an example of the first type of intervention: adjustment of the situation to the person with dementia's wishes (advocacy). This interference is comparatively unobtrusive. When it does not succeed, other stronger interventions may be applied.

Understanding as practical wisdom

A hermeneutic approach to dementia requires specific skills from caregivers. They have to be prepared to question their own definition of good care. This does not primarily mean they should discuss their own values in a debate. It means they should listen to critique, even when it is inarticulate or lacks argumentation. Emotional rejections to offers of care from persons with dementia, or passive reactions, should not be ignored. They should be regarded as an implicit form of critique that demands further attention. Apparently ill-founded resistance may indicate that the person with dementia does not accept the definition of good care of the caregivers. So the first requirement for all involved in the process of care (persons with dementia, their families, professional caregivers) is to be open to critique, implicit and explicit.

Being open to critique means being open to negative reactions from other people. It does not mean accepting that every rejection as justified. Confidence is a necessary prerequisite to a true discussion of one's opinion. It is essential to critical evaluation and the exploration of new ways of responding. Being open to Mrs C's negative reaction to the proposal of new clothes means not dismissing it because she is incompetent. Nor does it mean blind acceptance. Dirty and unkempt persons with dementia need care. The question is how to structure care so that the person with dementia accepts it and experiences it as care.

Meeting critique adequately presupposes the ability to find the right balance between tenacity and pliability. Those who are wedded too much to their own views tend not to listen to justified critiques from other persons. Those who are too flexible tend to lose sight of the worth of their insights. The competence of finding the right balance — the golden middle — is characteristic of wise people, according to Aristotle. The kind of wisdom involved here is primarily practical. Aristotle calls this practical insight *phronesis* (Widdershoven-Heerding 1987). Important about phronesis is not a mathematical calculation of the right middle nor a logical argumentation about it. To possess phronesis, one has to show it in one's actions, situated in time, place, circumstance, and history.

Practical wisdom implies the capability to handle matters and to avoid extremes. This means, in caring for persons with dementia, knowing when pressure is needed, but also knowing when to hold back. In Mrs C's case, it is wise not to give up the plan to change her clothes, while finding ways of motivating her to go along with this. Putting Moody's above-mentioned scale of interventions into practice in a responsible way requires practical wisdom. It is always possible to question whether some intervention is too severe or not forceful enough. This should be judged in such cases not by the success of the intervention, but by its suitability. Does it fit the situation? Does it help to reach an answer to the common question of what is good care?

According to Aristotle, practical wisdom, phronesis, is a virtue. This means that this type of wisdom includes a certain attitude, a certain condition, obtained by practice. Virtues are based on education and training; they are acquired in the process of acting and living. Virtues grow from experience. Only those who have had to deal with numerous ethical questions, and have a practical knowledge of it, may possess practical wisdom. Understanding dementia is in the end a practical matter, a matter of being experienced.

References

Agich, G. J. (1993). *Autonomy and Long-term Care*. Oxford: Oxford University Press.

Bernstein, R. J. (1983). *Beyond Objectivism and Relativism*. Oxford: Oxford University Press.

Emanuel, E. J. and Emanuel, L. L. (1992). Four models of the physician–patient relationship. *Journal of the American Medical Associatioan*, **267**: 2221–6.

Feil, N. (1984). Communicating with the confused elderly patient. *Geriatrics*, **39**(3): 131–2.

Feil, N. (1989). Validation: an empathic approach to the care of dementia. *Clinical Gerontologist*, **8**(93): 89–94.

Folsom, J. C. (1968). Reality orientation for the elderly mental patient. *Journal of Geriatric Psychiatry*, **1**: 291–307.

Gadamer, H.-G. (1960). *Wahrheit und Methode*. Tübingen: J. C. B. Mohr.

Moody, H. R. (1992). *Ethics in an Aging Society*. Baltimore: Johns Hopkins University Press.

Tronto, J. C. (1993). *Moral Boundaries. A political argument for an ethic of care*. New York: Routledge.

Widdershoven, G. A. M. (1999). Care, cure and interpersonal understanding. *Journal of Advanced Nursing*, **29**: 1163–9.

Widdershoven-Heerding, C. (1987). Medicine as a form of practical understanding. *Theoretical Medicine*, **8**: 179–85.

Section 4   A New Kind of Psychology

7 Meaning and causal explanations in the behavioural sciences

Derek Bolton

Legacies from the history of ideas

Since the beginnings of modernity, mind and its place in nature have been problematic. The problems were expressed by Cartesian dualism: the theory of two distinct substances, *res extensa* and *res cogitans*, that accompanied the development of the modern scientific world picture (Burtt 1932; Copleston 1960; Descartes 1641). The world described by the new physics was material, geometrical, independent, and objective. Mind, by contrast, was immaterial, non-spatial, and essentially subjective. This modern dualism effectively split the human being in two. The human body was conceived as matter like the rest of nature, and then mind comprised everything human that could not be construed as material. In this way not only was the spiritual or rational soul distinguished from the body and from nature, but so also from sensation, perception, appetite, and will, which would seem so clearly to be bodily qualities and functions, except in so far as the body, like the rest of nature, had been stripped of all sensitivity and life. The modern distinction between matter and mind raised many problems, including the problem of causal interaction. It always was unclear how immaterial mental processes could causally influence the material body, or vice versa. Although Cartesian dualism was transformed by subsequent developments, particularly in Kantian philosophy, in other contexts it survived, for example as a formative influence on psychological science in the closing decades of the nineteenth century. The core tenets of dualism — the subjectivity of mind, the mechanical nature of the body, the apparent impossibility of causal interaction between the two — defined two paradigms for the new psychological science that were mutually exclusive and exhaustive: introspectionism and behaviourism.

Further, a new problematic was emerging during the same period. The last decades of the nineteenth century witnessed not only the beginnings of psychological science, but also the emergence of sciences, such as history and sociology, that had as their subject matter the expression of mind in society. To the extent that these new *Geisteswissenschaften* had their philosophical roots in post-Kantian German idealism, rather than in seventeenth-century dualism, mind was not a problem for them; rather, the activity of mind in culture and society was a given. But there arose then a fundamentally new problem, which remains ours, namely, that knowledge of mind and its expression in activity does not conform readily to the methodological assumptions and rules of the natural sciences. The tension found expression in the celebrated distinctions between *meaning* and *causality*, and between *understanding* and *explaining* (von Wright 1971). Human activity is permeated by meaning, understanding of which is a fundamental aim of the cultural sciences. Meaningful phenomena, however, and the way they are known, seem to be different in fundamental ways from the subject matter and methods of the natural sciences. Meaningful phenomena (such as a historical event or a cultural practice) are singular or even unique, whereas natural science deals with repeated and/or repeatable phenomena. Another, connected, contrast is that physics seeks and uses general causal laws in its explanations, whereas the cultural sciences produce diverse meaningful accounts of diverse events. A third contrast is that understanding seems to be subjective, to draw on empathic abilities that vary from person to person, while the methods of observation in the natural sciences are objective and the results are meant to be the same for all.

The problems of mind and meaning have to do with a tension between meaningful phenomena and scientific method, the method used by the hugely successful paradigm of knowledge, modern natural science. They are distinct from the problems associated with dualism, such as the problem of causal interaction and the epistemological privacy of mind. On the other hand it was inevitable that the two sets of problems became muddled up. This is especially true in psychology and psychiatry, where both the mind–body issues and the problems of meaning and scientific method are of central relevance. The Cartesian framework remained enormously influential, in philosophy and in the sciences, including the new psychology. The older Cartesian problems of mind and body then overlapped and combined with the new problems of mind, meaning, and scientific method, both contributing to the idea that mean-ingful mental states and the meaningful behaviour associated with them have no clear place in the scientific world picture. The conflict here was genuine and profound, and has been resolved by splitting: causality as opposed to meaning, explanation as opposed to understanding, behavioural science as opposed to hermeneutic non-science.

The problem of meaning in relation to scientific method and explanation as it arose at the turn of the twentieth century was recognized immediately as relevant to the new psychiatry by Jaspers. His *Allgemeine Psychopathologie* (Jaspers 1923) attempted to construct a psychiatry that could embrace both causal explanation in terms of material events and empathic understanding of non-causal meaningful states of mind, but the tension between the two methodologies was covered over rather than resolved. Jaspers' problem was psychiatry's problem. He anticipated what was to become a split within psychiatry between explanation of disorder in terms of brain pathology and understanding in terms of (extraordinary) meanings: on the one side appeared medical psychiatry, along with experimental psychology, and on the other was psychoanalysis, championing meaning on behalf of its many offspring.

There were two main battles fought over this ground in the middle of the last century. Psychiatry was criticized for invalidating, medicalizing, and brutalizing the meaning in mental disorder (Foucault 1963; Laing 1960; Szasz 1961). At the same time psychiatry, joined by scientific psychology and latter-day empiricist philosophy of science, rounded fiercely on psychoanalysis for being pseudo-science. These battles of the 1960s were inevitable, highly charged, and highly symmetrical. The split between science and meaning was bound to lead to assault by the one side against the other for excluding it: sympathy with meaning led to outrage against scientific psychiatry, and adherence to science led to contempt for speculations about meaning. This mutual outrage was a sign that the split had become intolerable; dialectical synthesis was already in the making.

The cognitive paradigm in psychological science

In psychology and the behavioural sciences generally a paradigm shift was underway: behaviourism was being replaced by a new kind of psychological science, in which mental states with apparently semantic properties played centre stage. This was of course the 'cognitive revolution' in psychology, which began roughly in the 1960s and which continues apace (Baars 1986; Gardner 1985). The new paradigm posits mental or cognitive states as implicated in the regulation of behaviour, and this because they essentially carry information. Further, what matters in this context, the regulation of behaviour, is *semantic information*, information with *content*, which is about the environment and specifically organism–environment interactions, which is correct or incorrect, and so on. Cognitive states have to carry this kind of information if they are be of any use in the regulation of action, and they are encoded in the acting being — specifically in the brain.

The new paradigm, specifically the proposals that semantic states have a causal role in the regulation of behaviour and are encoded in brain states, effectively marks the downfall of the two great old dichotomies. It collapses not only the meaning–causality distinction, but also the mind–matter distinc-tion, because it affirms, first, that meaningful states are causal and, second, that the brain as *res extensa* is also *res cogitans*.

Implications for physicalism

A view consistent with dualism is that ultimately *all causing goes on at the physical level* or, again, that the causal laws invoked in causal explanations are ultimately physical laws. This view, part of contemporary physicalism, places sharp constraints on what can be said about causality that seems to involve semantic states. There is pressure not only to adopt mind–brain identity theory as soon as mental causation has been acknowledged, but also to find interpretations of mind–brain causation that either eliminate meaning without ceremony (Stich 1983), or that reduce mental to neural causation (Fodor 1975, 1987), or that at least underpin mental causation by physical causation according to physical laws (Davidson 1970). What physicalism cannot envisage is the idea that the causal explanations of a viable science should invoke laws that essentially involve reference to semantic, non-physically defined, states and processes. But this is what is happening in the contemporary cognitive behavioural sciences that have concepts of information processing at their core. This new explanatory paradigm is in a sense consistent with the physicalist principle that ultimately all causation is at the physical level, in so far as it posits no immaterial (e.g. Cartesian mental) causal objects, but it undermines the presumption that all causal explanations must ultimately be a matter of physics (or physics and chemistry). Rather, the implication is that the logic of explanation in the new information-processing paradigm is distinct from what we find in physics and chemistry, invoking systemic function regulated by semantic states. The position is that we find in the biological sciences upwards a form of causal explanation that in critical respects is unlike what we find in the sub-biological natural sciences. Causal explanations in biology upwards deal in the regulation of systemic function by information, a form of causation that may be called 'intentional causality' in contrast to the more familiar 'non-intentional causality' invoked in the physical sciences (Bolton and Hill 1996). The notion of encoded information is crucial here, to explain how events that are non-local in time have causal effects — analogous to 'potential energy' in physics. Indeed, the implication is that encoded information is a kind of potential energy, consistent with the principle that there are content-based causal processes (Bolton 1997a).

A further characteristic of the causal principles belonging to the biobehavioural sciences that distinguishes them from those of physics is that they are *more local* and *less general*. In phylogenesis, living beings are increasingly differentiated and (what comes to the same) they become sensitive to increasingly diverse aspects of the environment. Indeed the notion of environment itself becomes accordingly more differentiated and diverse. The physical environment, which is essentially the same for all, accounts for less and less of the variance in behaviour. Thus the biological, zoological, and ethological textbooks typically deal not with living beings in general but with the behaviour and information-processing systems of this or that species, or species–environment niche. In human beings differentiation and specificity are elaborated further in ontogenesis, associated with high capacities of learning. Individuals as well as species learn, and this individualism is reflected in increasing specificity of the rules governing behaviour. There are by all means generalities, for example that the experience of serious loss depresses mood and activity, but what these generalities amount to in particular cases may be highly specific, applicable, in the limiting case, to just one case. What counts as 'serious loss' and the extent of depression caused will depend on many inner and outer circumstances, some common and some individual.

Implications for post-modern semantics

While mind and meaning appear forever hardly real from within the modern scientific world picture, they appear as the most obvious given in positions deriving from post-Kantian idealism, phenomenology, and other expressions of post-modernity. A core assumption of post-modern theories of meaning and language is that they are grounded in language in social activity and discourse (e.g. Gadamer 1960; Habermas 1971; Merleau-Ponty 1945; Wittgenstein 1953). But now, just as the new cognitive science paradigm is problematic from the point of view of materialism and physicalism, so too it can appear highly suspect to post-modern semantics. In so far as meaning and language are grounded in social activity, the whole information-processing paradigm in the biobehavioural sciences, with its apparent assumption that meaning is 'in the brain', seems old-fashioned, conceptually confused, and wrong (Gillett 1999; Hacker 1987; Harré 1994).

However, the claim is not that meaning is in the brain, but that it is *encoded in* the brain. Moreover, attributions of encoded meaning are made on the basis of learning history and of the activity that is regulated by the content, and this is consistent with a functionalist approach to the definition of mental content, in terms of inputs and especially in terms of behavioural outputs. In this way the notion of encoded meaning is not incompatible with the view that what is encoded has to be defined in terms of activity, including social activity. The language of neural encoding need not, and does not, imply that in some way everything semantic is in the brain. On the contrary, if meaning (representation, cognition) is anywhere, it is in the whole interaction between the living being and its natural and social milieu.

There is another, related, difficulty between the cognitive science paradigm and post-modern semantics. Meaning viewed from within idealism, phenomenology, or the cultural sciences is essentially bound up with reason, consciousness, and language. This point of view is highly resistant to the suggestion that the 'information' posited in cognitive science has much or anything to do with *meaning*, because it applies to preverbal children, animals, bodily systems, and indeed to cells and to artificial computers, lacking any essential connection with reason, consciousness, and language (McDowell 1994; Searle 1990; Thornton 1997). As against this, as argued earlier, the concept of information required in cognitive science does seem to be genuinely semantic and intentional, because it has the required properties of *aboutness*. However, it is plain enough that there are differences in these respects between preverbal children, animals, bodily systems, cells and artificial computers, and mature human beings. It is plausible to affirm a distinction by saying that meaning or intentionality has to be associated with reason, consciousness, or language, but this has two drawbacks. First, as already noted, phenomena that seem to have defining features of meaning and intentionality, such as aboutness, do seem to occur below the level of mature human beings, in the absence of reason, consciousness, or language, and, second, this demarcation is hopeless from the point of view of the biopsychological sciences, which have to explore continuities and development as well as discontinuities and differences in phylogenesis and ontogenesis.

An alternative way of drawing the required distinction is to grant that core features of intentionality are to be found throughout biological and psychological systems, but to note also the appearance of *second-order intentionality*, involving the representation of (first-order) intentional states, which plausibly is a capacity associated with reason, consciousness, and language (Bolton 1995; Bolton and Hill 1996). In these terms it may be that the expression 'meaning' is best reserved for content linked to second-order intentionality, while 'information' may be used for either first- or second-order intentional content. In this way necessary distinctions may be drawn between the whole mature human being and the rest of the biopsychological realm, but without making a radical break between the two. There is a transition between intentionality and second-order intentionality, studied in developmental psychology, for example, under the heading of development of theory of mind (Davies and Stone 1995; Whiten 1991). This framework does posit a radical discontinuity, but it appears much earlier, with the appearance of intentionality in biological systems as opposed to the just physical. Having said that, there are links at that origin between the intentional and the physical, because intentionality is achieved by exploiting the physical properties of the system and is always constrained by those properties (Dennett 1996).

The various issues considered so far is this section are all a matter for negotiation, for reasoning one way or the other, taking into account the phenomena as well as appropriate use of terminology. However, there is a more ideological, *a priori*, issue in the background, one anticipated in the first section, as to whether meaningful phenomena, which include all human mentality and activity, can or cannot be brought with the domain of the sciences. Exactly the point of the early distinctions between meaning and causality was that the answer to this question is 'no' while all we have under the heading 'science' is the unreconstructed methodology of the natural sciences of the seventeenth to nineteenth centuries. But contemporary science has changed in fundamental ways; for example, the new physics envisages measurement as an interaction between what is measured and the measure, as being in this sense (among others) relative, and comprising 'subjectivity'. At the same time biology has established itself, after the physical sciences, with its study of systemic functional activity, goal-directed, regulated by information, according to 'local' laws, specific to systems and their environments. And so on. The question of whether there can be a 'science of meaning' has been transformed by the appearance of many post-modern scientific paradigms, of which indeed the cognitive revolution in psychology is just one of the latest, with the explanation of human behaviour as its specific subject matter. That this new psychological science has semantic states figuring in its explanations of behaviour is neither surprising in itself, reflecting as it does our familiar pre-scientific 'folk' psychology, nor is it incompatible with other contemporary, post-modern, scientific paradigms.

The theory that elucidates the meanings that regulate behaviour is firmly grounded in biological–evolutionary theory and in developmental psychology, but it also draws on the cultural sciences. Cognitive–behavioural semantics seeks to track the development of living beings grounded in evolutionary nature and elaborated in culture. It is impossible to know what meanings are regulating behaviour without understanding culture. Superficially the same event may have very different meanings between societies. A certain kind of practice may be innocent according to one set of values, but a sin to be avoided or concealed in another, and so on. Of course, all this is obvious. What alone has ever been controversial is whether or not these socially constructed meanings have anything to do with the 'hard science' of causally explaining and predicting behaviour. The argument here is that meanings are encoded in the brain and are thereby implicated in the causation (regulation) of behaviour, and this point is all the same whether the meanings be cultural or biologically determined drives and preoccupations. The benefits of having meaning within the scientific domain include being able to handle continuities and well as discontinuities between biology, psychology and the social, and in human development, and being able to envisage meaningful processes as one kind of cause of behaviour, along with other kinds. Nowhere are these issues more pressing than in psychopathology and mental health services.

Implications for psychopathology

As indicated in the first section, modern psychiatry was born into the splits between meaning and causality, understanding and scientific explanation, and they determined its form for the first half of the twentieth century. The cognitive revolution upsets the foundations of the old dichotomies, by placing explanations in terms of meaningful mental states at the core of the scientific paradigm. This revolutionizes psychology, but the implications for psychiatry are inevitably just as profound.

It always is a *possible* explanation of disordered mental states that they are caused by a lower-level disruption of normal information processing. 'Lower level' means by a physical or chemical lesion interfering with the information-processing function of biological systems. Cerebral atrophy, electrical discharges, and psychotropic drugs are examples of this 'bottom-up' type of causal explanation, and they have nothing to do with meaning. This is the paradigm explanation for the so-called 'medical model' in psychiatry (Szasz 1961). It is supported by the discovery of physicochemical causes, but also by an *a priori* line of thought, as follows: 'Even if meanings are normally causes of behaviour they cannot be in the abnormal case, because in the abnormal case meaning has run out. So we have to look at lower level causes, brain-behaviour relationships after all.'

But this line of thought raises the question of where the limits of meaning lie. Generally there are meanings in abundance over and above what is available to any one individual or culture at any one time, and they regulate activity. They include what readily feels familiar, but also meanings that are not, or that are hardly, comprehensible to us. The limits are vague and nego-tiable. This, of course, feels like hermeneutics and sociology, and makes the scientific mind uncomfortable. However, the implication of assumptions being explored here is that if we want the best scientific explanation of human behaviour — not just to understand the behaviour, but to give causal, predict-ive explanations — then we have to investigate the systems of beliefs, the world pictures, that guide and regulate the behaviour. This applies all the same whether the behaviour and beliefs are ours or not, whether they be scientific experimentation, or the practices of tribal magicians. Some would reject such a prospect for behavioural science, but the grounds are specious. But, specifically, the fact that meaning has run out for any particular person or group so far says as much about these observers as about the cognitive processes regulating the other's activity.

Alternatives to the medical model in psychiatry suppose that meaning is disrupted not by lower-level causes but by *more meaning*. They typically invoke intrusion by cognitive–affective states, usually resulting from earlier traumatic, forgotten, or atleast unaccommodated, experiences. This was the psychological model of explanation of mental disorder envisaged at the start by Freud, and in a much simpler way by Watson. Crucial to this kind of approach is that the mental states that regulate behaviour are not necessarily conscious (amenable to self-report). The idea that they should be is just a hangover from the Cartesian concept of mind, and has nothing to do with the cognitive–behavioural explanatory paradigm. What matters in this paradigm is that cognitive–affective states regulate behaviour. Articulation in language — in what was earlier called 'second-order' intentionality — is altogether a different issue (Bolton 1995; Dennett 1991; Gopnik 1993; Nisbett and Wilson 1977). Hence it is possible for unconscious mental states to intrude into conscious-ness, and into behaviour, without the person having a clear idea how or why, the result being experienced as a meaningless intrusion into normal mental life, as incomprehensible as an epileptic fit.

That it is possible to explain mental disorder in these two sorts of ways has long been known, but the problem has been the split between them. The effect of the cognitive revolution in psychological science is only partly to produce radically new types of explanation of psychological disorder. It does do this; for example, disruption of action may be caused not just by the intrusion of cognitive–affective states, but also by problematic second-order appraisals of cognitive–affective states, of the kind emphasized in the new cognitive therapy models (Beck 1976; Clark and Beck 1999). However, in addition to producing new approaches to complement previous ones, the main philosophical effect of the cognitive revolution on the science of psychopathology is that explanations in terms of meaning are to be regarded as just as causal, and just as much part of the science, as explanations in terms of physical or chemical lesions. These and other forms of explanation that link them, for example in terms of genetics, can now be discussed within the one conceptual space. This opens up indefinitely many possible models of mental distress that include varieties of different kinds of causal processes and interactions between them. The effect on aetiological theory is thus more diversity and much more complexity. These points are evident in current theorizing about various disorders, such as schizophrenia, Alzheimer's disease, and post-traumatic stress, to be considered in turn below.

Current models of schizophrenia implicate a primary early neurodevelopmental disturbance, disruption of the ordering and hence prediction of experience by learnt regularities, and strategies for dealing with this, including restriction of experience by behavioural means, or cognitive, perhaps by 'delusions', all this against the background of genetic and social risk factors (Garety *et al.* 2001; Hemsley 1994; Murray 1994). The cause of schizophrenia is not one thing, not, for example, one physicochemical lesion, or gene, or type of interpersonal experience. Rather, current models of the conditions or class of conditions known as schizophrenia implicate many causes and many kinds of cause, among which are the meaningful, for example the person's attempts to overcome adversity. What makes the connection between the neurological aspects of such models and the meaningful is the cognitive psychology paradigm: disruptions to neural processing mean disruption to information processing and hence to action, which leads in turn to functional, meaningful, compensatory strategies.

This line of thought suggests that whenever there is a lower-level physical disruption to mental processing, meaningful processes will still be part of the causal model of the phenomenology. The symptomatology will be a mixture of direct effects of the disruption together with attempts to adapt. This would apply in cases where the primary cause of the disorder is frankly organic, as in Alzheimer's disease. There remains the question as to the meaning of the patient's behaviour and words, and as to whether attending to this may affect the ability of the patient to cope with the illness, and even to some degree its course (Greenberg 1994; Hope 1994; Miller and Morris 1993; Sabat and Harré 1994).

As a third example of the interplay between types of causal process, let us consider a syndrome in which meaningful processes are plainly involved: post-traumatic stress. There is a variety of recent theories about the development and maintenance of post-traumatic stress, but they are generally involve variations on the following themes: the traumatic experience conflicts with basic expectations, causing the memories of it to repeat unaccommodated; both the experience and the repeated remembering lead to massive fear responses involving selective attention to danger signals and re-experiencing in relation to new stimuli the fear associated with the original event (Power and Dalgleish 1997). The various models are all within the broad cognitive psychology paradigm, and they all turn on the meaningfulness of experiences and responses to them. The cognitive psychological aspects can then be related to the brain. Neuropsychological theory suggests that event memories are generally encoded in sensory non-verbal form in the non-dominant hemisphere, and in verbal form in the dominant hemisphere. In the case of traumatic stress reactions, it may be that memories of traumatic events are atypically processed and encoded, for example in the non-dominant hemisphere with no or less representation in the dominant; there is some recent evidence consistent with this hypothesis (Hagh-Shenas 1996; van der Kolk 1994). Now, it may be that atypical encoding is the non-meaningful reason for the persistence of post-traumatic re-experiencing, especially in chronic cases. On the other hand, the failure of integration of the traumatic experience into conceptual structures, at the cognitive level, may be best explained staying within the cognitive level, as would be the working assumption of any form of psychotherapy. Which of these forms of explanation applies, in which cases, remains an open question.

There is, on the other hand, pressure to keep alive something like the old science–hermeneutics distinction. For example, Wiggins and Schwarz (1997) argue in the case of a person with manic depression that, even if a lower-level causal explanation applies, it remains a distinct enterprise to construct a meaningful narrative linking life experiences to the illness. This may be so, but the implication that meaningful narrative is not in the business of causal explanation is misleading: in some disorders, such as post-traumatic stress, perhaps also manic depression, meaningful processes may be all or part of the causal story (Bolton 1997b). Post-traumatic stress is a key case for psychological, meaningful explanation of disorder, just because it manifestly does involve meaning, and recovery typically involves the construction of new meanings incorporating the traumatic experience within the life story of the individual. It has been argued that the hermeneutic approach to post-traumatic stress differs fundamentally from the cognitive psychological and the cognitive therapeutic (Widdershoven 1999), but the crucial similarity is that they both deal with meanings and their reconstruction. The crucial difference is likely to lie more in the meta-theory: hermeneutics, unlike cognitive psychology and therapy, construes interpretation and reinterpretation of meaning as distinct from the scientific enterprise, uninvolved with causation, explanation, and prediction (McMillan 1999).

Preservation of the old science–hermeneutics distinction tends to lead to retrogressive claims — basically repetitions of what is familiar in the history. On the one side there are assumptions to the effect that the most important (basic, fundamental) science consists of studying the brain and brain–behaviour relationships *as opposed to* meaningful mental states. Then the future lies in the new and ever more sophisticated neurotechnologies, or in behavioural and ultimately molecular genetics, which will tell us about the fundamental causal processes. Never mind, then, about mental meaningful states and the quite distinct methodologies they require, such as textual analysis, or conditions of acceptance of interpretations, or theoretical work on meaning, personal and cultural. Why should a *scientific* research council fund that sort of thing? And so on. The problem with this old way of looking at things is that it neglects the role of meaning in (causally) regulating behaviour, and causal models of the behaviour that omit this fact will be so far drastically inadequate. On the other side of the same coin, there are the claims that personal, family, and social meanings are a matter for hermeneutics *as opposed to* causal science, and are out of reach of scientific theory and investigation. According to this line of thought, understanding a semiotic agent (one for whom meaning matters) has nothing to do with science, which can only misrepresent and distract from what really matters, which is fundamentally a matter of relating, and so on. One sign of the problem in all this is that the study of meaning is left stranded, isolated from the rest of science. There is no clear way that we might set out from here to study, for example, adult sequelae of childhood adversity, or how one kind of risk factor for the development of psychopathology interacts with others, or with protective factors, and so on.

By contrast, the prospect that opens up following deconstruction of the old dichotomies — mind–body and meaning–causality — is of an integrated biopsychological and social science in which meaning plays a crucial role, in both order and disorder.

References

Baars, B. (1986). *The Cognitive Revolution in Psychology*. New York: Guilford.

Beck, A. T. (1976). *Cognitive Therapy and the Emotional Disorders*. New York: Penguin Books.

Bolton, D. (1995). Self-knowledge, error and disorder. In *Mental Simulation: Evaluations and Applications* (ed. M. Davies and A. Stone), pp. 209–34. Oxford: Blackwell.

Bolton, D. (1997a). Encoding of meaning: deconstructing the meaning/causality distinction. *Philosophy, Psychology and Psychiatry*, **4**: 255–67.

Bolton, D. (1997b). Response to the commentaries on 'encoding of meaning'. *Philosophy, Psychology and Psychiatry*, **4**: 283–4.

Bolton, D. and Hill, J. (1996). *Mind, Meaning, and Mental Disorder: The Nature of Causal Explanation in Psychology and Psychiatry*. Oxford: Oxford University Press.

Burtt, E. A. (1932). *The Metaphysical Foundations of Modern Physical Science*. London: Routledge and Kegan Paul.

Clark, D. A. and Beck, A. T. (1999). *Scientific Foundations of Cognitive Therapy and Therapy of Depression*. New York: Wiley.

Copleston, F. (1960). *A History of Philosophy*, vol. iv. London: Burns and Oates.

Davidson, D. (1970). Mental events. In *Experience and Theory* (ed. L. Foster and J. Swanson). Cambridge, MA: MIT Press. Reprinted in Davidson, D. (1980). *Essays on Actions and Events*, pp. 207–27. Oxford: Clarendon Press.

Davies, M. and Stone, A. (ed.) (1995). *Mental Simulation: Philosophical and Psychological Essays*. Oxford: Blackwell.

Dennett, D. (1991). *Consciousness Explained*. Harmondsworth, UK: Penguin.

Dennett, D. (1996). *Kinds of Minds*. New York: HarperCollins.

Descartes, R. (1641). Meditations on first philosophy. In *The Philosophical Works of Descartes* (trans. E. S. Haldane and G. R. T. Ross). Cambridge: Cambridge University Press, 1911; reprinted 1967.

Fodor, J. (1975). *The Language of Thought*. New York: Crowell.

Fodor, J. (1987). *Psychosemantics*. Cambridge, MA: MIT Press.

Foucault, M. (1963). *Madness and Civilization*. New York: Random House.

Gadamer, H. G. (1960). *Wahrheit und Methode*. Tübingen: J. C. B.Mohr.

Gardner, H. (1985). *The Mind's New Science: A History of the Cognitive Revolution*. New York: Basic Books; reprinted 1987 with new epilogue.

Garety, P., Kuipers, E., Fowler, D., Freeman, D., and Bebbington, P. (2001). A cognitive model of schizophrenia. *Psychological Medicine*, **31**: 189–95.

Gillett, G. (1999). *The Mind and its Discontents*. Oxford: Oxford University Press.

Gopnik, A. (1993). How we know our minds: the illusion of first-person knowledge of intentionality. *Behavioral and Brain Sciences*, **16**: 1–14.

Greenberg, W. M. (1994). Commentary on the Alzheimer's disease sufferer as a semiotic subject. *Philosophy, Psychiatry, and Psychology*, 1: 163–4.

Habermas, J. (1971). *Knowledge and Human Interests* (trans. J. J. Shapiro). New York: Beacon Press.

Hacker, P. (1987). Languages, minds and brain. In *Mindwaves. Thoughts on Intelligence, Identity and Consciousness* (ed. C. Blakemore and S. Greenfield), pp. 485–505. Oxford: Blackwell.

Hagh-Shenas, H. (1996). Cerebral lateralization in processing of trauma-related information in post traumatic stress. PhD thesis, University of London.

Harré, R. (1994). The second cognitive revolution. pp. 25–40. In *Philosophy, Psychology and Psychiatry* (ed. A. Phillips-Griffiths). Oxford: Blackwell.

Hemsley, D. (1994). Perceptual and cognitive abnormalities as the bases for schizophrenic symptoms. In *The Neuropsychology of Scizophrenia* (ed. A. David and J. Cutting), pp. 97–116. Hove: Lawrence Erlbaum.

Hope, A. (1994). Commentary on 'The Alzheimer's disease sufferer as a semiotic subject'. *Philosophy, Psychiatry, and Psychology*, 1: 161–2.

Jaspers, K. (1923). *Allgemeine Psychopathologie*. Berlin: Springer. (Hoenig, J. and Hamilton, M. W. (trans.) (1963). *General Psychopathology*. Manchester: Manchester University Press.)

Laing, R. D. (1960). *The Divided Self*. Harmondsworth, UK: Penguin.

McDowell, J. (1994). The concept of perceptual experience. *The Philosphical Quarterly*, **44**:190–205.

McMillan, J. (1999). Cognitive psychology and hermeneutics: two irreconcilable approaches? *Philosophy, Psychiatry, and Psychology*, **6**: 255–8.

Merleau-Ponty, M. (1945). *Phénoménologie de la perception*. Paris: Gallimard.

Miller, E. and Morris, R. (ed.) (1993). *The Psychology of Dementia*. Chichester: Wiley.

Murray, R. (1994). Neurodevelopmental schizophrenia: the rediscovery of dementia praecox. *British Journal of Psychiatry*, **165**: 6–12.

Nisbett, R. and Wilson, T. (1977). Telling more than we can know: verbal reports on mental processes. *Psychological Review*, **84**: 31–59.

Power, M. and Dalgleish, T. (1997). *Cognition and Emotion: From Order to Disorder*. Hove: Erlbaum.

Sabat, S. R. and Harré, R. (1994). The Alzheimer's disease sufferer as a semiotic subject. *Philosophy, Psychiatry, and Psychology*, **1**: 145–60.

Searle, J. R. (1990). Consciousness, explanatory inversion, and cognitive science. *Behavioral and Brain Sciences*, **13**: 585–642.

Stich, S. (1983). *From Folk Psychology to Cognitive Science*. Cambridge, MA: MIT Press.

Szasz, T. S. (1961). *The Myth of Mental Illness: Foundations of a Theory of Personal Conduct*. New York: Harper and Row.

Thornton, T. (1997). Review article: Reasons and causes in philosophy and psychopathology. With peer commentary. *Philosophy, Psychology, and Psychiatry*, **4**: 307–22.

van der Kolk, B. A. (1994). The body keeps score: memory and the evolving psycho-biology of posttraumatic stress. *Harvard Review of Psychiatry*, **1**: 253–65.

von Wright, G. H. (1971). *Explanation and Understanding*. London: Routledge and Kegan Paul.

Whiten, A. (ed.) (1991). *Natural Theories of Mind: The Evolution, Development and Simulation of Everyday Mindreading*. Oxford: Blackwell.

Widdershoven, G. (1999). Cognitive psychology and hermeneutics: two approaches to meaning and mental disorder. *Philosophy, Psychiatry, and Psychology*, **6**: 245–53.

Wiggins, O. P. and Schwartz, M. A. (1997). Commentary on 'Encoding of meaning' *Philosophy, Psychiatry and Psychology*, **4**: 277–82.

Wittgenstein, L. (1953). *Philosophical Investigations* (ed. G. E. M. Anscombe and R. Rhees, trans. G. E. M. Anscombe). Oxford: Blackwell.

8 Subjectivity and the possibility of psychiatry

Rom Harré

Introduction

We lay folk have a touching faith in psychiatrists, in that we believe that they are much concerned with finding out how matters appear to those who consult them. They take reports of private miseries, of fears and anxieties, of voices counselling unwise actions, of impulses to ruin careers by propositioning the secretaries or shouting obscenities in public places, of strange bodily feelings and so on, seriously. The stories told by the curious characters that haunt the consulting room of the good doctor Oliver Sacks (1985) are intelligible to him and, by virtue of his skill as a raconteur, eventually intelligible to someone like myself. *This* is how it is with the one who sits in the client's chair or lies on the client's couch. 'Tell me . . .', is the psychiatrist's characteristic invitation. But what must be presupposed in assuming that he or she understands?

Patients complain of 'chronic fatigue syndrome' (CFS) and when physical medicine can find no lesions, nevertheless doctors now tend to believe what they are told. The person complaining does feel utterly banjaxed. In many psychiatric textbooks the authors generally go on as if everything one is told *qua* psychiatrist could be readily understood, at least to a first order of approximation, although deeper significances may need to be sought for. Even for that more fundamental exploration of the psyche of the other to be possible, the client's utterances must be intelligible. How is that possible? What conditions must be met by all concerned, and by the situation itself, for understanding to be achievable? Why is this a problem? Do not we all understand one another perfectly well?

We can discuss the truth conditions and the deeper significances of what is said only if there is at least a minimal common ground of shared meaning. Put all this in terms of the currently popular word 'subjectivity' and it is easy to persuade oneself that understanding someone else, when he or she tells us how it is with them, is a hopelessly speculative enterprise. It has been likened to translating from a strange language for which there is no dictionary. From whence comes this scepticism? It has to do with an ancient puzzle, the problem of access to other minds when one is resident only in one's own. The experiences others report are private in the radical sense that they are never present in the public perceptual domain to serve as exemplary referents for coordinating what we all, each and every one of us, might mean by the common words of our language, for instance the common vocabulary of feelings. The troubling words can be as mundane as 'itch' and as exotic as the vocabulary of Sufi mystical poetry.

Here is a clue. Some of the work of communication is done by pointing to a public situation, 'How I felt *after the flu*' or by displaying a gesture, a hand drooping flaccidly from the wrist. Now I have some idea as to the meaning of 'I'm banjaxed' in the mouth of someone who is moving into CFS. Can this clue be expanded into a full-scale theory of the possibility of psychiatric communication? The argument of this paper is directed towards a prolegomenon to just that enterprise, drawing on the fundamental insights of Wittgenstein (1953) and Vygotsky (1978).

'Subjectivity'

Recent writings on health psychology make a great deal of use of the word 'subjectivity'. The expression is particularly common among feminist authors, for instance Carla Willig (2000). Expressing one's subjectivity is a commonly described project and accomplishment. What would be presupposed by someone who used one of the discourses of subjectivity and by one who found such discourses intelligible?

There seem to be three overlapping uses of the word, forming a typical Wittgensteinian pattern of 'family resemblances', a semantic field. All emphasize some aspect of the personal:

1. In the vernacular an accusation of being subjective is roughly equivalent to the suggestion that one is biased. Here we have something personal in the sense of seeing things from only one point of view. The implication of this usage seems to be that 'point of view' should be taken as a metaphor for personal opinions and prejudices rather than literally as the place from which the scene is perceived visually. In this sense to accuse someone or some discourse style of subjectivity is to allege bias.

2. We also seem to mean whatever is or could be known only to the one who makes the knowledge claim — the hues of colours as they are experienced by an individual or the unpleasant sensations of a painful bruise, or the pleasant sensations of a sip of Chardonnay on a hot evening in France. In Russell's terminology such matters are known to the author of the reports by acquaintance, but to everyone else, indirectly, by description. In Russellian philosophy, knowledge by acquaintance is greatly to be preferred to knowledge by description, but its transpersonal and intersubjective unattainability is one of the great problems of philosophy. In this sense subjectivity is 'logical' privacy, the character of experiences that could not be had by anyone else.

3. A new sense of the word 'subjectivity' has appeared in feminist writings. It is defined by Willig (2000, p. 558) as: 'what it feels like to be constructed and positioned in certain ways'. Women's subjectivity is then something like this: the kind of experiences typical of those moments when one's status, position, nature, or characteristics as a member of the category 'woman' are attended to explicitly. In contrast to sense 1, this sense expresses a point of view, but, although particular, it is not a reflection of bias. In conformity to sense 2, while it may be unknowable by anyone who cannot, for various reasons, be constructed or positioned in the relevant ways, it is an experience encountered by many women.

It is worth noting that the use of the word 'feels' in the definition of sense 3 is broad, including bodily sensations, say 'nauseous', and opinions or judgements, such as that a certain action by someone else is condescending, and, in addition, the hybrid experience of bodily sensation and judgement that we describe as 'humiliation'.

Sense 1 does not seem to offer a foothold for philosophical problem-mongering, only moral complaint. Sense 2 is the locus of all sorts of philosophical problems, not least the perennial problem of the grounds for treating words such as 'pain' or 'itch' as having robust common meanings, publicly learnable. Clearly there is a foothold for the problems traditionally associated with sense 2 when we come to reflect on sense 3. Under what conditions is a telling of 'how it is with me' intelligible to anyone else?

Willig's characterization of sense 3 invokes two relatively new notions. Her way of explaining what subjectivity in sense 3 is to cover has the implication that people are constructed, made, manufactured, and are not natural objects, or at least not wholly natural objects. However, she also invokes the idea of someone 'being positioned'. This is a new concept in social psychology (van Langenhove and Harré (1999)) and will need to be spelt out. As a preliminary sketch one can take positioning to be a social process by which each actor in a complex interaction is assigned a certain limited set of rights and duties with respect to the kinds of speech-acts that are acceptable and proper for that person to contribute to the interaction. Positioned as a parent, one can rebuke a child. Positioned as a supplicant, one must accept the decision of the tribunal, and so on. Positioning is a dynamic process and positions are generally ephemeral.

How one is positioned is not subjective in sense 2 above. Positioning is a sociodiscursive process through which rights and obligations are mutually established, whether or not those who are positioned are contented with their lot. However, how one feels about how one has been positioned does have an important subjective sense 2 aspect, for example if one took oneself to have been humiliated by the public act of positioning. It is also important to bear in mind that public displays of 'being humiliated' or 'being embarrassed' run according to well established sets of local conventions. The conceptual structure of Willig's sense of subjectivity is complex. In the course of this analysis the major components will be brought out and discussed. My thesis is simply this: that the problem of the conditions of understanding in psychiatry is more or less the same problem as that thrown up by Willig's third sense of subjectivity.

The problem of problems

None of the above, let alone the practice of psychiatry as conversation, would make any sense unless 'how it is with me' can be understood by you when I *tell* you how it is, or *show* you by some suitable performance.

Here are two ways of formulating the problem:

1. How is it possible to sustain the public intelligibility of an account from an irreducibly personal point of view, and the feelings that are expressed, as the account of a privileged narrator, without re-erecting the barrier between the subjectivity of a person as the domain of logically private experiences and the public voice of objectivity?

2. Or, to put the matter in another way: how can reporting how it is with me as I become aware of how I am being constructed and positioned be made intelligible and plausible to others?

The problem is first of all one of meaning, and only if that is solved can questions about truth be raised. The source of the problem is this: if the exemplars of meaning are private, how can there be a common public discourse that is mutually intelligible to all involved? This question seems intractable if we assume that meanings are, or are determined by, the entities denoted by the word in question. Thus if 'itch' denotes a private feeling, how could it be learned? The teacher's itchy feelings are not available to the learner (as the teacher's horse might be), nor are the learner's itchy feelings available for checking by the teacher. So, if the feelings are the meanings or the sources of the meanings of the word 'itch', how can anyone manage to learn the word?

One does learn these words. There must, therefore, be both an error in the reasoning sketched above and some condition, the satisfaction of which makes the mastery of this part of the lexicon possible.

Two ways of framing our investigations

Cartesianism: the two substances theory

For most of the last four centuries, reflections on the mental life of human beings have been framed in a conceptual structure, which had its most striking expression in the writings of Descartes (1641). The metaphysics of the

Cartesian frame required the acknowledgement of two radically different sub-stances conjoined, somehow, in each human being. According to Descartes, the body consisted of material stuff and the mind of mental stuff. Even those who repudiated this ontology retained one of its foundational assumptions, that the mental–material distinction could be mapped on to the metaphor of two domains, the inner and the outer. Mental states, including feelings, memories, images, and so on, were 'inside' the person, whereas movements of the body, even if expressing these inner states, were on the outside. It is amazing how deeply this metaphor has become embedded in both common speech and in the writings of psychologists.

The Cartesian frame is enriched by mapping the distinction between subjective and objective points of view on to the inner–outer distinction. It is completed by the claim that a person's inner, subjective, and mental life can be known only to that person, while anyone can be acquainted with the outer, objective, and mater-ial aspects of a person. Now we have the traditional epistemological impasse that is easily fatally conjoined to the seeming paradox of the impossibility of establishing public meanings for those parts of our working vocabularies that refer to inner states and processes.

We have reached a moment in the development of the philosophy of psychology that, when coupled with a positivistic refusal to countenance the unobservable as part of a science, gave birth to behaviourism and its empiricist descendants.

Vygotsky and the priority of the public domain

In the 1930s there were three Russian psychologists, Luria, Leontiev, and Vygotsky, whose insights into the foundations of psychology provided a thorough-going alternative frame to the long-standing Cartesian way of think-ing about the mental life. From the point of view of this discussion, the work of Vygotsky is crucial. In essence his developmental psychology was built on the principle that the realm of private mental activity was shaped by the appropriation of structuring forms from the public realm within which a child, from earliest infancy, was embedded.

Mature forms of thought and action were present in inchoate and rudimentary form — in the 'zone of proximal development', as he called it. A child attempts to carry out some project, be it ever so simple, and the adults and elder siblings engage with the child's performance in two ways. They define more sharply what the project should be, and they supplement the child's inadequate actions to complete what is required to bring off the project. All this is in the public domain. The child imitates the supplementary performances, thus acquiring competence. The child's form of thought and action as engaged in this project is now no longer in the zone of proximal development, but part of the standing repertoire. Eventually children learn the trick of thinking, speaking, emoting, and so on, privately and individually.

The essential insight is that, although thought and language have different roots, the one physiological and other social, as far as meaningful and normatively constrained activities go the social domain pre-exists the personal domain. Culture pre-exists mind for any actual individual, in the sense that the inchoate flux of thought and feeling is given form by what the individual appropriates during the many episodes of psychological symbiosis that dominate its life. Mental and material actions are shaped by the child's appropriations of adult contributions. The whole thing has been called 'psychological symbiosis'.

Well and good, but how does embedding the pattern of family resemblances that delineate the complex semantics of the word 'subjectivity' in the Vygotskian frame solve the problem of the meanings of the relevant 'how it is with me' vocabulary? It serves to highlight the way that a publicly intelligible language pre-exists its private or subjective use — that is sense 2. However, in order to tie this in with Willig's sense of 'subjectivity' (how it is with me when I am aware of having been positioned), we need to solve another and consequential problem. What are the circumstances in which the mutual understandings that are presupposed in episodes of psychological symbiosis are possible? For the answer to this question we must turn to the well known, but sometimes not well presented, 'private language argument' of Ludwig Wittgenstein in §244 of his *Philosophical Investigations* (Wittgenstein 1953).

Wittgenstein's insight

Let us first pose our question in the form that it has traditionally taken:

> How can *reporting* 'how it is with me' be intelligible to anyone else, if the exemplars from which I must have learned the meaning of the words for describing my private feelings and reactions cannot be shared by teacher and learner?

Wittgenstein saw that there were two errors in this formulation.

The first mistake is to assume that when I convey to you how it is with me I must be describing what I am experiencing. When I am making known to you how I feel, I am not describing what I feel but expressing it. I shall set out in some detail how Wittgenstein establishes this subtle, but immensely telling, distinction between describing and expressing.

The second mistake is to assume that establishing meanings must always follow the pattern of the baptismal ceremony, pointing to the object signified and saying its name. There are all kinds of ways of showing how a word is to be used, of which this is only one. In particular, the way to use words that refer to how it is with me are learned in a different way, a way that is nicely adjusted to their role in expressions of feeling and opinion rather than in impossible descriptions of what I am thinking or feeling.

Expression and description

In his characteristic way, Wittgenstein makes both points set out above in the course of the one flow of argument and analysis. Here is the famous §244:

> This question [how can I understand what other people tell me about their private thoughts and feelings] is the same as: how does a human being learn the meaning of the names of sensations? — of the word 'pain' for example. Here is one possibility: words are connected with the primitive, the natural expressions of the sensation and used in their place. A child has hurt himself and he cries, and then adults talk to him and teach him exclamations and later sentences. They teach the child new pain behaviour.
>
> "So you are saying that the word 'pain' really means crying?" — On the contrary the verbal expression replaces crying and does not describe it.

So the use of the sentence 'I am in pain' does the same communicative and expressive work as groaning, crying, and rubbing where it hurts. But how is groaning and writhing related to feeling pain? Here we have the concept of expression, as opposed to description.

A description and what it describes can exist independently of one another. A state of affairs need not be described, nor must a description always 'hit' an appropriate state of affairs. Descriptions can be true, but they may be false.

However, expressions and what they express are not independent. What it is to be in pain is, among other things, to have a tendency to groan, to cry, and to rub the injured place. If one has a tendency to laugh and sing, in the primordial condition of life, the life as an infant lives it, whatever it is that one is experiencing it is not pain. Pain and the natural means of its expression are, as philosophers say, internally related. When a verbal expression replaces a natural expression, it is still 'grammatically' a means of displaying or expressing how it is with the sufferer.

This is how we learn our feeling vocabulary, through the replacement of a basic set of natural expressions by verbal expressions. Exemplars are not required for the words to be learned as ways of displaying how it is with me. Of course, once established, all sorts of metaphorical and metonymic extensions of the root vocabulary into culturally diverse lexicons of feeling can be made.

As Wittgenstein puts it in his usual epigrammatical way, it cannot make sense to say, 'I know I am in pain'. That sort of remark admits of the possibility that I might be wrong, might have misdescribed my experience, which was, let us say, really one of great joy. All we can say is, 'I am in pain'. Prefixing 'I know . . .' can only be a cognitively empty means for enhancing the force of the expression.

A display of 'subjectivity', à la Willig, must therefore be expressive — it must be a way of displaying rather than describing how one takes one's situation. All avowals of how it is with me, my logically private experience, must be expressive.

The kind of 'subjectivity' to which Willig and other feminist authors have drawn our attention is just the kind of subjectivity with which psychiatrists routinely deal. Whatever the context, mutual understanding presupposes an ethology of feeling. Does it also presuppose an ethology of resentment, humiliation, pride, and other emotional states relevant to positionings?

The Willig sense of subjectivity surely suggests that it must. The Wittgensteinian solution to the semantic problem of other minds suggests that it does. Our common human form of life includes natural capacities to express our own private and personal reactions, and to understand the expressions of the private and personal reactions of others to events in their lives.

It is important to see the scope of Wittgenstein's insights. The issue that he is tackling directly is the viability of the idea that a language could be based on a system of meanings established by a kind of private pointing or attending to feelings, hues, and other sensory states, which, by hypothesis, only the private linguist could be acquainted with. His argument is directed to showing that no such language is possible. The issue I am using Wittgenstein's insights to tackle is, at a first level, the age-old question of if and how I can know what you are thinking and feeling. How do I even know what you are doing if I do not have access to your intentions? The obvious answer, that I know these things by what you tell me and what I see you do, works only if I can understand what you tell me and if your gestures and other bodily displays make sense to me. This is why Wittgenstein's hints as to how a common public language of feeling can be established are so fundamental for the philosophy of both psychology and psychiatry. His solution rests upon the assumption that there is a common human ethology, a repertoire of displays that pre-exists the establishment of languages and the cultural refinements of our ways of life. By coupling these insights with the Vygotskian frame in which, for each human individual, the social is prior to the individual and the public to the private aspects of mature cognition, we arrive at a full-scale alternative to the vicious subjectivity of the Cartesian frame. At the same time we are provided with an account of the conditions that must have been satisfied for subjectivity in Willig's sense to become a topic for discussion. As this is the kind of subjectivity on which the possibility of psychiatry itself rests, the Wittgenstein–Vygotsky pairing is fundamental for the philosophical grounding of psychiatry itself.

Let us now turn to look more closely at the second novel concept in this discussion: the concept of a 'position'.

Positioning

Willig's brief account of subjectivity, in the third sense, is couched in terms of two major contemporary concepts: *construction* and *position*. The former is now familiar to most people acquainted with recent developments in psychology as a way of summing up the Vygotskian approach to cognitive development.

We can think of the processes of psychological symbiosis as ways of constructing psyches. Mature human beings are largely artefacts. Families are people factories. More needs to be said about the concept of 'position'.

One useful way of establishing the concept is by contrast with two complementary concepts: 'role' and 'footing'. Role theory played a large part in social psychology in the twentieth century, in relating individual performances to the exigencies of a local social order. A role was psychologically founded on a set of rules, customs, and conventions, adherence to which maintained a consistent pattern of behaviour and a coherent presentation of self. Thus the professions could be understood social psychologically in terms of such specific concepts as the 'role of policeman', and such general concepts as the 'role of mother'.

However, Goffman (1959) in particular, and others, pointed out the many ways in which roles were less stable and less fully articulated in real life than in the formulations of social psychology. Turning his attention to the microdynamics of conversations as exemplary social interactions, Goffman (1981) introduced the idea of 'footing'. Not everyone present on an occasion has the right to enter into a conversation as a proper participant who would be heard and understood. One has to have or to establish a footing in the group of conversants. In so doing one is accorded or achieved certain rights and duties in respect of what one can and may then do.

However, this concept turned out to be too generic. Gaining a footing was all very well, but the concept did not suggest the fine grain of the acquired rights and duties. Yet 'role' seemed too formal and too pre-established to capture the way that right and duties to say and do things were established, lost and gained momentarily in the give and take of real social interactions. Hollway (1984) appropriated the concept of 'position' to refer to the dynamic equilibria of real interactions. Positioned as so and so, certain types of actions were open to one and others were not. Positions could be challenged and reassigned in the course of an episode. So the phenomenon of positioning became a focus of study (Davies and Harré 1990).

The concept of 'position' can be tied to two other important concepts from the philosophy of language and from narratology, namely *speech-act* and *story-line*. To take up or to be assigned a position determines how what one says is heard as a social act. An uttered sentence is socially efficacious as a speech-act in ways that often exceed its literal meaning. A commonplace example is the use of a question format to issue an invitation: 'Why don't we have a picnic on Sunday?'. Relative to how one is positioned, one's utterances are taken as the performance of this or that speech-act. Episodes of everyday life are usually orderly, and often the source of that order is a cultural pattern of narrative, a story-line. It might be as grand as a heroic quest shaping something as mundane as shopping. It may be something as banal as the 'nurse–patient' game shaping something as momentous as home care of the seriously ill.

Thus specific positions are always tied in with specific repertoires of speech-acts and specific story-lines. Change any one member of the interlinked triad and the others change with it. Thus one can see how important acceptances of and challenges to positionings are.

There is a further consequence. The same set of utterances, sentences spoken by the members of a group in conversation, or the actions that occur in some other form of orderly social interaction, may be taken by different members differently, in so far as it is possible that some may position each other differently from the way others position the members of the group. There may be more than one conversation going on, although only one set of sentences has been uttered. The same sentence can express more than one speech-act depending on the positionings assumed by the various people who hear it. It follows, too, that there will be more than one story-line unfolding in the flow of utterances and other potentially meaningful actions.

We can now return to look once again at Willig's brief presentation of the third sense of subjectivity.

Subjectivity as 'how it is with me'

It seems that this important and contemporary concept lies on the cusp between the available repertoire of Wittgensteinian expressions, verbal and non-verbal, and the long- and short-term positionings that constrain the possible scope of access to the repertoire, and thus to what can be meaningfully manifested by anybody at any time. We have identified at least some of the conditions that must be satisfied if subjectivities in this sense are expressible in such a way that others can have access to how it is with me. These include the existence of a natural repertoire of expressive displays, internally related to the experiences they serve to make publicly visible and audible, in short a human ethology. They also presuppose that the methods by which vocabularies of words and gestures are acquired are in Vygotskian moments of psychological symbiosis. These, one may remark, can occur at any time in one's life!

Some insights

What does the discursive, constructionist approach to psychology mean for psychiatrists? As I emphasized in the beginning of this chapter, they hardly need encouraging to listen to what people say and, generally, to take this talk as expressive of 'how things are' with someone. That is the business of psychiatry. But doing something about what they hear is also the business of psychiatry. The normative underpinnings of any ameliorative action have often been remarked upon. However, with the discursive insight that cognition is a matter of using symbol systems according to local norms and conventions, another dimension of 'correctness' opens up. This is the dimension of the standards of 'proper' discourse.

From this point of view it is not so much what the discourses of the troubled express that is the root of the matter, but the troubled discourse itself. Another role for the psychiatrist emerges, to repair defective forms of talk, and to recover and enhance intimations of correct discourse in those who might be thought to have drifted out of the local discourse community altogether. I want to round off this introduction to the discursive point of view by briefly running over two examples of what I mean.

When Morton Prince (1905) took on the problem presented by Miss Beauchamp's 'multiple personality' presentations — her tendency to talk as if she were inhabited by three distinct persons — he recorded her non-standard ways of using personal pronouns as the means by which this expression was managed. Towards the end of his book about the case, he describes a therapy of great general interest. He pressed her to *repair* her use of the person pronouns. He tried to get her to use pronouns in reporting her life and announcing her plans in the ordinary way current in standard American middle-class English. According to those conventions, if the same body is involved in various events, past, present, and future, the correct pronouns for the one speaking in the identity determined by that body are 'I', 'me', 'mine', and 'myself'. According to the discursive, constructionist point of view, repairing grammar *is* repairing the mind.

The work of Steven Sabat (2001) on bringing to light the experience of those who are troubled by Alzheimer's condition also emphasizes the role of pronouns. He has shown how, in the seemingly disordered speech of those who suffer from word-finding problems, the use of personal pronouns, particularly and significantly the first person, remains robust. According to Wittgenstein's 'expressive' account of the uses of language, the personal pronouns express one's sense of self in relation to others. Thus, Sabat's finding shows that the sufferer has retained a sense of self. This insight allowed him to develop ways of recovering and enhancing that sense. Since other matters of importance, such as a sense of personal worth, go along with the generic sense of self, Sabat's work not only illustrates the way that a surviving cognitive function, the expression of personhood, can be enhanced, but also how the place of a person in the social world can be recovered. The rule might be: listen to the pronouns as they shine through the otherwise tangled threads of defective efforts at communication.

How do we know what standards we ought to be attending to in listening to such matters? This can come only from close attention to the *local* standards of correct usage. For example, although Standard English has almost wholly lost grammatical gender, it has been retained or perhaps reinvented in certain dialects. In Australian working-class English, grammatical gender is systematically involved in 'correct' uses of words for tools, for large and small objects, for machinery, and so on. Whose standard is in question? Clearly it is that of the speaker — not as an isolated individual, but as a member of a loosely bounded speech community.

These are some of the important insights that can be gained from a shift of attention from the meaning to the message itself.

References

Davies, B. and Harré, R. (1990). Positioning: the discursive production of selves. *Journal for the Theory of Social Behaviour*, **20/1**: 43–63.

Descartes, R. (1641). Meditations on the first philosophy. In *The Philosophical Writings of Descartes* (trans. J. Cottingham, R. Stoothoff, and D. Murdoch) (1984). Meditations Two and Six, pp. 16–23, 50–62. Cambridge: Cambridge University Press.

Goffman, E. (1959). *The Presentation of Self in Everyday Life*. New York: Doubleday.

Goffman, E. (1981). *Forms of Talk*. Philadelphia: University of Pennsylvania Press.

Hollway, W. (1984). Gender difference and the production of subjectivity. In *Changing the Subject: Social Regulation and Subjectivity* (ed. J. Henriques, W. Hollway, C. Urwin, L. Venn & V. Walkerdine). London: Methuen.

Prince, M. (1905). *The Dissociation of Personality*. London: Kegan Paul.

Sabat, S. (2001). *The Experience of Alzheimer's*. Oxford: Blackwell.

Sacks, O. (1985). *The Man Who Thought his Wife was a Hat*. London: Duckworth.

van Langenhove, L. and Harré, R. (1999). *Positioning Theory: Moral Contexts of Intentional Action*. Oxford: Blackwell.

Vygotsky, L. S. (1978). *Mind in Society* (ed. M. Cole, V. John-Steiner, S. Scribner and E. Souberman). Cambridge, MA: Harvard University Press.

Willig, C. (2000). A discourse-dynamic approach to the study of subjectivity in health psychology. *Theory and Psychology*, **10**(4): 547–70.

Wittgenstein, L. (1953). *Philosophical Investigations* (trans. G. E. M. Anscombe). Oxford: Blackwell.

9 Form and content: the role of discourse in mental disorder

Grant Gillett

The centrality of mind

The human mind is a central topic in philosophy, psychology, and psychiatry, and an adequate science of the mind is of interest to all these disciplines. Jaspers famously argued that meaningful and causal features of life history played somewhat different roles in mental disorder, and he has widely been interpreted as saying that the form of a disorder is a matter of causal forces acting (presumably in the brain) whereas the content (of delusions, obsessions, etc.) is explicable by appeal to life history (Jaspers 1913). The particular disorder that I will use to illustrate my discussion of form and content is anorexia and its relation to the hunger drive, which, in humans, has a critical feature that allows it to operate as we would not expect it to in non-discursive animals. In coming to grips with the operation of this desire or drive in anorexia, we can therefore expose a fallacy that has driven a great deal of work in biologically motivated psychiatry. The fallacy is that any mental faculty that operates in human beings can be understood in the same way (and therefore by using comparable experiments and experimental results) as it is understood in non-discursive animals. I want to argue that both the form of the disorder and its content are best understood by mixing an appreciation of biology with that of culture. In the case in point, this involves the cultural expectations on young men and women in relation to sexuality and their relationships in adult life.

I should begin by openly espousing the Aristotelian thesis that the mind is a configuration of characteristic functions of human beings and is not a special object or substance within human beings. Mental functions are distinguished from others in the way that is central to phenomenology, that is by their intentionality or aboutness — they take objects and features of the world as topics or contents and direct the activity of human beings through the meaning or significance central to some or other intentional content associated with them. Because desires or drives as instanced in human minds must therefore be understood not only as forces causally impelling us towards certain ways of thinking or acting, but also as themselves potential topics (in fact of second-order thoughts) that have a significance to us, they can operate in ways that are hard to understand when we consider only their biological function. On this basis I will argue that the mental origins of psychiatric disorders are affected in both their structure and their operation by the way that our own mental acts can become foci of intentional attitudes. As such they are informed by the productive and evaluative aspects of inter-personal relations and cultural evolution. This comes about because human beings formulate mental contents which they communicate to one another and are, in so far as they do, *mind-makers* as much as mind-exhibiters. As human groups who share a language and cultural heritage, we perform these functions collectively in regard of each human being who comes amongst us. What is more, each of us individually plays an autobiographical role in shaping his or her own life history and thus in mind-making for the self (Gillett 2000*a*).

The particularly challenging implication of this view is that the object or topic of our study — the human mind — is itself directly shaped or affected by the concepts and conceptions that we use to characterize it. People regard themselves as having souls, or personalities, or intelligence, or unconscious thoughts, or psychiatric disorders as a result of discourse concerning the nature of human beings. All such discourse takes shape in a cultural context replete with myths and meanings that shape our images of what it is to be human. Therefore, an important part of human discourse is its evaluative content relative to the norms of one's culture — and human beings are exquisitely sensitive to evaluations. Thus, it is only by laying bare the evaluative and symbolic content of cultural conceptions of food and its associated need-state that we can understand the phenomenology of anorexia in which the narrative and discursive essence of self is critical in moderating the form and content of what is seen clinically.

Wittgenstein (1953, §124) remarked, 'philosophy leaves everything as it is'. If he is right, we ought to be somewhat sceptical about getting beneath the 'surface' of our modes of understanding of ourselves to discover the true essence of mind (as, for instance, science might reveal the true essence of coal). What is more, as we investigate the mind we also modify it by chang-ing the discourse through which it understands itself.[1] In fact, every descrip-tion that we produce is a signification or categorization that records a certain way of looking at a phenomenon. On this view phenomena such as electron talk, calcium-channel talk, serotonin-reuptake talk, neurone talk, action-potential talk, brain circuit talk, information talk, thought talk, attitude talk, and so on each embody ways of categorizing things. Our categories them-selves each make a distinct contribution to our attempts to account for the workings of the world. It is, however, tempting to regard certain concepts as more basic because they deal with more scientifically measurable (or natural)

---

[1]Ian Hacking (1995) refers to this as 'the looping effect of human kinds'.

features of the human organism. But we should recall in any discussion of metaphysical basicness, that the talk concerned necessarily sets aside the remarkable fact that our understanding is framed in terms of human concepts, which themselves are products of human minds, and therefore they attest that we are *not* just like other (non-discursive) denizens of the world. Thus, the basicness of biological terms such as 'neurone' is derived from factoring out the differences that make us (as distinct from other biological things with neurones) able to devise such terms. This must inform our metaphysics of the mind and should alert us to the fact that it is unlikely to be simple.

My view of the metaphysics of mind begins with the thought that we exist as thinking beings in a world of objects and that conceptualizing the world is an interactive process. We use concepts to categorize things. Our categories enable us to do things that otherwise we could not do. We make discoveries when something we come across is marked by a concept that records a new way of thinking about things around us. One obvious example would be the way in which concepts of electricity allow us to construct a simple light source from a battery, a bulb, and wire connections. The discovery that wire is a conductor becomes able to be known only once we have concepts about electricity, but once the concepts are in play the conductivity of wire is an objective fact.

Concepts empower us by identifying regularities and connections between the different situations we find in the world (Gillett 1992b). For human beings, our ways of thinking are shared and promulgated through language and embody discursive techniques that help us to identify aspects of the world relevant to the diverse interests evident in human activities (Wittgenstein 1953, §570). Wittgenstein's remarks on 'language games' highlight the fact that it is through language and related activities that we elaborate the rules governing our use of concepts. One might say that understanding a concept is more or less equivalent to engaging successfully in the use of that segment of a natural language in which the concept is expressed — a thesis usually attributed to Michael Dummett (1981).

It is evident that the mental structure basic to success in any domain of activity has two aspects:

1. a set of classifications that give us a good way of ordering our interactions within the domain; and
2. the perceptuomotor and cognitive techniques required to engage with features of that domain.

The result of activity based on these two sources is a 'cognitive map', the attainment of which by any thinker or group of thinkers yields a fairly straightforward sense in which a thought could be true or false; it is true or false depending on whether it represents the world as it would appear in the relevant segment of the map (in accordance with the rules governing the relevant concepts).

As engaged subjects we ourselves appear on our maps along with the contents of the mind, including our desires. What is more, the map is intrinsically value-laden; its terms are conditioned by our interests. Thus, when we seek to understand a disorder in which desire figures prominently, such as anorexia, we need to understand that our responses to the world depend not only on what the desire impels the subject towards doing but also on the significance for that subject's life project that is attached to the desire as it figures on the subject's cognitive map. At this stage we can enunciate an important principle.

The principle of duality of content states that any mental state or occurrence will affect me through its biological or causal role in the mind, and also by virtue of its role as a signal which says something about me.

Intentionality, objects, and causality

Jaspers' two types of understanding are directly relevant to understanding the principle of duality of content in that one involves tracing the causal origins of various psychic events and states, and the other involves discerning their meaning to the patient. The former kind of understanding marks the natural sciences where we seek biological explanations. The latter kind of understanding, which concerns the meanings of events for human beings, is crucial in our understanding of intentionality or the contents of the mind. Those contents crucially concern objects in the world but, as Brentano, Husserl, and Frege, among many others, have noted, the contents important in psychological explanation are not given by merely specifying the objects concerned. We have to find out how the subject thinks of the thing concerned in order to understand the thought and the significance that the subject attaches to it. Think, for instance, of the thought, made famous by Frege, that the morning star has risen. One could think this and not realize that the planet Venus was visible in the sky or that the evening star could be seen, whereas in fact these three thoughts all concern the same object. The significance of any event or object to a subject is what features in an explanation of their actions.

Jaspers claims that meaningful or intentional explanations of human thought and action are based on evidence gained 'while we gather experience in our contact with human personalities' (Jaspers 1913, p. 84). He further distinguishes between 'rational' and 'empathic' understanding, claiming that the connections revealed by the former can only reveal contents as they are governed by the 'rules of logic', whereas the latter bring us into contact with a person's individual psychology (or autobiographical narrative). When we pursue psychological connections empathically, we engage with the person's thought and address ourselves to them as a person. In this we appreciate the rule-governed and meaning-giving nature of the person's cultural context and his or her engagement in it. We do not merely seek 'objective' evidence about the forces acting on a person, but rather we seek to understand how the person understands what is happening to them. Thus, to understand the significance of food to an anorexic patient, we would need an appreciation of how she positions herself in relation to the world that evaluates and makes demands on her. We would then begin to discern what content might be attached to eating and hunger in her particular evolving life story.

Casual theories of intentionality

Peter Strawson (1974) has argued that there is a fundamental conceptual divide between the type of explanation implicit in reactive attitudes such as praise, blame, and resentment (e.g. *He did that because he felt the insult deeply*) and objective attitudes such as those involved in causal explanation (*He was caused to do that by his high levels of testosterone*). He argues that the reactive attitudes are inextricably tied to the ways in which we relate to each other as moral beings and that these relationships inform the descriptions of others that constitute the common currency of everyday life.[2] Bolton and Hill (1996) attempt to go beyond Strawson's claim about the essential difference between these two approaches and argue that mental explanation is a subtype of causal explanation. They argue that mental states are realized by (or encoded in) brain states, which are the medium of the organism–environment interactions qualifying as intentional. In this they follow a well-established philosophical literature defending the thesis that to explain a thought, intention, or action is to provide its causal history. What is more, the relevant causal connections are most plausibly thought to lie in an underlying cognitive architecture that works according to the laws of neuroscience. Therefore we can short-circuit some of the more complex metaphysical discussion by asking: 'Can we explain human cognitive neuroscience entirely in its own terms?'. I have argued a contrary position based on the cultural and discursive embedding of the development of neurocognitive structures (Gillett 1999, 2000b). I claim that a non-causal men- tal and social understanding of mental phenomena is indispensable for mental explanation. To be fair, Bolton and Hill also argue that a reduction of mental explanation in psychiatric disorder to a more fundamental level is not likely to be possible because of the importance of what is being encoded. I want to argue for a more radical view: that, in fact, a genuine explanation needs to recognize that the brain does not provide a level of basicness for psychiatric explanation at all and that discursive explanation has an epistemically and metaphysically coeval status.

We can examine this claim by turning our attention to the concepts needed to make sense of intentional content.

---

[2]For most people, testosterone level would not be a moral difference.

The brain and intentionality

The brain is the repository of meanings; it is the physical medium in which mental content is realized, and throughout life the brain stores information partly in terms of the meanings that have structured a given individual's experience. These meanings draw on rules shaped in human discourse so that there is a deep relation between the language that a community speaks and the classifications used by members of that community in dealing with the world (Gillett 1992a). In fact, the role of words in forming and refining our thoughts is becoming increasingly clear from theoretical, clinical, and experimental work in cognitive psychology (Luria 1973; Vygotsky 1978; Karmiloff-Smith 1986, 1992).

Words mark significant groupings of stimulus features and cognitive associations so that they can be conveyed from one thinker to another. Words therefore convey 'good tricks' (Dennett 1995) of environmental adaptation between individuals who are co-linguistic or inhabit the same culture. The word and the encounters with the environment that ground its meaning interact in such a way that there is constant negotiation between variations in stimulus pattern, the connections of the word to other words, and the purposes and interest of the individual in the total context of use. The word helps to organize the search and detection patterns that focus on the features of a situation that would warrant its use in that context, and its meaning draws on those conditions. Therefore, words help to shape and not merely to express our thoughts in the same way that the rules of chess help to shape moves and strategies in a game of chess.

The way in which words operate to fulfil their cognitive role and organize brain function can be explained by certain features of neural network theory and practice, which I have discussed elsewhere (Harré and Gillett 1994; Gillett 1999). In brief, a neural network can be used to register certain configurations of activity that have been associated with significant objects. At its most simple, the network registers the co-occurrence of patterns of excitation, which may arise from anywhere. Obviously patterns that consistently arise from an object in the environment are likely to be packaged together or internally associated with one another. However, other associations may be used to advantage. For instance, if a characteristic sound pattern is consistently produced in relation to an object then that sets up a cognitive connection. Strings of signs can also be constructed where the occurrence of one pattern will tend to evoke another depending on the multiple contextual constraints acting on (and within) the information system at a given time. This simple principle of connectivity means that the system is plausibly able to become capable of associating words with repeated features of the world. If those objects have been picked out and remain linked to words in common usage then the combination of arbitrary sound pattern and input from the object can form what we might call a 'semantic complex', which is the kind of capacity we need in the brain to develop a cognitive map or picture of the world. We find exactly this kind of thesis expressed in the writings of both Luria and Freud.

Intentionality and discourse

Freud discusses the fact that an 'object presentation' is formed in the mind as a result of experience and that this comprises two components, both of which are complex patterns of association — one verbal, the other situational or experience-based:

> A word is thus a complex presentation . . . there corresponds to the word a complicated associative process into which the elements of visual, acoustic and kinaesthetic origin . . . enter together (Freud 1986, p. 182)

We can plausibly regard meanings as marked by signs that are used within human discourse to structure different activities. On this view, meanings are stimulus patterns and connections between stimulus patterns are associated with signs (as captured in a segment of language). In fact, Luria (1973, p. 306) characterizes a word as a 'complex multidimensional matrix of different cues and connections'. Neural network theory enables us to see that meanings, construed in this way, shape or influence the microprocessing structure of the brain by forming connections between different world-related patterns of information.

In the real world, connections between patterns of information arise both socially (through the signs accompanying information from objects and events in the environment) and individually (direct organism–world interactions). Humans clearly do modify their behaviour as a result of motivational information, such as the availability of food or other physical gratifications, and have innate propensities to respond in certain ways. The most important of these, in the human case, is that the infant or child imitates and learns from the responses of other human beings in any situation so that 'any view which . . . construes the child as a solitary inquirer attempting to discover the truth about the world must be rejected' (Hamlyn 1973, p. 184). It is as if the responses of other people cue the learner as to what is worth attending to (Gillett 1999). These facts allow us to outline a connectionist approach to causality and explanation that provides an adequate springboard for discursive theories of mind.

On the discursive view, we begin with the fact that words and their meanings or passages of discourse have a formative effect on the contents of the mind and the connections that underpin mental life. We use words as a powerful means to affect each other. Harré remarks:

> Conversation is to be thought of as creating a social world just as causality generates a physical one (1983, p. 65).

In a similar way to the causes operating in the natural order, words have an existence and force in part independent of the individual who uses and is influenced by them.

The thesis is that language is a joint project partly given before the advent of any individual and partly modified by all the individuals who use it. We all contribute to language through our discourse by using the words we have inherited. A lexicographer charts this shared and evolving process when he or she marks the changes that affect the meanings of our words. What is more, we are formed into English thinkers, American thinkers, French thinkers, Hungarian thinkers, or Mandarin thinkers by our immersion in a sociocultural context. This fact has important consequences for the metaphysics of mind. Only by taking seriously the shared project of meaning that defines each of us as a thinker can we arrive at a view that is adequate to understand the form and content of psychiatric disorder.

Discourse and the brain

Bolton and Hill (1996) espouse what they call an 'encoding thesis', according to which 'the brain encodes meaning' (p. 76) by realizing information that mediates brain–world interactions according to functional specifications structuring the subject's reaction to the environment. Their summary claim is as follows:

> the brain can be said to encode meaning or information, though not because there is a one–one correspondence between meaningful states and neural states. The language of meaning and of encoded meaning is based in organism–environment interactions, and can be applied to the brain only in so far as the brain serves in the regulation of those interactions (Bolton and Hill 1996, p. 116)

On the basis of this claim, they make the further claim that mental explanation is causal explanation, resting that argument almost entirely on the predictive power of such explanation.

This theory-driven predictive power apparently makes unavoidable the conclusion that explanations involving meaningful mental states are in some sense causal, and it lies at the basis of replies to all arguments to the contrary (Bolton and Hill 1996, p. 118).

This is an argument that seeks to overturn any non-causal account of explanatory power. It is antithetical, for instance, to Wittgenstein's rejection of the causal view in favour of a rule-following account and, in fact, it is vulnerable to any account of predictive power that does not rely on causal chains. Wittgenstein himself often used the analogy of chess to point out the difference between mental or rule-governed and physical or causal explanation, such as that which accounts for natural regularities (e.g. cardioregulatory responses; Bolton and Hill 1996, pp. 221ff).

Rules that govern meaning give me techniques for talking and thinking about objects in the environment that my human group has found to be tried and true. However, the rules of language do not merely cause me to respond thus and so, they allow me to construct patterns of action and thought — just as the rules of chess do not cause me to move the pieces in a certain way, but they do provide narrow constraints within which I can make a legal move. By contrast, a cardiorespiratory reflex causes my body to react in a certain way — albeit one that suits my purposes. The discursive view focuses on the power conferred by following the rules of human discourse. It identifies positions and moves in the game of life that these rules make available, and conceives of mental explanation as locating a person in relation to a sphere of discourse. When one sees the meanings being deployed by a person, one can identify the subjective relationships holding between the person and the context. This understanding reveals what choices for perception and action present themselves to that person in a given situation: it is therefore an empathic mode of understanding. This, in turn, illuminates relationships of power, reveals the content of any significations used to organize behaviour, and renders intelligible (not merely explicable) the activity of the person concerned; it is as if one were successfully to locate a person on a map so that you and they both remarked, 'Ah, now I see where I am!'. This, I have argued, is not causal explanation, but does have a great deal of explanatory and predictive power (Gillett 1993*a,b*). In fact, it may yield explanations where an objective viewpoint yields none. We can now compare the discursive approach to the causal view characteristic of the natural sciences.

Bolton and Hill argue that mental explanation is a species of causal explanation. Their basic argument for this view, as Millikan expresses it, is that for those who want to see psychology as a natural science like biology: 'the only alternative to biological design, in our sense of "design", is sheer coincidence, freak accident'(Millikan 1995, I, p. 262). However, the discursive view is an account that offers us to a real alternative to this stark choice.

Discourse and explanation

I would argue, in agreement with Bolton and Hill, that successful creatures are likely to develop cognitive mechanisms that track or are linked to external or environmental objects and features, rather than internal ones. This implies that their actions are intentional, in a phenomenological sense, in that they are essentially directed upon objects in the environment outside the mind. This claim embodies, in fact, a kind of externalism. Tyler Burge, in this vein, remarks:

> [a]n illuminating philosophy of psychology must do justice . . . to psychology's attempt to account for tasks that we succeed and fail at, *where these tasks are set by the environment and represented by the subject him- or herself.* The most salient and important of these tasks are those that arise through relations to the natural and social worlds (Burge 1995, I, p. 201)

I have already suggested that the evidence of neuroscience tends to make this commitment, and its implicit socially relativized externalism, quite attractive in that we find in the brain many circuits designed to lock on to environmental targets and track them. Burge has drawn our attention to the importance of both the natural and social worlds in yielding the objects represented in mental content. Thus we need to devise a mode of explanation that combines and moderates causality and connectionism in a way that does justice to discursive psychology. In this we can take note of the fact that many of the most important elements of our mental world are socially or interpersonally mediated, things like a sense of belonging, the fact that others like or loathe me, the occurrence of guilt, a sense of rejection, and so on.

The inescapable conclusion seems to be that the realm of words or signification, and therefore sociocultural reality, and the environmental or physical determination of content combine to shape the processing structure of the brain. The causal forces at work here can, at one level, be understood by shifting distributed patterns of information in the brain which fit themselves to the influences discussed above, namely words used, objects present, and contexts or projects that are current. However, at another level, the forces that have moulded those processing patterns can be discerned only by looking at discourse, and therefore at society and culture. Therefore, if we want to understand psychological explanations we will need to take into our surview regularities that become evident at many levels of understanding.

In the face of this conclusion, we are justified in turning to discourse and pointing out that brain-processing networks are quite plastic and therefore might be expected to realize within them the artefactual saliencies that arise in human forms of life (such as the Brooklyn Bridge, classical music, and my family traditions) and that these artefacts should, on any decently Aristotelian theory of mind, be represented in configurations of brain activity. Given that many of the things we think about are profoundly cultural in nature, even when they are physically realized as objects in the world, the prospects for a self-contained physicalism that produces explanations totally in terms of biological kinds look grim.

I have argued that discourse — exchanges with other human beings — is the milieu in which human cognition is shaped. I have then argued that this implies that the domain of the personal is the basis of understanding and meaning. We are constantly adapting, refining, and shaping our thoughts about what is around us on the basis of the responses of others to us. Thus their attitudes and reactions shape what I think about this or that object or situation. Therefore, a human being's growing conception of how the world actually or objectively is cannot proceed independently of the effects of other persons on the shape and coherence of his or her thinking. This is equally true both of my conception of what is *out there* and of what is *in here*, so that my conception of who and what I am is sensitive and responsive to the effects of others on me both through their actions toward me and their conceptualizations of me. The effects of others on me is, however, not straightforwardly causal in that they impart norms or values to me (semantic and psychological), which I can obey or disobey as I choose and which do not causally compel me to do certain things as a result of antecedent events.

The discursive nature of the production of the mind has quite significant implications for the explanation of psychological events and processes. The major implication is that a discursive explanation locates the subject in relation to the discourse in which that individual is embedded. That, in turn, reveals the position of the individual with respect to the power relations obtaining in the discourse, which allows us to understand the subjectivity at the centre of an experience and the significations that are available to organize patterns of thought and action. This becomes highly significant in relation to the idea of the unconscious, in that the unconscious is traditionally conceived as being the locus of processes that cause behaviour but are not consciously chosen or even accessible to the thinking subject. The discursive approach emphasizes the multilayered meanings configuring the experience of the subject and that certain meaningful or intentional configurations, particularly those that escape rational or conscious control, can deeply affect a person. Discursive explanations, in a way that differs from causal explanations, put the self-forming relational subject at the centre of all mental explanations.

The style of explanation found in discursive theory is genealogical explanation, which trades in the power relations and discursive positions occupied by a subject. We might therefore expect that many of the most important influences on subjectivity have their origins in early childhood, when intentionality is being constructed. Human beings cue their offspring in terms of their own responses to things around them; they also greatly extend the range and productivity of the child's information-gathering by imparting to the child a set of shared concepts.

Discursive explanation, psychology, and psychiatric disorder

The study of genealogy, in the sense used by Nietzsche and Foucault, overturns the thesis that any particular set of discursive formations and the significations that make them up is privileged. Thus there is no progressively pure and scientific story to tell about the human condition that leads us to a single view of the nature of reality (as is assumed by traditional metaphysics in general and by scientific realism in particular). There is instead a concept of truth that is prefigured by Nietzsche when he describes truth as 'a mobile army of metaphors' that capture our minds so that we see the world in certain ways. Some of these, as a result of the power relations in human discourse, come to be widely seen as legitimate, and others as heretical. Therefore, when we try to understand human beings, a fluid conception of the requisite knowledge is suggested. This knowledge is under certain constraints, the nature of which, particularly on the postmodern view, is more likely to be found by observing and deconstructing human practices of knowledge, creation, and validation than by trying to discover some 'match' between our representations and the real world.

We need not subscribe to postmodern ways of thinking to understand the power of this view in recasting what passes as knowledge in the social or moral sciences. We need merely to observe that our conceptions of what the mind is and of what people are like influence the way we are. This effect has been called 'the looping effect of human kinds' (Hacking 1995, p. 21), and it highlights the formative role of myths and images in my conception of what I am. The fact is that human beings are the kinds of creature that do shape their own life stories in the light of the attitudes and evaluations that surround them and to which they commit themselves. For this reason psychology, medicine in general, and psychiatry in particular do not merely describe human nature and its variations: they also influence it.

The form and content of anorexia

Analytical tools — such as discourse, subjectivity, position, power, signification, evaluation, legitimation, and so on — allow us to make visible the interaction between human thoughts about humanity and the nature of the human beings thinking those thoughts. These tools explain human activity by mapping it on to a world structured by human discourses. That mapping reveals points at which we can predict what somebody would do and understand why they have done certain things that otherwise would puzzle us. The resulting knowledge is important not only for psychology but also for any discipline that tries to understand influences, whether 'normal' or 'pathological' on the human mind. For this reason psychiatry can benefit from discursive explanation just as it can from causal explanation; indeed, the two should complement one another as, in fact, Jaspers surmised. What is inescapable is Jaspers' conclusion that without empathic knowledge or the discursive pattern of explanation in which empathy has its natural home we will not understand why people act as they do. This is nowhere as evident as in the understanding of the eating disorders.

Recent research in young women with anorexia has suggested that there are hormonal disturbances in the hypothalamus that cause a malfunction in the satiety centre and suppress eating behaviour. Even if this were true, it would explain only one feature of the phenomenology of this puzzling disorder. In addition to the dramatic suppression of eating, we need to try to answer a number of other questions.

- Why are such young women are often exquisitely sensitive, at the time they develop the disorder, to remarks about their weight?
- How can their perception of their own bodies can be so disordered that they do not realize how dangerously thin they are?
- Why is there an association between anorexia and other self-destructive behaviours?
- Why does the anorexic demonstrate such iron resolve in carrying out her project of weight loss and alteration of her own physique?
- Why are so many anorexic patients obsessed with food and its preparation?
- Why do these young women react with such horror when they discover they have made weight gains?

These questions take us beyond the organic cause that potentiates reduced eating and into a set of meanings that inform the psyche of the young woman who is caught in this disorder. We need to consider the loss of autonomy inherent in certain conceptions of the woman's role, resistance to physical development and maturity as a woman, the sociopolitical cult of thinness, the mixed messages surrounding food and goodness for young women, and the layers of meaning associated with each of these features of a young woman's adaptation to the transition from child to adult.

Both the phenomenon and the phenomenology of anorexia are illuminated by these considerations, which many therapists have found indispensible in mounting effective programmes to restore anorexic patients to health (Orbach 1993; McCarthy and Thompson 1997).

In anorexia we encounter a young woman who sees herself, when she is hungry or eating, as not being in control of her life or destiny. Food is a sign of her dependency on the mother who has charted a motherly life to be lived, and yet also food is the threat that means that she may not be attractive enough to find a man who will allow her to live the womanly role. But does she want to live out that role, with its loss of autonomy and pressures to be attractive to others who may not share her dreams and goals? Can she defer this entry into a conflicted state of living in which she is expected to be good at food and yet not allow it to do bad things to her? Hunger and eating are signs of this conflict — this narrative autobiographical problem that must be solved. Time is pressing and menses are a sure indicator that the problem is imminent. But then starvation keeps her childlike, defers the problem, stops her menstruation, indicates her control over her own life, emphasizes the clean purity of her own body as not needing and being cloyed up by relationships with others. A non-answer to the too-difficult problem is now born with the onset of a pattern of food refusal or (in bulimia) a disempowerment of food so that it is purged from the system and cannot shackle her with the chains of nature. The human mind is locating the subjective body, the lived autobiography on a cognitive map of the world, and finds one way to resist the forces that seem inexorably to drive the young female towards the tricky choices that await her in womanhood. This place on the map seems like a haven, and all that reveals its deadly location is the very nature and wisdom that surrounds her and that she is resisting. Why, her actions have reversed the natural change of menses, so why should the other inevitable, predictable things be any more powerful? This myth as lived is powerful.

The style of inquiry that allows these questions to be broached and these insights to be explored is, in Jaspers' terms, concerned with meaningful connections between behaviour and life history. The relevant connections are investigated, appreciated, and confronted empathically, and cannot otherwise be understood. Anorexia is just one example in which that crucial discursive feature of the moral sciences holds such deep lessons for psychiatry that, without it, we can only limp haltingly in our search for a surview of the mind and its discontents.

References

Bolton, D. and Hill, J. (1996). *Mind, Meaning and Mental Disorder*. Oxford: Oxford University Press.

Burge, T. (1995). Individualism and psychology. In: *Philosophy of Psychology: Debates on Psychological Explanation* (ed. C. Macdonald and G. Macdonald), pp. 173–205. Oxford: Blackwell.

Dennett, D. (1995). *Darwin's Dangerous Idea*. London: Penguin.

Dummett, M. (1981). *The Interpretation of Frege's Philosophy*. London: Duckworth.

Freud, S. (1986). *The Essentials of Psychoanalysis* (ed. A. Freud). London: Penguin.

Gillett, G. (1992a). Language, social ecology and experience. *International Studies in the Philosophy of Science*, **5**: 1–9.

Gillett, G. (1992b). *Representation, Meaning, and Thought*. Oxford: Clarendon.

Gillett, G. (1993a). Actions, causes and mental ascriptions. In: *Objections to Physicalism* (ed. H. Robinson), pp. 81–100. Oxford: Clarendon.

Gillett, G. (1993b). Free will and mental content. *Ratio*, **VI.2**: 89–108.

Gillett, G. (1999). *The Mind and its Discontents*. Oxford: Oxford University Press.

Gillett, G. (2000a). Moral authenticity and the unconscious. In: *The Analytic Freud* (ed. M. Levine), pp. 177–92. London: Routledge.

Gillett, G. (2000b). Dennett, Foucault and the selection of memes. *Inquiry*, **42**: 13–23.

Hacking, I. (1995). *Rewriting the Soul*. Princeton, NJ: Princeton University Press.

Hamlyn, D. (1973). Human learning. In: *The Philosophy of Education* (ed. R. S. Peters), pp. 178–94. Oxford: Oxford University Press.

Harré, R. (1983). *Personal being*. Oxford: Blackwell.

Harré, H. R. and Gillett, G. (1994). *The Discursive Mind*. Thousand Oaks, CA: Sage.

Jaspers, K. (1913 [1974]). Causal and meaningful connexions between life history and psychosis. In: *Themes and Variations in European Psychiatry* (ed. S. R. Hirsch and M. Shepherd). Bristol: John Wright.

Karmiloff-Smith, A. (1986). From meta-process to conscious access: evidence from children's metalinguistic and repair data. *Cognition*, **23**: 95–147.

Karmiloff-Smith, A. (1992). *Beyond Modularity*. Cambridge, MA: MIT Press.

Millikan, R. G. (1995). Biosemantics: Explanation in Psychology. In: *Philosophy of Psychology: Debates on Psychological Explanation* (ed. C. Macdonald and G. Macdonald), pp. 253–76. Oxford: Blackwell.

Luria, A. R. (1973). *The Working Brain*. Harmondsworth, UK: Penguin.

McCarthy, A. and Thompson, M. (1997). *The Hungry Heart*. Auckland: Hodder, Moa Beckett.

Orbach, S. (1993). *Hunger Strike*. London: Penguin.

Strawson, P. (1974). *Freedom and Resentment and Other Essays*. London: Methuen.

Vygotsky, L. S. (1978). *Mind in Society*. Cambridge, MA: Harvard University Press.

Wittgenstein, L. (1953). *Philosophical Investigations*. Oxford: Blackwell.

10 Meaning and causes of delusions

Michael Musalek

The meanings of 'delusion'

Our world is characterized by the precariousness and misunderstandings produced by the ambiguity of languages. Language can never convey absolute meaning, and therefore the interpretation of our words and world(s) can never be definitive (Derrida 1978, 1982). The same word, a particular term, can be understood in many different ways; the same literal expression may produce various cognitive associations and emotional reactions. This applies particularly to the term delusion, which derives from the Latin word 'deludere', meaning 'to put on an act for someone', 'to lead someone to believe in something', 'to pull the wool over someone's eyes'. From the observer's point of view, the deluded person seems to be confronted with an unreal world; that is to say the observer and others decide what is real and unreal.

Closely connected with the term delusion is the diagnosis of paranoia. This term emphasizes the existence of a disorder of relations to reality (Störung des Realitätsbezuges) in contrast to 'common reality'. 'Noos' means reason, insight, and knowledge, and paranoia therefore means para-reason or para-knowledge, an insight that does not meet commonsense, or widely accepted experiences and interpretations.

In French psychiatric terminology we find the term 'le délire' instead of delusion. This expression goes back to the Latin 'de lira ire', which means, literally translated, 'to come off the track', 'to leave the furrow', and focuses particularly on withdrawal from common social life leading to social isolation and alienation ('das aus der mitmenschlich gemeinsamen Welt Herausgerückt-sein', das 'Verrücktsein'; Scharfetter 1991).

In German, delusions are called as 'Wahn', a term that derives from the indo-germanic root 'wen', meaning 'to look for something', 'to ask for', 'to desire', 'to expect', 'to assume'. The term 'win' may derive from the same word-stem. Sometimes 'Wahn' is confused with 'Wahnsinn' (Musalek 2000). In contrast to 'Wahn', the latter term stems from the radical 'wan', which is closely connected with the gothic word 'vans' and the Latin term 'vanus, vastus' meaning 'empty'. In English we may find the term 'vain' as a leaf of the stem 'wan'. 'Wahnsinn' therefore means, literally translated, 'empty of sense', 'empty of reason'.

All of these different meanings of delusion may be found in everyday usage of the word delusion in non-professional talks and discussions, leading to various misunderstandings, but professional medical terminology is also characterized by ambiguity and precariousness. Today, no commonly accepted definition of delusion is available (Kisker and Wulff 1999). Various psychopathological — and sometimes not even pathological — features and phenomena are summarized under the term delusion. For this reason it seems worthwhile to start this section on the meaning(s) of delusion with some words regarding its definition. These introductory remarks cannot be taken as an extensive discourse on definitive problems in this field, but should help to make clear what is being talked about (and not talked about) in what follows.

In recent decades the definition of delusion as a false belief reappeared in the psychiatric literature, despite its use having been considered inappropriate since the beginning of the last century (Ayd 1985). For many theoretical as well as practical reasons, the value of this definition in clinical practice is questionable. The assumption that a delusional idea represents a false belief would mean that, in clinical practice, the psychiatrist has to judge what is right and what is wrong, what is the true and what is not. But psychiatrists are clearly not trained to make in these judgements: it cannot be the responsibility of a psychiatrist to decide whether a statement is correct or not. With respect to delusions of persecution or jealousy, for example, this would mean that the diagnosis of a delusion does not depend on the medical, psychological, and psychopathological knowledge of the psychiatrist, but much more on his or her criminological abilities (or disabilities).

Another argument against this and similar definitions is the fact that such definitions are based on exclusion: one may produce false *or* right interpretations. According to the findings of post-modern and post-structuralistic philosophical research, leading to the main conclusion of a multifaceted truth (Derrida 1986; Kristeva 1981; Lacan 1966; Lyotard 1979), such a diagnostic position seems highly problematic today. Furthermore, such a position implies that, for example, proof of being persecuted would prohibit the diagnosis of a delusion of persecution — which stands in contrast to the fact that persecuted people tend to develop delusions of persecution much more often than non-persecuted individuals. The same would be true for delusions of jealousy: proof of being betrayed by the partner may protect the diagnosis of a delusion of jealousy; or, conversely, a person could avoid being betrayed by developing a delusion of jealousy.

Other critics have focused on the term 'belief' (Fulford 1991). Again, this term has different meanings, one of which is found in the term 'religious or political beliefs'. However, deluded individuals do not *believe* that they are persecuted, they do not believe that the persecutor is a persecutor, they *know* that they are persecuted, they know that they are betrayed, they know that they are suffering from a severe disease, they know that the persecutor is a persecutor — just as we do not only believe, but know, that the priest in the church is a priest, the teacher at school is a teacher, and the grocer at the corner shop is a grocer. Delusions represent a particular kind of knowledge, and not beliefs.

Early in the twentieth century, similar considerations led to the replacement of the definition of delusions as false beliefs by the Jaspersian criteria for delusions (Jaspers 1975). Jaspers emphasized that, besides the criterion of impossibility of content ('Unmöglichkeit des Inhaltes'), it is mostly the extraordinary degree of conviction concerning particular ideas ('unvergleichlich hohe subjektive Gewissheit'; Jaspers 1975) and the outright rejection of alternative explanations ('Unkorrigierbarkeit'; Jaspers 1975) that are the crucial signs of a delusion. Berner (1982) pointed out later that the last two criteria are obligatory for the diagnosis, whereas the impossibility of content is only an accessory criterion: if present, it strengthens the diagnosis of delusion, but its absence does not prohibit the diagnosis. The content of delusions may be possible in principle (Sedler 1995). This means that patients suffering from delusional parasitosis, for example, may be also infested by real parasites (Musalek 1991).

When discussing the diagnostic guidelines of delusions, we should not forget that the great certainty and its incorrigibility represent only the final point of a continuum. From this point of view, delusions can no longer be considered as a discrete diagnostic category but as located on the uncertainty–certainty continuum. The greater the degree of certainty, the greater the likelihood of the diagnosis of delusion. As we are quite often confronted in daily life by such high and incorrigible certainties, it does not make sense to classify all such delusional states as pathological features. Only when the great certainty and incorrigibility influence the thinking and actions of the person in a particular way may he or she become a patient. In other words, delusions in a narrower sense (as pathological features) are characterized by a loss of 'degrees of freedom' ('Verlust von Freiheitsgraden'). The patient suffering from delusional ideas is no longer able to decide what he or she wants to do: the delusional convictions move the patient. These so-called 'polarized delusions' are the opposite of 'delusions in juxtaposition', incorrigible convictions without decreased degrees of freedom (Berner and Musalek 1989). Again, we are confronted with a continuum with blurred edges. The greater the loss of degrees of freedom, the more pathological the feature; or the greater the degree of polarization, the greater the certainty that the delusional ideas represent a pathological process. Below, the term delusion is used only in this narrower sense, to signify meaningful constructs that consist of delusional ideas characterized by particularly great certainty and its incorrigibility, and leading to a significant loss of degrees of freedom.

Occurrence of delusions

Delusions may thus be considered as ideas with meaningful content character-ized by extraordinary conviction and the outright rejection of alternatives, leading to a significant loss of the individual's degree of freedom. This raises three crucial questions for research on the pathogenesis of delusions:

1. The question of the origins of a particular delusional theme
2. The question of the constellations of conditions giving rise to the incorrigible conviction
3. The question of the factors increasing the degree of polarization.

The first question deals with the problem of why a particular person chooses a particular theme and not another one. For example, why is one person suffer-ing from delusions of persecution and not from delusions of jealousy, and why is another person suffering from hypochondriacal ideas and not from ideas of persecution or jealousy? During the last decade an increasing number of empirical studies were carried out to answer these questions. The results of these studies indicate that the choice of the particular delusional theme is caused by a complex interaction of factors such as age, gender, social situation (particularly social isolation and alienation) and so-called 'key experiences'. Prevailing problems for males and females in particular life periods, as well as the content of actual crises, reappear in the delusional themes (Kretschmer 1966; Musalek *et al.* 1989; Rümke 1951).

The second main concern in pathogenesis research is the elucidation of the constellation of conditions that are responsible for the occurrence of a incorrigible conviction. Why is the deluded patient so sure that his or her interpretations are right? Why does he say that he *is* persecuted? Why does not he say that he is probably persecuted, or that he assumes himself to be persecuted? Why does not he accept any other interpretation? According to recent studies, different factors are responsible for the fixation of a particu-lar theme (for the occurrence of the incorrigible conviction) than for the choice of a delusional theme. Cognitive disorders in the frame of organic or schizophrenic psychoses on the one hand, and emotional disorders as observable in the course of affective psychoses on the other hand, result in the high certainty and incorrigibility of convictions (Musalek and Kutzer 1989). There is some evidence that, in some cases, personality disorders and social isolation may also be of importance in connection with the develop-ment of delusional fixation, but further studies are necessary to clarify their role in the pathogenesis of delusion. So, we may conclude that various psy-chological and social factors are involved in the development of a particular delusional theme, whereas physical factors such as cognitive and emotional disorders are the indispensable basis for the occurrence of the incorrigible conviction.

Concerning the third crucial question, it was thought for a long time that the higher the degree of certainty and incorrigibility, the higher the degree of polarization. However, this assumption stands in contrast to the empirical finding that in clinical practice we may find patients (or, rather, clients) with incorrigible convictions but without a significant loss of 'degree of freedom'. The degree of polarization of a delusion is not a pre-existing sign of a delusion; it is much more an effect of the so-called 'Wahnarbeit' — the client's work producing delusional convictions. Other factors that may be responsible for the increased polarization are discussed in the following section.

Persistence of delusions

The classical studies on the pathogenesis of delusions have been based mainly on Zubin's (1977) concept of vulnerability, and have focused on the various physical, mental, and social factors that lead to mental disorder. The classical vulnerability concept derives from the assumption that an increased vulnerability for mental disorders (genetically caused or acquired in early life periods by so-called 'predisposing factors') leads to a manifest disorder only when appropriate triggers occur ('triggering factors'). However, as has been shown in recent studies, vulnerability of delusions cannot be considered as a static manifestation but represents a dynamic process ('dynamic vulnerability hypothesis'; Falloon *et al* 1984). In other individuals with low vulnerability, intensive triggers are necessary to trigger the same disorder. Physical, mental and/or social factors that act as predisposing factors are responsible for the degree of vulnerability (Musalek *et al.* 2000).

In the light of to the dynamic vulnerability hypothesis, delusions can no longer be reduced to psychopathological manifestations once established and therefore persisting for long time. We live in a 'world of things' ('verdinglichte Welt'). Such a virtual world of things produces the illusion of a stable world and gives us the feeling of security. But a human being is not a thing like a house that, once built, exists for a long time: human existence is a permanently unstable process that requires maintaining factors for its prolongation. Therefore, disorders in general, and delusions in particular, are not things but processes, which need disorder-maintaining factors for their prolongation. As well as the occurrence of a delusion being due to a process based on dynamic vulnerability, the delusional symptomatology itself is a dynamic process that will persist only if disorder-maintaining factors become effective (Musalek and Hobl 2001).

The distinction between predisposing, triggering, and disorder-maintaining factors is not of only theoretical interest, but also of practical importance. Predisposing and triggering factors undoubtedly provide us with the indispensable basis for effective prophylactic and long-term treatment, but with respect to acute treatment they are of no or minor value. Treatment of the acute state has to be based on an accurate differential diagnosis of the disorder-maintaining factors. The following example may serve to illustrate these relations.

> H.M. is sitting in a pleasant mountain lodge in the Austrian Alps. After having some drinks he is putting on his skis and going downhill. Stimulated by the alcohol, he is skiing very fast (which does not really matter, because he is a well trained skier). While doing so and looking around, he suddenly notices a pretty young woman, who glances at him — obviously admiring his professional skiing. This motivates him to show off, and he skis faster and faster. Overestimating his abilities, he is going to loose control and, just at that moment, a little hill appears and the following very impressive jump ends with a terrible crash. Unfortunately the ski binding has been fixed too tightly and our overmotivated man is now suffering from a broken leg.

Analysing this situation, we find some predisposing physical, psychological, and environmental factors for the broken leg: the alcohol consumption, the self-overestimation, the effect on the man of a pretty young woman admiring him, the fast skiing, the ski binding being fixed too strongly. As a triggering factor, we remember the little hill that provoked the impressive jump and led finally to the physical damage to the leg, which is the disorder-maintaining factor. None of us would think that the best way to help the patient with the broken leg is to work on the predisposing and triggering factors. None of us would think that the best help is to talk with our man about his alcohol consumption while skiing. None of us would discuss with our man his reaction to pretty young women or his tendency to overestimate himself in order to treat the broken leg. None of us would think that advising him to ski more slowly would help him in his situation, and none of us would think that he might recover faster by planing and straightening the downhill course. The first step of treatment, of course, has to be attention to the physical damage, the disorder-maintaining factor — the broken leg. The first step of treatment has to be to set the bones and fix them in plaster. Of course, in case this was not H.M.'s first severe skiing accident, it makes sense to discuss with him the effects of alcohol consumption or of his success-oriented relation to young women — at least that it would be wise to adjust the ski binding in order to avoid further accidents. In other words: the prophylaxis is dependent on the predisposing and triggering factors.

For many decades, psychiatric treatment strategies have been determined merely by the assumption that the patient will recover from a disorder if pre-existing pathogenetic factors are overcome. Finding the pre-existing 'real cause' — the 'final explanation' — has been the main diagnostic focus. In some cases such an approach succeeds; in others it fails. In cases where the predisposing and triggering factors are the same as the disorder-maintaining factors, treatment strategies that influence predisposing and triggering factors may be successful, but also in these cases it is, in fact, not the predisposing but rather the disorder-maintaining factors that provide the basis for effective treatment of the actual symptoms. And, as previous clinical psychopathological analyses have shown, disorder-maintaining factors are not necessarily the same as predisposing and triggering factors (Musalek *et al.* 2001).

Accordingly, we have to ask the question: 'What are the disorder-maintaining factors of delusions?'. Of course, all of the physical, psychological, and social predisposing and triggering factors mentioned above in the discussion of the occurrence of a delusion may persist, and then act also as disorder-maintaining factors. In particular, the persistence of cognitive disorders and emotional deviations, which provide the basis for the occurrence of delusional convictions, may prolong the delusional symptomatology. But, in addition, there are some factors that may prolong a delusional conviction. Not least, the observation that a delusion may persist even though the emotional disorder responsible for its occurrence has disappeared led to search for other factors that underlie and cause the persistence of delusional convictions (Musalek 1989).

To date, two further disorder-maintaining factors have been found: (1) the meaning of delusions and (2) the 'self-dynamics of delusions' (Musalek 2000; Musalek and Hobl 2001). Both factors are due to and dependent on the existence of delusional symptomatology, and therefore they cannot be considered as pre-existing pathogenetic factors. They are both not only effects of the delusional symptomatology, but also become effective themselves in the pathogenetic frame of delusions.

Meaning of delusions and its impact on the delusion's persistence

What is the meaning of delusions? An illness does not exist only in its *pathos*; it does not exist only in its symptomatolgy, it presents itself also in its *nosos* — in its particular meaning (Glatzel 1978; Fulford 2001). Mental disorders, in particular, have special meanings. Suffering from a gastrointestinal disorder and suffering from a mental disorder is not the same — does not have the same meaning — and patients are often affected much more by the meaning of the mental disorder than by the symptoms of the disorder itself. In the early stages of cancer, for example, patients may be suffering much more from the meaning of the disease (e.g. chronic disease leading to death) than from its symptoms. Patients with mental disorders in general, and patients with delusion, often suffer more from being told they have a mental disorder than from the disorder itself.

Before discussing the particular meanings of delusion and their impact on the persistence of the disorder, we need to consider the different approaches concerning meaning. One of the central problems of the philosophy of the twentieth and twenty-first century has been the work on meaning.

Summarizing the manifold publications on the theory of meaning we are confronted with three main approaches (Rohmann 2001):

1. the referential approach;
2. the propositional approach;
3. the hermeneutic approach.

The main thesis of the classical referential approach is that the meaning of a word is its referent — the object the speaker is referring to. For example, 'delusions', 'delire', 'delirio', and 'Wahn' all have the same referent and hence mean the same. This approach derives from the 'mythic notion, shared by many cultures, that word and object were once a unity that has been broken into two' (Rohmann 2001).

In contrast, proponents of the propositional approach focus not on individual words but on sentences or propositions: words are arbitrary symbols with conventional connotations, which gain meaning through their interrelationships (de Saussure 1960). Chomsky (1993, 1995) emphasized that meaning derives from the syntactical structure of words in a sentence. Frege maintained that a word has meaning only in the context of the statement of which it is part (Geach and Black 1980). According to 'formal semantic theory' the meaning of a statement is identical to the conditions under which it is true, and according to the 'verifiability theory', a modern version of the propositional approach (Rohmann 2001), only those statements that are subject to analytical or empirical verification are meaningful. Even more radically, Wittgenstein (1956) considered meaning as a social phenomenon: the meaning of an utterance depends on how it is used in social intercourse, not on any formal qualities ('Die Bedeutung eines Wortes ist sein Gebrauch in der Sprache': 'The meaning of a word is its use in language').

The hermeneutic approach represents a further remove from classical referential theory. The basic assumption of this approach is that meaning can be asserted only within a broad historical and cultural context. Any shift in the context inevitably produces a shift in meaning.

To these three classical approaches we should add a fourth one, which we will call 'interactional behavioral approach'. The transfer of meaning is dependent not only on words and their relations but also on para-verbal aspects, such as timbre, volume, speed, interruptions, sound, pitch of the voice, mimicry, gestures, and postures. As well as the literal language ('world of words'), a behavioural language ('world of non-verbal interactions') exists. It is the tone that makes the music. In recent publications Derrida has proposed a preference for the term 'phonocentrism' rather than 'logocentrism' (Sim 1999). We are able to say much more with the spoken (and non-spoken) word than with the written word. More than that: we may change the meaning of words or sentences only by changing the intonation or the accompanying behaviour. The interactional behavioural approach, which considers also para-verbal and non-verbal means of communication and their manifold interactions with verbal expressions, plays only a minor role in today's philosophy of language, but has a major role in our (and therefore also our patients) everyday life communication. In patients suffering from delusion such non-verbal or para-verbal interactions, and the resulting misunderstandings, may even become disorder-maintaining factors.

What are the meanings of delusions? In principle, delusions have three kinds of meaning:

1. the meaning(s) of the delusional content;
2. the meaning(s) of suffering from a delusion as a particular mental disorder;
3. the meaning of particular behaviour(s) of deluded patients.

Meaning of the delusional content

Delusions are content-dependent constructs. Every delusion has its special theme. Of course, it is not the same to be persecuted by drug dealers, members of the CIA, work colleagues, neighbours, or a husband; of course, it is not the same to be certain that you are suffering from an incurable illness or from unrequited love, to be God, or to be betrayed by your partner. In addition, the same theme and thematic presentation do not necessarily mean the same thing to different people. For example, being persecuted by a neighbour may not mean the same for everybody. Being infested by parasites may represent the incarnation of filth for one person, whereas for others it may mean the presence of a severe illness, or imprisonment in parasitic infestation, or an inescapable persecution (Musalek 1991).

These differences of meaning often result in multiple misunderstandings. Sometimes we do not understand the sense of our patient's delusional convictions — which does not mean that the delusion represents non-sense. Every delusion makes sense to the person concerned by it. Sometimes we are not able to follow the ideas of our patients (and we then call these forms of delusional idea bizarre delusions; Stanghellini and Rossi-Monti 1993), but for the patient they always make sense. Delusional ideas are produced by patients themselves, and therefore they are always part of their world of ideas (Roberts 1991). In every case the chosen theme has its particular meaning for the deluded patient; usually it stands for a particular (unsolved) problem of the patient. This basic concern is often covered by the presented delusional convictions what might become another source for misunderstandings.

It is we who create our world, but we do not create our world independently from our surroundings. What we are doing is not a work of poetry, in the sense of arbitrary inventions, but an attempt to translate extensive and intensive psychological processes into communicable events. Patients suffering from delusions are also cosmo-poets: they also create their world. It is a more or less understandable world, it is a world that is more or less similar to the world of the non-deluded, but in any case it is an unambiguous world. Stanghellini (2001) maintained that, in contrast to the Age of Enlightenment's triad of *liberté–fraternité–egalité*, the maxim of the post-modern world is the triad of *'liberté–flexibilité–precarité'*, which rhymes with *anxieté'*. Thrown into a risky world characterized by ambiguity and precariousness, our lifelong journey is to look for islands of safety. Such an island of safety may represent delusional ideas. To create and establish an unambiguous, stable, delusional world may be considered a form of defence from the highly uncertain and ambiguous world in which we all live.

The presentation of the delusional world may lead again to misunderstandings. Language, as we ordinarily use it, is imprecise and ambiguous. Hence our referents cannot always be determined unequivocally. Putting together all these considerations we may conclude that patients suffering from delusions (as well as their relations) are living in a world of misunderstandings. These misunderstandings provide the ideal basis for the reinforcement and prolongation of delusional convictions, and in this way they increase the degree of polarization as well as the duration of delusional ideas.

Meaning(s) of suffering from a delusion as a particular mental disorder

The second meaning of the delusion is that of a psychopathological phenomenon, of a particular mental disorder. As mentioned above, every psychiatric disorder has its particular meaning — and that applies especially to delusions. Suffering from a delusion is the paragon of being crazy. This fact alone may make patients defend their ideas with all the arguments they can find. One of the most commonly heard phrases in clinical work with deluded patients is: 'Doctor, I am not crazy'. Patients are fighting against being recognized as mentally ill, and this fight leads to an intensification of the delusional conviction. They have to defend their ideas with all available means to avoid being given the label 'lunatic'. This defensive work becomes 'delusional work' ('Wahnarbeit'), and results in the reinforcement and prolongation of delusional convictions. In this way the meanings of delusions may become disorder-maintaining factors.

However, delusions do not have a particular meaning only for patients. Delusions and their meanings do not remain restricted to patients, they also gain importance for members of the patient's social network. More than that, according to Wittgenstein's social theory of meaning, meaning derives from social intercourse (Wittgenstein 1953). Mind is not located within the individual but in the individual–social relationship. Following Sartre's saying that we are damned to be free (Sartre 1962), it might be said: 'We are damned to communicate'. As social beings we are sentenced to communicate. It is impossible not to communicate; even if we withdraw ourselves from communication with others, this is only a special form of communication. Patients with delusions often try to avoid communication, and this withdrawal from social life also gives their ideas and behaviours a special meaning. But the patient's relations also bring their experiences, ideas, and prejudices into the picture — and the meanings of delusions given by relatives may differ significantly from those given by patients. Suffering from delusions has, in any case, a special meaning for the relatives, for people living closely with the patient, for people of the patient's social network.

As we are suffering not from facts but from the meaning of facts, patients often suffer much more from the meaning of their disorder than from their delusional ideas. They suffer much more from the prejudices of their relatives, working colleagues, bosses, and so on, than from their own interpretations. Nobody objects to having a medical doctor suffering from gastroenteritis, but in our society we would object greatly if confronted by a medical doctor suffering from delusions of persecution, even if we knew perfectly well that the doctor's delusional ideas had no influence on his or her work. The same would be true for teachers, nurses, or politicians. Prejudices encountered by patients in their social network may enhance and prolong their delusional ideas. In this way members of the patient's social network may become disorder-maintaining factors. In this context it has to be emphasized that medical doctors and psychotherapists are (at least should be) part of the patient's social network and therefore they, too, may become disorder-maintaining factors.

Communications and social contacts are not stable and permanent factors. People come and go; relationships may not be sustained. Only rarely we are able to experience feelings of stability and permanence — and such feelings always remain a relatively short-lived illusion. Today's world is characterized not only by the expression 'anything goes' (Feyerabend 1975, 1978): its keynote is *anything goes away*. Also opinions concerning delusions or deluded patients are not stable, which may result in amplifying ambiguity and precariousness. The prejudices of relations may change, which sometimes means that new weapons are introduced in the fight of ideas.

But it is not only the prejudices of members of the social network that patients with delusions are suffering from. Today truth and meaning may be seen as culturally determined constructions, not as absolutes (Foucault 1961, 1972). Mental disorders in general, and delusions in particular, have particular meanings in every society. Some of the meanings of delusions were described in the opening section of this chapter on the roots of the term delusion and related words in some other languages. These 'cultural meanings', resulting in the prejudices of individuals living in the particular social context, may also have an effect on the suffering of the patient, thereby reinforcing and prolonging the disorder. As we all are members of our society, all of us may become reinforcement and disorder-maintaining factors. The greater the counter-productive influence of the social network on the patient, the greater the reinforcement of delusional ideas, resulting in an increasing loss of the degree of freedom and prolonging the duration of delusional convictions.

Meaning of the behaviour of deluded patients

The third meaning of delusions represents the meaning of the behaviour of deluded patients (see above, *behavioural interactional approach of meaning*). The patient's behaviour and the resulting para-verbal and non-verbal inter-actions play a major role in the frame of so-called 'self-dynamics of delusions', described as (interactional) reinforcement processes specific for particular psychopathological features — in the present case, delusional ideas. These reinforcement processes are induced by the delusional symptomatology itself and they lead to an increasing loss of the degree of freedom and to a prolonga-tion of delusional symptoms. They thus represent typical disorder-maintaining factors.

For example, patients suffering from delusions of persecution are usually suspicious about the people surrounding them and suppose them to be possi-ble persecutors. Uncertain as to whether these people are persecutors or not, patients suffering from delusions of persecution interact with them not only verbally but also para-verbally and non-verbally, in a very special way. The behaviour and communication style of the patients may lead to particular reactions in people they relate to. People who are usually very open and friendly with others may react to the deluded patient also with some reserva-tion and resentment because of the patient's suspicious behaviour. This serves to reinforce the suspicions of the patient. In this manner a vicious circle may be established, amplifying and prolonging paranoid behaviours and ideas. Similar mechanisms may be found in interactions with a patient suffering from delusions of jealousy. The patient accuses their partner of betrayal. The partner's defensive reaction in protesting their innocence, accompanied by uncertainty as to whether the solemn affirmation will be accepted or not, may then induce a reinforcement and prolongation of the patient's cnvictions. In patients suffering from hypochondriacal delusions it is usually the fear that the multiple complaints are not being taken seriously by the doctor on the one hand, and the particular behavioural reactions of medical doctors (character-ized by haste and impatience) to hypochondriacal patients on the other hand, that help to establish a similar vicious circle.

Common to all these self-dynamics of disorders is that the meaning of the particular para-verbal and non-verbal information and interactions provides the basis for the establishment of reinforcement circles, resulting in an increased polarization (loss of degrees of freedom) and prolongation of delusional ideas. In conclusion, both the meaning of written or spoken opinions and prejudices, and also particular behaviours and non-verbal aspects of communication, may be considered to be important disorder-maintaining factors.

Non-verbal communication plays a central role in the expression of emotions and feelings. As not only ideas but also (much more importantly) feelings create and determine our world (Musalek and Hobl 2001), so too the world of deluded patients in particular is constructed by feelings and emotions based on and induced by the meaning of para-verbal and non-verbal interactions. The greater the intensity of emotions, the greater the loss of degrees of freedom; the longer the duration of the emotional engagement, the greater the prolongation of delusional convictions. In any case, it is interactions between individuals that promote the occurrence and, in particular, the persistence of delusions. Delusions, as a product of emotions and ideas, are not located within the individual but in the individual-in-social interaction. These social interactions, in connection with accompanying emotions resulting in reinforcement and prolongation of delusional ideas, may therefore become disorder-maintaining factors. These social interactions again produce meaning, and in this way suffering. Usually we are not suffering from facts but from the meanings derived from facts. Also, our patients with delusions are much more suffering from the meaning of their disorder than from the symptoms themselves. And, because we are all imprisoned in such social interactions effecting the production of meanings in general and the meanings of delusions in particular, we may all become disorder-maintaining factors and the cause of suffering.

Conclusion

With regard to the significance of meaning in the diagnosis and origin of delusions, delusions may be considered to be content-dependent constructs with different meanings for patients and their relatives, leading to a more or less increased loss of degrees of freedom. The meanings of delusions include three aspects: the meaning of the delusional content, the meaning of the particular mental disorder, and the meaning of the behaviour of deluded patients. In particular, the last two aspects of meaning come into force in the pathogenetic frame of delusions. Acting as important disorder-maintaining factors, they become responsible for the amplification (loss of degrees of freedom) and persistence (chronicity) of delusions. The manifold social interactions on verbal as well as para-verbal and non-verbal levels, and the accompanying emotions and feelings, produce the particular meanings of the delusions and usually result in increased suffering for the patient, which may also become an important disorder-maintaining factor. Knowledge of the meanings of delusions and their interactional effects for patients and their relatives is not only of theoretical interest but also of the utmost practical importance. As meanings of the disorder and the resulting suffering represent important disorder-maintaining factors, they provide the indispensable basis for treatment (in particular psychotherapy) of the acute delusional symptoms. Further pathogenetic and psychotherapeutic research is needed to clarify the significance of the various meanings of delusions in the pathogenesis of delusional states and their effects as disorder-maintaining factors, in order to provide the basis for the development of new effective treatment strategies for patients with delusional syndromes.

References

Ayd, F. J., Jr. (1985). *Lexikon of Psychiatry, Neurology and the Neurosciences*. Baltimore: Williams & Wilkins.

Berner, P. (1982). *Psychiatrische Systematik*. Bern: Huber.

Berner, P. and Musalek, M. (1989). Schizophrenie und Wahnkrankheiten. In: *Handbuch der Gerontologie. Band 4. Neurologie und Psychiatrie* (ed. H. Platt), pp. 297–317. Stuttgart: Fischer.

Chomsky, A. N. (1993). *Language and Thought*. Wakefield: Moyer Bell.

Chomsky, A. N. (1995). Language and Nature. *Mind*, **104**: 1–61.

Derrida, J. (1978). *Writing and Difference*. London: RKP.

Derrida, J. (1982). *Margins of Philosophy*. Chicago: Chicago University Press.

Derrida, J. (1986). 'Shibboleth'. In: *Midrash and Literature* (ed. G. Hartmann and S. Budick). New Haven: Yale University Press.

de Saussure, F. (1960). *Course in General Linguistics*. London: Peter Owen.

Falloon, I. R., Boyd, J. L. and McGill, C. W. (1984). *Family Care of Schizophrenia*. New York: Guilford Press.

Feyerabend, P. K. (1975). *Against Method*. London: NLB.

Feyerabend, P. K. (1978). *Science in a Free Society*. London: NLB.

Foucault, M. (1961). *Histoire de la Folie*. Paris : Librairie Plon.

Foucault, M. (1972). *The Archaeology of Knowledge*. New York: Harper & Row.

Fulford, K. W. M. (1991). Evaluative delusions: their significance for philosophy and psychiatry. *British Journal of Psychiatry*, **159**(Suppl.14): 108–12.

Fulford, K. W. M. (2001). 'What is (mental) disease': an open letter to Christorpher Boorse. *Journal of Medical Ethics*, **27**: 80–5.

Geach, P. and Black, M. (1980). *Translations from the Philosophical Writings of Gottlob Frege*. Oxford: Oxford University Press.

Glatzel, J. (1978). *Allgemeine Psychopathologie*. Stuttgart: Enke.

Jaspers, K. (1975). *Allgemeine Psychopathologie*. 8. Aufl. Berlin: Springer.

Kisker, K. P. and Wulff, E. (1999). Wahn. In: *Psychiatrie, Psychosomatik und Psychotherapie* (ed. W. Machleidt *et al.*), pp. 320–4. Stuttgart: Thieme.

Kretschmer, K. (1966). *Der sensitive Beziehungswahn*. 4. Aufl. Berlin: Springer.

Kristeva, J. (1981). *La Langage, Cet Inconnu*. Paris : Seuil.

Lacan, J. (1966). *Écrits I et II*. Paris: Editions du Seuil.

Lyotard, J. F. (1979). *La Condition Post-moderne*. Paris : Minuit.

Musalek, M. (1989). Les indicateurs psychopathologiques et biologiques pour la thérapeutique des délires chroniques. *Psychologie Médicale*, **21**: 1355–9.

Musalek, M. (1991). *Der Dermatozoenwahn*. Stuttgart: Thieme.

Musalek, M. (2000). Die Bedeutung des Wahns in unserer Gesellschaft. In: *Paranoia und Diktatur* (ed. H. G. Zapotoczky and K. Fabisch), pp. 156–72. Linz: Universitätsverlag Rudolf Trauner.

Musalek, M. and Hobl, B. (2002). Der Affekt als Bedingung des Wahns. In: *Affekt und affektive Störungen* (ed. C. Mundt and T. Fuchs), pp. 231–42.

Musalek, M. and Kutzer, E. (1989). The frequency of shared delusions of parasitosis. *European Archives of Psychiatry and Neurological Sciences*, **239**: 263–6.

Musalek, M., Berner, P., and Katschnig, H. (1989). Delusional theme, sex, and age. *Psychopathology*, **22**: 260–7.

Musalek, M., Griengl, H., Hobl, B., Sachs, G., and Zoghlami, A. (2000). Dysphoria from a transnosological perspective. *Psychopathology*, **33**: 209–14.

Musalek, M., Hobl, B., and Mossbacher, U. (2001). Diagnostics in psychodermatology. *Dermatology Psychosomatics*, **2**: 110–15.

Roberts, G. (1991). Delusional belief systems and meaning in life: a preferred reality? *British Journal of Psychiatry*, **159**(Suppl. 14): 19–28.

Rohmann, C. (2001). *The Dictionary of Important Ideas and Thinkers*. London: Hutchinson.

Rümke, H. C. (1951). *Signification de la Phénoménologie dans l'Etude Cliniques des Délirantes. I. Psychopathologie des Délires*. Paris: Hermann.

Sartre, J. P. (1962). *Das Sein und das Nichts*. Reinbeck: Scharfetter.

Scharfetter, W. (1991). *Psychopathologie*. Stuttgart: Thieme.

Sedler, M. J. (1995). Understanding delusions. *Psychiatric Clinics of North America* **18**: 251–62.

Sim, S. (1999). Jacques Derrida. In: *One Hundred Twentieth-Century Philosophers* (ed. S. Brown, D. Collinson, and R. Wilkinson), pp. 43–5. London: Routledge.

Stanghellini, G. (2001). Anthropology of anxiety. Lecture held at the symposium 'Anxiety'. AEP-Section Psychopathology, Paris, April 2001.

Stanghellini, G. and Rossi-Monti, M. (1993). Influencing and being influenced: the other side of 'bizarre delusions'. 2. Clinical investigation. *Psychopathology*, **26**: 165–9.

Wittgenstein, L. (1953). *Philosophical Investigations* (ed. G. E. M. Ascombe and R. Rees). Oxford: Blackwell.

Zubin, J. (1977). Vulnerability — a new view of schizophrenia. *Journal of Abnormal Psychology*, **86**: 103–26.

Section 5 A New Kind of Phenomenology

11 The phenomenology of body dysmorphic disorder: a Sartrean analysis

Katherine J. Morris

Introduction

Body dysmorphic disorder (BDD) — also still known by its older name 'dysmorphophobia'[1] — is often characterized, loosely, as 'a distressing and impairing preoccupation with an imagined or slight defect in appearance' (Phillips 1998), 'imagined ugliness' (Phillips *et al.* 1994) or an 'ugliness complex' (Schacter 1971). Although BDD has been known to the psychiatric community for a long time, this puzzling condition is still little known by members of the general public.[2] Since BDD was named as such (and included in DSM-III under that name) there has been a burgeoning of psychological and psychiatric attention to this condition.[3]

However, BDD has yet to capture the attention of philosophers.[4] My own philosophical approach to it will be phenomenological, although I am using the term 'phenomenology' *not* in the sense commonly used in the psychological literature (where it refers simply to descriptions of patients' experiences) but in the strict philosophical sense where it refers to a *method* (invented by Husserl, taken up and modified by Heidegger, Sartre, Merleau-Ponty, etc.) by which the *essence* of what is experienced is revealed. BDD occupies a significant position at the intersection of two central dimensions of human experience: our

---

[1]One or two studies refer to it, quite incorrectly, as 'body dysmorphia'.

[2]Katharine A. Phillips' (1996) book *The Broken Mirror*, aimed at sufferers and their friends and family rather than the medical community, has undoubtedly contributed greatly to what public awareness there is. The present article makes fairly substantial use of this one book, for which I make no apology: Phillips is one of the leading players in the BDD field, having published many scholarly articles on the subject, and my own survey of the literature supports her summaries; hence I do not in general cite other literature except in where it brings out something that her book does not.

[3]For example, in the period from 1984 to 1987 there were 13 items listed in the Psychological Abstracts; interest peaked in the (shorter) period 1996–1998, when 84 items were listed; there are already 59 items in the period 1999–2001.

[4]The Philosopher's Index to date lists nothing on this topic. There are, I suspect, complex historical and cultural reasons for this.

experience of our own bodies and our experience of other people. This point of intersection is one that Sartre highlighted as 'my existence "for myself as a body known by the Other"'.[5] BDD can specifically be described as a disorder of *this* dimension of the 'lived body'.[6]

Background

These are the DSM-IV diagnostic criteria for BDD:

1. Preoccupation with some imagined defect in appearance. If a slight physical anomaly is present, the person's concern is markedly excessive.

2. The preoccupation causes clinically significant distress or impairment in social, occupational, or other important areas of functioning.

3. The preoccupation is not better accounted for by another mental disorder (e.g. dissatisfaction with body shape and size in anorexia nervosa).

Like most psychiatric 'definitions', this one is vague in places as well as being contestable. Moreover, although 'dysmorphophobia' was deemed to be a single diagnostic entity in DSM-III, DSM-III(R) and DSM-IV in effect divide it into two subtypes: 'body dysmorphic disorder' and 'delusional disorder, somatic type', where the latter is defined as: 'Delusions that the person has some physical defect or non-psychiatric medical condition'. This distinction, as the DSM-IV Casebook notes, is itself contestable: 'It appears that the degree of insight may be more appropriately conceptualised as spanning a spectrum that ranges from good insight to delusional thinking, along which the person's belief may move over time'. (As things stand, someone who 'lacks insight' receives *two* diagnoses: 'BDD' and 'delusional disorder, somatic type'.) Further questions revolve around the categorization of BDD: much of the literature considers BDD to be an obsessive–compulsive spectrum disorder, yet in DSM-IV it is classified as a somatoform disorder (together with conversion disorder, hypochondriasis, and so on), while obsessive–compulsive disorder (OCD), as well as phobias (including social phobia),[7] are classified as anxiety

---

[5]Sartre's own remarks on this 'dimension' are brief and notoriously bewildering (Sartre 1969); an investigation of BDD might therefore have the collateral effect of illuminating a dark corner of Sartre scholarship.

[6]The only other study of this nature to my knowledge is Enzo Agresti and Mario Taddei (1970); the English summary in Psychological Abstracts indicates the conclusion that 'on the phenomenological level the dysmorphophobical manifestations indicate a change of the "co-existence" which concretizes itself in the esthetic-formal sphere'.

[7]BDD's earlier name 'dysmorphophobia' classified it as a type of phobia (an abnormal fear of deformity), although this classification was criticized early on, for example in Schacter (1971) and Liberman (1974). Intuitively, it is not so much a *fear* of deformity as an unfounded *conviction* of deformity.

disorders.[8] ICD-10 classifies it as a type of hypochondriasis, and the comparable Japanese manual classifies it as in the same category as social phobia. (Some questions about these classifications will be addressed below.)

Much of the psychological and psychiatric literature on BDD focuses either on treatment (the most promising treatments being widely held to be serotonin-reuptake inhibitors and/or some form of cognitive–behavioural therapy)[9] or on the relationship of BDD with other mental disorders, in particular OCD, hypochondriasis, eating disorders, social phobia, depression, and schizophrenia. Psychiatrists typically compare these disorders by looking at such factors as symptoms, male : female ratio, age at onset and course, co-occurrence, family history, and treatment response (see Phillips 1996, p. 214). For example, eating disorders show a high female : male ratio, whereas 'Preliminary evidence suggests that Body Dysmorphic Disorder is diagnosed with approximately equal frequency in women and in men' (DSM-IV); although BDD sufferers very commonly also experience major depression at some time in their lives, the converse is far less frequent (Phillips 1996, pp. 335–6); and, although schizo-phrenia and BDD may sometimes share certain symptoms (in particular, referential thinking), they rarely co-occur. BDD and social phobia are adjudged very similar on all dimensions apart from treatment response (for example, beta-blockers, often helpful with social phobias, are ineffective with BDD) (Phillips 1996, p. 219). BDD and OCD are very similar on all these dimensions and it is often concluded that they are closely related disorders (Phillips 1996, p. 213ff.).

From the point of view of phenomenology, however, the dimension that is most significant is that of symptoms; the symptomatic relationships between BDD and these other disorders will be more fully explored below, after a sketch of some relevant phenomenological distinctions.

Phenomenology: background and basic distinctions

The phenomenologists, far more than their Anglo-American counterparts, have focused philosophical attention on the human body. In so far as Anglo-American philosophers have thought about the body at all, they have tended to think of it as a physical or physiological or biological *object*. Of course, it *is* these things too. We might label these 'dimensions' thus:

(1) **The body-as-physical-thing**. The human body is a solid object with a certain weight and height that, like other physical objects, is subject to the law of gravity, and so on.

---

[8]Eating Disorders — which one might be inclined to think of as 'somatoform' — constitute a category of their own.
[9]The evidence is summarized in Phillips (1996), Chapters 13 and 14.

(2) **The body-as-physiological/biological-object**. The body is an organism with nutritional needs, capable of reproducing, subject to disease, and all the rest.

However, these are not the *only* dimensions; and it is the other dimensions of the human body that the phenomenologists have stressed.[10] Some of these other dimensions — in particular (4) and (5), discussed below — are referred to collectively by psychologists by the term 'body image'.[11] Hence BDD is sometimes described as involving a 'distorted body image'. One implication here (although this conclusion is hardly original) is that the term 'body image' stands in need of refinement: it covers a wide variety of *very* different things.

(3) **The body-of-the-other (the body-as-meaningful-object)**. In the first place, we do not normally encounter the bodies of *other human being* primarily as physical, physiological, or biological objects but as '*psychic* objects' (cf. Sartre 1969, p. 305) or 'meaningful objects' (cf. Sartre 1969, p. 344).[12] A man and the park bench he is sitting on are utterly different types of objects. The man is on the bench in a different sense from that in which his newspaper is (he *is sitting* on it); the lawn is in front of the man in a different sense from that in which it is in front of the bench (he may be contemplating its verdancy with pleasure, it presents an opportunity for stretching out if he wishes to risk the outrage of the *guardien*), etc.: he, unlike the bench, has a perceptual and instrumental 'world' which is organized around him (cf. Sartre 1969, p. 254). If he grows red and shakes his fist at the dog that snatches his sandwich, we do not perceive his gestures either as 'mere movements' or as *signs* of a 'subjective and hidden anger': we see *his anger* (Sartre 1969, p. 294, cf. p. 346), etc.

(4) **The lived-body-for-itself**. In our ordinary engagements in the world (writing an article, playing tennis, watching a circling hawk), our own bodies are not encountered as objects, 'meaningful' or otherwise; indeed they are not *encountered* at all. Rather than itself being perceived or known or utilized, the body-for-itself functions as the unperceivable *centre* of the field of perception and the unutilizable *centre* of a field of instruments (i.e. things that hinder or aid our projects), although 'referred to' by the order and orientation of these fields. The specific properties of the body-for-itself, be they transient (having one's legs crossed, having a pain in the foot) or relatively permanent (being

---

[10]Sartre has been sometimes accused of *ignoring* the body as physical, biological, and physiological object altogether. This is not wholly fair; to the extent to which he *emphasizes* the other dimensions, it is by way of corrective to a long philosophical tradition of ignoring them.

[11]Indeed the phenomenologists, in particular Merleau-Ponty, have contributed to some extent to their conceptions of the body image. See, for example, Gallagher (1995).

[12]Although this is of course contestable, one might suggest that the oft-cited 'absence of a theory of other minds' found in autism and Asperger's disorder would be better characterized as a disorder of this dimension of bodily experience. The term 'theory' invites just the sort of cognitive or intellectualist construction that the phenomenologists — surely rightly — would want to resist here.

tall, being fat) are referred to by the properties of the lived world; for example a tall person 'lives' her tallness by living in a world where low doorways are potential obstacles and items on high shelves are within reach.

The lived-body-for-itself can become either the 'object' of reflection[13] or the object of cognition; so to do is (temporarily) to *cease* 'living' the body, and consequently (although Sartre does not do this) one might distinguish two further dimensions:[14]

- To reflect on the body-for-itself is to become *explicitly* aware of what was formerly in the background: to *focus* on the position of the limbs (as opposed to the tennis ball), on the pain in the foot (as opposed to the terrain), on the phantom arm (as opposed to the piano), etc.

- To cognize the body-for-itself is to bring our *knowledge* or *understanding* to bear on this explicit awareness. For example, we understand the pain as the result of a blister caused by overtight shoes. In some cases there will be a discrepancy between what we are aware of in reflection and what we know or learn. For instance, we might learn (as often happens in tennis lessons!) that the 'felt position' of the limb is not its actual position.

(5) **The lived-body-for-others**. Just as the body of the other is a meaningful object in my world, my body is a meaningful object in *his* world; and awareness of this very fact — a necessary aspect of living in a world populated by others — radically alters my 'lived experience' of my own body. When I live my body when on my own, the perceived and utilizable world 'refers' to my body as *subject*: the piano is to be played *by* me, the terrain to be crossed *by* me. This changes drastically when another enters the scene and looks at me. I am suddenly in the startling position of being both a subject and an object.

Sartre (1969) has a famous description of one such transformation of lived experience: 'Let us imagine that moved by jealousy, curiosity, or vice I have just glued my ear to the door and looked through a keyhole . . . But all of a sudden I hear footsteps in the hall. Someone is looking at me!' (pp. 260–1). 'I shudder as a wave of shame sweeps over me' (p. 277). Here I am actually

---

[13] Anglo-American philosophers are liable to object to the term 'reflection' here; they are inclined to restrict that term to the mind's awareness of its own operations. If they are then pressed to say how it is that we, say, know that we are in pain or know the position of our limbs, they are inclined either to mentalize (so that pain itself comes to be seen as something *mental*) or to posit 'bodily senses' in addition to the usual five. (Thus Descartes, rather than mentalizing pain, hunger, and thirst as modern philosophers are wont to do, thought of these as conditions of the body and posited internal senses whereby we perceive them; modern psychologists often speak of proprioception as an 'internal sense' whereby we perceive the position and motion of our limbs, and so on.)

[14] Some 'body image' researchers make a distinction that partially parallels the distinction between living and cognizing. See, for example, Tiggemann (1996).

doing something 'shameful' ('peeping'); yet 'shame is nothing but the original feeling of having my being *outside* . . . not a feeling of being this or that guilty object but in general of being *an* object . . . ' (p. 288). This might seem to suggest that we *always* experience shame when looked at, *whether or not* we are doing something 'shameful', or perhaps that the very fact of being an object just *is* shameful. Or it might be felt that Sartre is here playing with words: using the word 'shame' to mean now the experience of being a shameful object, now that of being an object *tout court*. Yet his choice of words is not arbitrary, and BDD sufferers will find it peculiarly *apt* for their way of living their bodies-for-others. '[S]hame is so common in BDD, it may even be intrinsic to the disorder' (Phillips 1996, p. 82). ' "The one word I associate with my body is shame" ' (Phillips 1996, pp. 82–3). 'Shame became the mirror through which she experienced her body'.[15]

This is one powerful indication that it is *this* dimension of the body that is *uniquely* affected in BDD. (In any case, 'preoccupation with appearance' implies it: 'appearance' just *means* 'the appearance of *my body* to *others*'.) This dimension is explored in more detail later in this chapter. (As we will see there, distortion of this dimension may imply distortion of dimension (3).)

Just as the body-for-itself could be reflected on and cognized, so too can the lived-body-for-others. Again, to do so is no longer to *live* the body-for-others. (And again, we *could* treat these as *separate* dimensions of the experience of the body.)

- To reflect on the body-for-others is to become explicitly aware of one's body as an object for others. Instead of simply being immersed in the semi-paralysis of shame, I may become explicitly aware of, say, my nose or my skin as 'being stared at'.

- The cognized body-for-others brings knowledge or understanding to bear on reflection and, as with the body-for-itself, there may be a mismatch between reflection and cognition: just as the amputee may be able to say that her 'felt' limb is not a physical or biological limb, a BDD sufferer may be able to say that despite her 'awareness' of the other staring at her nose, she is not actually doing so. (What characterizes the 'poor insight' of persons with 'delusional disorder, somatic type' is the inability to achieve this understanding.)

---

[15]Kathy Davis's (1995) book *Reshaping the Female Body* deals with a different, but undoubtedly overlapping, set of people: women seeking cosmetic surgery (on the national health in the Netherlands). Although Davis says nothing about BDD in her book, the fact that many were seeking surgery for 'defects' that were invisible to others constitutes some *prima facie* evidence that these women may have been BDD sufferers. 'In the course of my field work, I watched fifty-five people . . . enter the room for various kinds of cosmetic surgery. With one exception . . . I was never able to guess what the person had come in for' (p. 70). Conversely, about 33% of BDD sufferers have sought cosmetic surgery (and a further 49% dermatological treatment) (Phillips 1996, p. 288).

BDD and other mental disorders

This initial orientation will help to focus a symptomatic comparison of BDD with certain other mental disorders. This discussion is not meant to be *exhaustive*. It has two aims: (1) to help to round out the overall picture of BDD, and (2) as a corollary, to comment upon the current classification of BDD in DSM-IV.

Comparison with OCD

BDD involves both obsessive thoughts and compulsive, often ritualistic, behaviours intended to alleviate the anxiety produced by the thoughts. Most BDD sufferers think about their supposed defects for at least an hour a day, and many for more than eight hours a day (Phillips 1996, p. 77). These thoughts are generally negative and distressing in content, for example ' "I have this tape that goes through my head that says 'I hate how I look' " ' (Phillips 1996, p. 132). Most sufferers feel that they have little or no control over these thoughts (Phillips 1996, p.79). Typical compulsive behaviours include comparing the hated body part with those of others, checking their appearance in mirrors, camouflaging the body part, seeking surgery or other medical treatment to repair the alleged defect, seeking reassurance from others, and excessive grooming (Phillips 1996, p. 98).[16] From this point of view, the principal difference between BDD and OCD is the content of the preoccupying thoughts (and consequently the specific form that the compulsions take): OCD concerns are not focused exclusively on the body, and even those that are focused on the body (e.g. symmetry preoccupations) are concerned not with the lived-body-for-others but with the body-as-physical-object (which, like other physical objects, may be asymmetrical).

Comparison with hypochondriasis

Although the concerns in both BDD and hypochondriasis are focused on the body, the focus of hypochondriacal concerns is illness (i.e. the body-as-(potentially diseased)-*physiological*-object), not appearance (the lived-body-for-others).

Comparison with eating disorders

Both BDD and eating disorders involve excessive concern about the body, but there are salient as well as less salient differences in the symptomatology.

---

[16]Many of these behaviours are shared with the (partially overlapping) group of candidates for cosmetic surgery discussed in Davis (1995).

First, whereas anorexics at least typically look *abnormal*, viz. abnormally thin, BDD sufferers, by definition, look normal.[17] Second, whereas BDD sufferers are *sometimes* concerned about their weight or the size of their waist or hips, the typical locus of concern is some part of the *face* — the skin, hair, nose, or eyes. Third, more subtle questions concern whether the so-called body-image distortions in eating disorders are distortions of the *same* dimensions of the body as in BDD. BDD, being an excessive concern with *appearance*, is by definition a disorder of the lived-body-for-*others*. It may be that at least some sufferers of eating disorders distort the lived-body-for-*itself*. On this hypothesis, such people would not so much feel that *others* find them repellent (because fat) as 'feel as if they are fat' in somewhat the sense that an amputee may 'feel as if he has a limb': we might almost say that they possess a 'phantom fat body' as the amputee may possess a 'phantom limb'. This hypothesis, however, requires further research.

Comparison with social phobia

Perhaps not surprisingly, many BDD sufferers are socially anxious or avoidant. '"I feel so ugly and unpresentable that I avoid parties and dates. I feel too anxious when I'm around other people. I think they're evaluating how ugly I am . . ."' (Phillips 1996, p. 138). But not everyone who is socially phobic is so because of BDD: although social phobics are typically preoccupied with others' views of them and fear negative evaluation, the 'views' and 'negative evaluations' in question are not necessarily about their *appearance*. (They may, for example, fear being judged as 'stupid' or 'boring', rather than 'ugly' or 'repulsive'.) What we may say is that social phobics, while preoccupied with their *being*-for-others, are not necessarily specifically preoccupied with their *body*-for-others.

Comparison with schizophrenia

Although it is clear that most BDD sufferers are not schizophrenic, or vice versa, there are certain interesting symptoms that often or occasionally show up in BDD and that also characterize some forms of schizophrenia. Most striking is 'referential thinking', the idea that not only is their alleged defect *visible* to others but these others are taking special notice of that defect.

---

[17]Actually, this is not strictly true: the parts of the body that are the *focus of concern* look more or less normal by definition. This is consistent both in theory and in practice with other parts of their bodies *not* looking normal; hence a woman with BDD who had concerns about 'her "sunken and dull" eyes, which other people considered attractive' did not worry at all about the 'large, deep, red ulcers on her legs', which she had as a result of a medical illness (Phillips 1996, p. 76).

(Although we need to distinguish between *ideas* of reference and *delusions* of reference, and note that most BDD sufferers do not have delusions, about 65% of Phillips' patients report referential thinking; Phillips 1996, p. 85.) 'When she walked down the street, she believed that people stared at her skin and thought "That poor girl — look at her skin. It looks terrible!" When she entered a restaurant she believed the acne and marks distracted people from their meals, and she could eat out only if she hid in a booth in the restaurant's darkest corner' (Phillips 1996, p. 86). Obviously most schizophrenics' referential thinking will not have this particular sort of content. Other symptoms include gaze avoidance[18] and auditory hallucinations (rare in BDD, but they do occur — for example the woman who 'thought that people said "She's ugly", or muttered "Dog!" under their breath as she walked by them'; Phillips 1996, p. 87).

A subsidiary conclusion here might be this: DSM-III created the category of 'somatoform disorders', continued in DSM-IV, specifically *on the basis of 'shared phenomenology'* (DSM-IV Options Book, B.18). Yet the 'phenomenology' lying behind it is, I think one may say, crude: it conflates concerns with phenomenologically very different 'dimensions' of the body. *If* it makes sense to create categories on the basis of shared phenomenology at all, one might suggest that they ought to be grounded in a phenomenology that learns from the phenomenologists.[19]

Indeed, it *might* even turn out that not everyone in fact diagnosed with BDD has a 'shared phenomenology'. Consider this alleged case of BDD: ' "The problem is that I'm totally obsessed that my nose is fragile and is going to break . . . I worry all day long that I've damaged it. Whenever I bump it or brush against something, I panic" ' (Phillips 1996, p. 72). Fragility has nothing to do with *appearance* but rather concerns the body-as-physical-object; one might question whether this ought to be counted as a case of BDD. There may well be other, less obvious, cases. Although *some* self-descriptions of appearance clearly refer to the lived-body-for-others ('ugly', 'looking like a dork' (cf. Phillips 1996, p. 17), 'looking like a nerd' (Phillips 1996, p. 68), none of which would make *sense* independently of the perceived responses of others), others are more ambiguous. We noted already that the self-description 'fat' *could* equally refer to the lived-body-for-*itself*; 'too tall', 'too small', but also 'deformed', 'misshapen' (i.e. 'dysmorphic') and so on, exhibit the same ambiguity. A great many BDD sufferers do describe their preoccupations in unambiguous being-for-others terms. However, without more careful questioning and more sensitive psychological testing instruments, it may simply be

---

[18]This does not seem to have been studied systematically in BDD; Doerry and Brockington (2000) describe only two patients.

[19]Obviously the same problem arises with the subcategory of 'delusion disorder, somatic type', if the idea is that 'delusional BDD', 'delusional hypochondriasis' and pseudocyesis are grouped together on the basis of shared phenomenology!

unclear whether someone's concern with being 'fat' or 'tall' or 'small' is a concern with *appearance* or with the lived-body-for-itself.

BDD and the 'lived-body-for-others'

We need now to look more closely at the idea of the 'lived-body-for-others'. I want to bring out five interrelated aspects that may help to illuminate the phenomenology of BDD in more detail, and may help to stimulate ethical reflection on this disorder.

Sartre, as we noted, offers shame as one paradigm of lived awareness of being looked at — a paradigm with a peculiar centrality for BDD sufferers. Sartre connects shame with three further concepts that will likewise resonate with BDD sufferers:[20] the 'longing for invisibility', 'nausea' and 'alienation'.[21]

'Longing for invisibility'

The man 'embarrassed by his own body' (for-others) 'longs "not to have a body anymore", to be "invisible" (Sartre 1969, p. 353). BDD sufferers will say, ' "My biggest wish is to be invisible" ' (Phillips 1996, p. 37). But what exactly *is* this longing? There seem to be two aspects. First, given that they continue to suppose themselves to be monstrously ugly and repulsive, they wish *not to be seen at all*, which explains the social avoidance so common in BDD. Second, what many of the behaviours of BDD sufferers are aimed at (camouflage, for example hats used to cover 'thinning' hair, long sleeves to cover 'repulsively hairy' arms, etc.; hiding in dark corners of restaurants; many hours spent grooming) and what they hope to achieve on a more permanent basis through cosmetic surgery or dermatological treatment is 'invisibility' in a different sense: 'They want to no longer look like the Elephant Man; they want to no longer stand out in a crowd' (Phillips 1996, p. 66). This might be called a *kind* of invisibility. As a woman who underwent cosmetic dental surgery put it: 'What I noticed right away was that no one noticed me. Now *that* was a great feeling . . . Finally, nobody is there looking at me' (Davis 1995, p. 102).[22] 'Invisibility' in this context means not being

---

[20]To the extent that social phobia is a distortion of one's *being*-for-others (although not the specific aspect of one's *body*-for-others), all of these apart from 'nausea' (specifically connected with 'flesh' in Sartre's analysis) will resonate with social phobics as well.

[21]These three negative-sounding concepts exhibit the same ambiguities as does 'shame': Sartre seems at times to suggest that the lived body for others is *always* alienated and nauseous and that we *always* 'long for invisibility'. As before, the choice of terminology is not *arbitrary* and the BDD sufferer will not find these words inapt.

[22]This woman was *not* a BDD sufferer as she had genuine dental defects. The example seems, however, to express the sort of 'invisibility' that BDD sufferers long for.

looked at by others. One might borrow Gilman's term '(in)visible' for this: what BDD sufferers want (again in Gilman's terms) is to ' "pass" as "normal" ' (Gilman 1999, pp. 22–3).[23]

Nausea

Sartre — infamously and exaggeratedly — refers to 'the nauseous character of all flesh' (Sartre 1969, p. 357). This 'nausea', when 'surpassed toward a dimension of alienation' (i.e. mediated through the look of the other), presents my body-for-others to me as 'disgust with my face, disgust with my too-white flesh, with my too-grim expression, etc.' (p. 357). These are *paradigmatic* BDD feelings, and the language of 'disgust' and similar terms are highly characteristic of BDD: ' "I'm afraid if people see me they might say to themselves 'Oh, gee, look at that guy. Isn't he gross-looking?" ' (Phillips 1996, p. 142); ' "I'm the ugliest thing in the world. I hate my skin and my hair . . . I feel repulsive" ' (Phillips 1996, p. 55); ' ". . . [I] look totally unappetizing. It's all so *unaesthetic*, so completely unacceptable — *dirty*" ' (Davis 1995, p. 74).

Alienation

The shy man 'is vividly and constantly conscious of his body not as it is for him but as it is for the other', and this is 'the apprehension of my body's alienation' (Sartre 1969, p. 353). This apprehension, says Sartre, 'can determine psychoses such as ereutophobia [erythrophobia] (a pathological fear of blushing); these are nothing but the horrified metaphysical apprehension of the existence of my body for the Other' (p. 353).[24] When this sense of alienation is reflected upon, it may express itself as the sense that the hated parts of the body do not belong to *oneself*: 'Prior to surgery, she saw her breasts as . . . a "pair of sagging knockers" that just "hang there", an alien piece of flesh which "sticks to your body" ' (Davis 1995, p. 74).[25] There might even be a paradoxical 'reverse alienation' wherein the BDD sufferer identifies wholly with the

---

[23]It should be stressed that the people dealt with in Gilman's (1999) book are *not* by and large BDD sufferers, but include people disfigured by disease or war and people from oppressed minority ethnic groups who want to minimize their visible differences from the oppressors, although the 'longing for (in)visibility' is surely parallel.

[24]Note that erythrophobia *may* be a feature of BDD, and it may well be that Sartre would have included BDD as one of the 'psychoses' 'determined' by 'the apprehension of my body's alienation', had the term then been invented. He no doubt knew about the phenomenon from Janet.

[25]Although, again, the people discussed by Davis (1995) are patients undergoing cosmetic surgery, who may or may not be suffering from BDD, BDD sufferers express themselves in similar ways. Phillips does not stress this particular aspect of BDD.

hated body part, i.e. they may 'view themselves in terms of the defect' (Phillips 1996, p. 165): ' "Before I got better with the medication, I was just one big pimple, without any feet or even any toes!" ' (Phillips 1996, p. 76).

Two further features of being-for-others in general might help further to illuminate some of the characteristic symptoms of BDD: 'inapprehensibility' and 'responsibility without control'.

Inapprehensibility

Shame reveals the certainty *that* there are other conscious subjects. At the same time, the nature of that object that we are is 'inapprehensible'. 'With the appearance of the Other's look I experience the revelation of my being-as-object . . . A me-as-object is revealed to me as an unknowable being . . . [My] "lived experience" becomes — in and through the absolute, contingent fact of the Other's existence — extended outside in a dimension of flight which escapes me' (Sartre 1969, pp. 351–2).

Most of us can find this undeniable fact about human existence disturbing; none the less there is a commonsensical response to it: that we can tell how we appear to others by the simple expedients of looking in a mirror, or *asking* them, or noticing how they react! But — and this is what grips the BDD sufferer — each of these ways of 'telling how we appear to others' falls short of *certainty*.

First, mirrors and people alike have straightforward temporal limitations. For example, if you look in a mirror at time *t*, it 'tells' you how you look *at time t*, but cannot tell you how you look after you have left the mirror.[26] Most of us don't worry unduly about this: we expect our appearance to remain relatively stable for at least a few hours. The compulsive mirror-checking and questioning characteristic of BDD sufferers (rather like the pathological doubts of OCD sufferers) takes off from the *logical* possibility of change.[27] It is fed, at least in the case of mirrors, by the fact that one's 'apparent appearance', if I may so put it, *can* change rapidly and drastically. (One woman, concerned about her freckles, said: ' "sometimes, they seem really bad. I look in a mirror and I panic. I think 'They really *are* that bad!' " ' (Phillips 1996, p. 91).)

Second, asking people how one looks has a further limitation: others can be biased, or inattentive; they can lie (whether maliciously, out of kindness, or out of duty), and they can change their minds. At the same time, most of us, by and large, do not doubt that what others tell us is true, unless there are *particular*

---

[26]Mirrors also have geometrical limitations; because of the simple fact that eyes are in heads, we cannot, even with three-way mirrors, get a complete view of our own bodies. (This point does perhaps not run deep; if the focus of BDD concern is a part of the body, for instance the hand or the penis, that can be seen without a mirror, it doesn't apply.)

[27]Penises are measured and remeasured in a similar way.

reasons for thinking otherwise. ('Aren't you shutting your eyes in the face of doubt? — They are shut.') BDD sufferers may *begin* from such 'particular reasons' for doubt: one woman 'sought reassurance at cosmetic counters to "get an objective view". As she explained, "My husband loves me, so he might have a biased view of how bad it is"' (Phillips 1996, p. 117). '. . . "if people said they didn't notice it, I wouldn't believe them anyway. I'd think they were just trying to be nice"' (Phillips 1996, p. 116). But the BDD sufferer's lack of trust is pathological: she continues to doubt what others tell her even in the absence of such special reasons (for example, the woman won't accept the cosmetic salesperson's reassurances *either*), or where the supposition that such 'special reasons' are present stretches credulity: 'Another young woman had been asked to work as a model, and as a child she'd been told that she would someday be Miss America; she, however, believed that such requests and statements were motivated by pity for her ugliness' (Phillips 1996, p. 35)!

Third, gestures, facial expressions, direction of gaze, and so on are also inherently limited sources of knowledge in yet a different way: they are sometimes ambiguous, and evidence for a given 'interpretation' is, in Wittgenstein's terms, 'imponderable' (Wittgenstein 1953, p. 228). In most cases, as non-BDD sufferers recognize, the context disambiguates, or at least we tend to consider alternative interpretations and put the most plausible construction on the glance or gesture. The referential thinking of BDD sufferers shows up in their construing these ambiguous glances and gestures as referring to them, and in a negative way: 'If someone glances in their direction, they assume they're being looked at in horror' (Phillips 1996, p. 85). The pathological distrust of others noted earlier — albeit over an extremely limited domain of discourse — together with the ideas of reference projected upon ambiguous gestures and glances constitutes a distortion of dimension (3) of the body (the body-of-the-other).

What the BDD sufferer is really after is something impossible: he doesn't simply want to *know* how others really view him, he wants *certainty*, beyond any possibility of doubt. Even the seemingly strange behaviour of trying to persuade others that his view of the defect is right (Phillips 1996, p. 118–19) is to be understood in this light: at least then he'd be *certain* of what they thought.

Responsibility without control

We are inclined to think of the primary scope of responsibility as free *actions*. Sartre overturns this common presupposition in two ways: first, by extending the scope of freedom to cover, for example, values and character traits, and, second, by extending the scope of responsibility to cover aspects of our being that are not in our *control*, viz. our being-for-others, which is ultimately in the control of *the other*. I am responsible for my being-for-others because I *am* it (*inter alia*) (*pace* the widespread conviction that 'the real self' is what is 'on the inside').

There is a temptation to see BDD as vanity gone wild. Many BDD sufferers feel *this* temptation very strongly: cf. Phillips' characterization of 'the "double whammy" of BDD': many patients feel 'selfish and vain for being so preoccupied with such "trivial concerns" . . . They feel ashamed of being ashamed' (Phillips 1996, p. 83).[28] ('"My father would have said 'Be happy that you have ears at all!' "' (Davis 1995, p. 86).) The usual reply is that 'BDD should be viewed as an illness like depression or anorexia nervosa or heart disease. It has a life of its own and doesn't reflect moral weakness' (Phillips 1996, p. 83). True though this may be, I want to suggest a different way of looking at it.

Consider the 'culture-bound syndrome' (DSM-IV) *taijin kyofusho* found in Japan: this is an 'intense fear that his or her body, its parts or its functions, displease, embarrass or are offensive to other people in appearance, odor, facial expressions, or movements' (DSM-IV). Here the central experience of this BDD-like syndrome is quite clearly *guilt*, because 'displeasing, embarrassing or offending other people' is a thought of as a *moral* failing.[29] Yet it is a moral failing that in an important sense is not in one's control: it is up to the *other* person whether she is displeased or offended or embarrassed. *Taijin kyofusho* sufferers evidently feel too heavily the weight of Sartre's 'responsibility without control'.

I cite this syndrome as a kind of counterweight to the 'vanity' picture: we might, and might encourage BDD sufferers to, see BDD as *more* like *taijin kyofusho* and *less* like empty-headed primping in front of the mirror. There is nothing 'trivial' or 'selfish' or 'vain' about being concerned about offending or displeasing other people! And their desperation for certainty about their lived-body-for-others might be seen as a desperate (although hyperbolic and misdirected) concern to take responsibility for their body-for-others.

Conclusions

What I have tried to argue here is that BDD is a *specific* disorder of the 'lived-body-for-others'. This makes it phenomenologically absolutely distinct from any other mental disorder. Many of its characteristic feelings and behaviours can be illuminated by looking at it in this way.

---

[28]Davis (1995, p. 85) independently uses the same phrase 'ashamed for feeling ashamed in the first place' in reference to women seeking cosmetic surgery. A strong theme in her book is the idea that feminism contributes to many of these women 'feeling ashamed of being ashamed' (see, for example, p. 86), and one aim of the book is to try to place an acceptable positive feminist spin on undertaking cosmetic surgery.

[29]There *might* be thought to be a similar motivation behind the so-called 'ugly laws', for instance those instituted in Chicago as recently as 1966, imposing fines on 'persons who appeared in public who were "diseased, maimed, mutilated, or in any way deformed so as to be an unsightly or disgusting object" ' (Gilman 1999, p. 24).

One conclusion already drawn was that, to the extent that categorization in DSM is to be done on the basis of 'shared phenomenology', the 'phenomenology' in question might do well to avail itself of the work of the phenomenologists.

A second conclusion might be is that it is deeply *phenomenologically* misguided (as well as empirically implausible) to attempt to offer a sociological explanation (e.g. in terms of media pressure to be attractive) for the occurrence of a disorder of a dimension of experience that is *essential* to embodied human beings living amongst others. Although the *content* of BDD concerns is *undoubtedly* influenced by culture, gender, and the media, its *occurrence* cannot be.

Finally, although it may be well true that BDD is to be viewed as an illness and that people are not to be blamed for illnesses, a deeper response to BDD sufferers' worries about being 'vain' or 'selfish' might be to see them as suffering from a pathologically heightened sense of *responsibility*: the responsibility we all have for our own being-for-others, even though it is not in our control.

References

Agresti, E. and Taddei, M. (1970). On the subject of dysmorphophobia: a clinical and phenomenological study. *Rivista di Psichiatria,* **5**(3): 224–48.

Davis, K. (1995). *Reshaping the Female Body: The Dilemma of Cosmetic Surgery.* London: Routledge.

Doerry, U. and Brockington, I. F. (2000). Gaze avoidance and baby gazing. *Psychopathology,* **33**(1): 11–13.

Gallagher, S. (1995). Body schema and intentionality. In: *The Body and the Self* (ed. J. L. Bermudez, A. Marcel, and N. Eilan), pp. 225–44. Cambridge, MA: Bradford/MIT Press.

Gilman, S. L. (1999). *Making the Body Beautiful: A Cultural History of Aesthetic Surgery,* Princeton, NJ: Princeton University Press.

Liberman, R. (1974). Dysmorphophobia in the adolescent. *Revue de Neuropsychiatrie Infantile et d'Hygiene Mentale de l'Enfance,* **22**(10–11): 695–9.

Phillips, K. A. (1998). Body dysmorphic disorder: clinical aspects and treatment strategies. *Bulletin of the Menninger Clinic,* **62**(4 Suppl. A): A33–48.

Phillips, K. A., Mc Elroy, S. L., Keck, P. E., and Harrison, C. (1993). Body dysmorphic disorder: 30 cases of imagined ugliness. *American Journal of Psychiatry,* **150**(2): 302–8.

Schacter, M. (1971). Dysmorphic neuroses (ugliness complexes) and the delusion or delusional conviction of dysmorphia: concerning the so-called 'dysmorphophobias' of the adolescent and young adult. *Annales Medico-Psychologiques,* **1**(5): 723–46.

Tiggemann, M. (1996). 'Thinking' versus 'feeling' fat: correlates of two indices of body image dissatisfaction. *Australian Journal of Psychology,* **48**(1): 21–5.

Wittgenstein, L. (1953). *Philosophical Investigations* (ed. G. E. M. Anscombe and R. Rhees, trans. G. E. M. Anscombe). Oxford: Blackwell.

12 Putting the *époché* into practice: schizophrenic experience as illustrating the phenomenological exploration of consciousness

Natalie Depraz

Introduction: the status of experience

If there is one feature that characterizes phenomenology with respect to other disciplines and other philosophical projects, it is surely the emphasis placed on lived experience, described with the greatest precision and in maximum detail, as accurately as possible. Phenomenological description is guided by intuition as the sole criterion of internal truth. Its criterion of validation is in the first person, i.e. the phenomenologist apprehends the phenomenon without reconstructing it in a speculative vision abstracted from its concrete presentation. The phenomenological description is all the more accurate and convincing in so far as it confines itself what is actually apprehended. To return to the lived subjective experience, to a description of this experience that is as complete as possible, and which is never filled out by unverified speculative hypotheses — these are the two correlative characteristics that make phenomenology an original and innovative discipline.

The first question that confronts us is: what should be understood by 'experience'? Even if it is agreed that the experience of which the phenomenologist speaks is lived experience (Erlebnis) by an individual subject, and not the experimentation (Experiment) performed by science using objective protocols that frame third-person observations and results, it remains true that this first-person experience covers an important diversity of types, qualities, and levels of experience.

In considering the perceptual visual experience of the apple blossom in the garden compared with the emotional, brutal, and shocking experience (albeit mediated by television) that I may have of the atrocities committed in a war-torn part of the world, there are commonalities regarding elements of subjective experience and discontinuities regarding the type of existential situations implied. In the first case, what is in question is an elementary action — local visual perception — that involves me alone; in the second case, the act is complex, at the same time emotional, intersubjective, and communal, implicating a historical setting in which I am not well versed.

But, over and above these types of experience (from an isolated local perception to a shared, existential, and generative situation), there are also different qualities of experience. Consider the daily experience of each morning's drive to my son's nursery school compared with the exceptional experience (which represents a limit-event) when I learn suddenly, by a telephone call, of the disappearance of a close friend. Or consider the familiar experience of supper together with the family, compared with the shock and ordeal experienced when I meet a person in the street who through moral and physical distress has lost his humanity. Experiences of the first type are situated on the plane of the everydayness and familiarity, which implies that, on the one hand, they often pass unnoticed because they go without saying for us. On the other hand, these experiences derive meaning from repetition and ritualization and, therefore, from their sedimentation into the individual history of each person. Experiences of the second type are characterized by their quasi-unique side: exceptional, unrepeatable, brutal, and unexpected, they pertain to the singular event. Finally, one could equally draw a distinction between communal experience, shared and shareable (the perception of the apple blossom, the everyday experiences already mentioned), and limit-experiences, which necessarily presuppose a thrown-into lived situation (the experience of the death of a close friend, becoming aware of the loss of humanity). The latter are more radical experiences, almost ontological. Between the two, there are intermediate experiences, like listening to a piece of music, or the olfactory appreciation of a perfume, or wine-tasting, which presuppose a certain apprenticeship and are not, in any event, available to everyone.

In short, there are standard-experiences about which most people can come to an understanding because they arise from a lived situation that is shared or shareable, and there are limit-experiences, which are difficult to communicate by virtue of being exceptional and reserved *de facto* — although not *de jure* — for a very few. A question that will function as a guiding thread through this maze concerns schizophrenic experience: to which type of experience is it to be referred? Intuitively, one would classify it as the second type, but we shall see that this classification implies an additional enquiry against the grain as to whether — and how — schizophrenia cannot equally belong to the first kind. In fact, the proposed distinction between standard-experience and limit-experience already contains a presupposition that there is a hermetic discontinuity between these two qualities of experience, even if one takes account of intermediate experiences that presuppose some training but are nevertheless accessible to only a small number of people.

Strikingly, Merleau-Ponty, but equally the majority of phenomenologists, has adopted this discontinuist position. They rest their case for the most part on examples that anybody could have lived: the example of the concert hall in *Phenomenology of Perception* (Merleau-Ponty 1945/1962), or again Sartre's example of the café waiter. Considering that the phenomenological reduction (i.e. the process through which we don't examine the object of consciousness but the act that constitutes it) cannot be performed completely, Merleau-Ponty notably makes it into an inaccessible experience, a limit-experience. Phenomenologists believe that schizophrenic persons have the capacity to perform the reduction much better than ordinary people: they show an enhanced aptitude to the *époché*. This is supposed to be one of the major features of the vulnerability to schizophrenia (Stanghellini 1997). People with schizophrenia can 'bracket' commonsense experience and have access to the way an object originally presents itself to consciousness and to the way consciousness appropriates the object to itself. This is not, for them, an achievement, but so to say a *natural experience*. Whereas for non-schizophrenic persons the *époché* requires an unnatural exercise, for people with schizophrenia it is part of the natural attitude situated in ordinary life. Following the guiding thread of the ambiguous hinge-experience of the schizophrenic reduction or *époché*, I would like to call into question the hermetic discontinuity that forms the phenomenologists' presupposition of the major understanding of experience. I raise this question in order to bring to light how an experience — in this case the cardinal experience of the *époché* — can be learned and cultivated until it becomes an everyday and familiar practice.

The *époché*: a limit-experience?

Is it possible to experience the transcendental *époché*?

In the preface to *Phenomenology of Perception*, Merleau-Ponty (1962, pp. xiv, xxi) writes these celebrated words: 'The most important lesson which the reduction teaches us is the impossibility of a complete reduction. This is why Husserl is constantly re-examining the possibility of the reduction. If we were absolute mind, the reduction would present no problems. . . The unfinished nature of phenomenology and the inchoate atmosphere which has surrounded it are not to be taken as a sign of failure, they were inevitable . . .'.

One might as well say that here confirmation is found, and has been for a long time, of the idea of the transcendental *époché* arising from a methodological requirement — undoubtedly the principal methodological requirement of phenomenology — but one that precisely cannot, de jure, be met. The reduction is *the* regulative ideal of the phenomenological approach, but only an ideal that is never in fact realized. Since Merleau-Ponty, we have never stopped repeating this *leit-motiv* of the constitutive incompleteability of the transcendental *époché*: an experience incomplete de jure. One cannot have a genuine experience of it; in short, one cannot practise it, if it cannot serve as a guiding thread situated at the indefinite horizon of experience, or at least an approximation of an ideal that is never fully realized.

Some might consider that the transcendental dimension of experience arises from pure ideality and returns to a myth. It then becomes a fiction, inaccessible to human experience. This transcendental *époché* corresponds to the ideal target of an experience, always aimed at but never actually lived. Or rather, the *époché* is lived only through the fact of this singular target of the ideal. But it is then accessible only by a reconstruction that sends us see-sawing in speculation, the very speculation which Husserl, in the *Crisis*, stigmatized as the 'mythical construction of concepts'. So understood, it involves a return to the transcendentality of experience with which German idealism was concerned in the last century. This transcendentalism was formalized as a speculative logic of experience for which there was no concrete description at all (compare in this regard with Goddard (1999)).

In the wake of the Husserl's apodictic approach, one could none the less understand the transcendental *époché* in a third sense: neither as a constitutively non-realizable ideal requirement, nor as a mythical and speculative reconstruction, but as a simple formal and theoretical method of *a priori* justification of knowledge. But such an understanding of the transcendental *époché* likewise evades all concrete description. The hypothesis that I would like to explore at this stage is this: to what extent could the schizophrenic *époché*, as much as the limit-experience, play the role of an incarnate (or embodied) transcendental *époché* because it is lived existentially (as opposed to being theorized like a method, with its de jure incomplete ideal requirement, or indeed reconstructed as mythical speculation)?

The schizophrenic *époché*: an existential analogon (or realization) of the transcendental *époché*?

In the midst of these three somewhat abstract interpretations of the transcendental *époché* (ideal of incompleteness, speculative construction, or theoretical method), the 'schizophrenic *époché*' presents as an experience that, all at once, introduces a rupture in our normal perceptions arising in what phenomenologists call the 'natural attitude', i.e. the sedimented 'taken-for-granted' world of the familiar and everyday[1]. The schizophrenic *époché* holds together the radical interruption of the experiential world in undertaking the most radical version of the Husserlian transcendental *époché*, in the midst of our most natural attitude. Whether one has here a matter of a 'loss of natural evidence' as in Blankenburg (1971*b*), or perhaps making evident the interval, the room for play (*aida*) in our intersubjective constitution as for Kimura

---

[1]The following case examples illustrate the schizophrenic *époché*, the loss of the familiar ground of experience in schizophrenia. In the first two examples, the effect of the *époché* is particularly evident in the realm of social life:

Case 1: 'P.S. is a forty-two-year-old man who has been affected by paranoid schizophrenia since the age of twenty. At the onset of his psychosis he was trying in various ways to *compensate for his difficulties in getting in touch with other people*. He had no secure ground to interpret other people's intentions. He lacked the structure of the rules of social life and systematically set about searching for a well-grounded and natural style of behavior. For instance, he was busy with an ethological study of the "biological" (i.e. not "cultural", not artificial) foundation of other people's behaviors through a double observation of animal and human habits. The former was done through TV documentaries; the latter via the analyses of human interactions in public parks. An atrophy in his knowledge of the "rules of the game" led him to engage in intellectual investigations and to establish his own "know-how" for social interactions in a reflective way.' (From Stanghellini 2000).

Case 2: 'Robert, a 21 year-old unskilled worker, complained that for more than a year he had been feeling painfully cut-off from the world . . . This experience of disengagement, isolation, or ineffable distance from the world, was accompanied by a tendency to observe or monitor his inner life. He summarized his affliction in one exclamation: "my first personal life is lost and replaced by a third person perspective".' (From Parnas 2000).

Case 3: This case is also primarily social but in a patient with mainly 'negative' symptoms (i.e. loss of motivation, of social engagement, etc.). It is a fragment of Blankenburg's famous report of the case of Anne Rau, the person who suggested the formula 'loss of self-evidence', with which he entitled his book on the phenomenology of 'symptomarmer' schizophrenia (i.e. schizophrenia with few and minimal symptoms):

'What do I really lack? Something little, funny, something important, but without which one cannot live . . . I need the support [*den Halt*] of the simplest everyday things. I am still too little, too little in my trust. I cannot do on my own . . . It is no doubt the self-evidence what I lack . . . All human beings must know how to behave, all human beings have a view, a way to think. Their behaviours, their humanity, their sociality, all these rules of the game they play: until now, I haven't been able to recognise them so clearly. I lack the basis.' (From Blankenburg 1971*a*).

Case 4: The final case illustrates a wider *époché* involving cognition. Taken from the French writer Antonin Artaud and reported by Sass (2001), it illustrates the radical extent of the schizophrenic *époché* or disintegration of 'first assumptions':

'. . . in every dominant state of consciousness there is always a dominant theme, and if the mind has not automatically decided on a dominant theme it is through weakness and because at that moment nothing dominated, nothing presented itself with enough force or continuity in the field of consciousness to be recorded . . .

'It so happens that this slackening, this confusion, this fragility express themselves in an infinite number of ways and correspond to an infinite number of new impressions and sensations, the most characteristic of which is a kind of disappearance or disintegration of first assumptions which even causes me to wonder why, for example, red (the color) is considered red and affects me as red, why a judgment affects me as a judgment and not as a pain, why I feel a pain, and why this particular pain, which I feel without understanding it' (From Sass 2001).

(1986), it is always within the lived natural attitude that the most radical existential disturbance comes to light and unfolds.

The schizophrenic *époché* thus combines the Husserlian intensity of the transcendental disturbance of familiarity upon which we depend every day, with the radical existential disturbance in that peculiar 'naturalness' that is the schizophrenic experience. This is what Schütz described in his *Collected Papers* (1962, 1964, 1966, 1996) as a 'natural *époché*'. But, for Schütz, to *propose* a 'natural *époché*' is to *oppose* oneself to all transcendental radicality, because the 'natural' and the 'transcendental' attitudes are irreconcilable. But the challenge of the schizophrenic *époché* consists precisely of holding together *transcendental radicality* and the *natural incarnation* in the world. Such a challenge implies that one ceases to consider the transcendental dimension as a simple requirement, a speculative myth or a theoretical attitude, and recognizes it as an experience properly so called, certainly radical, but accessible as such.

On these grounds the schizophrenic *époché* — and that which has recently been termed 'the hallucinatory *époché*' as a concrete form which the former could take (Naudin 1997) — corresponds to a possible concrete incarnation (or embodiment) of the Husserlian transcendental *époché*, to which it supplies a given empirical content, situated at the peak of methodological transcendental radicality. The limit-experience that is proposed by psychopathology has the incarnate intensity of the profound reductive experience, which is the transcendental *époché*.

The fruitfulness of the experience of the schizophrenic *époché* goes further still. It offers not only, downstream, an empirical illustration of the transcendental *époché*, but affects equally, and correlatively, upstream, the transcendental *époché* itself, to the point of shaking it up from the perspective of an incarnated reduction.

The schizophrenic *époché* provides a milestone towards an effective incarnation of the transcendental *époché*, inasmuch as (1) downstream, it makes the transcendental *époché* empirical on the plane of an existential natural experience, and (2) it effects in return its transcendentality in situating this on the plane, no longer of an idealism, but of a 'transcendental empiricism'.[2]

None the less, at this point the question that arises is this: is the experience of people with schizophrenia worthwhile only for its radicality, its limit-character, which appears to be completely adapted to the transcendental *époché* by virtue of being an incarnate existential analogon? Or is there not an everyday counterpart of the schizophrenic *époché*? If so, does this not imply, as Fink (1974) has often argued, the uprooting of the transcendental *époché* itself from its ontological dramatization, from its limit-experience radicality?

---

[2]Compare in this regard Landgrebe (1982) and, more recently, Depraz (2001*a*); cf. also 'De l'empirisme transcendantal: entre Husserl et Derrida' (Depraz, 2001*b*).

The *épaché*: a concrete act, an accessible praxis?

This second section takes its impetus from a proposed understanding of the transcendental *épaché* as an accessible praxis, ordinarily capable of cultivation. This account is aimed at establishing how such a new comprehension of the methodological *épaché* allows us to make sense of a schizophrenic *épaché*, itself situated just above the everyday or mundane. I therefore follow the inverse logic of that which was implied at the end of the last section. The aim is to define a circular causality, as Piaget put it, or perhaps a non-linear logic (on the analogy of contemporary dynamic mathematics), between the transcendental *épaché* and the schizophrenic *épaché*. The connection between these two épochai will shift in this second section, from the ontological radicality as a limit of experience, to its practical and accessible everydayness. In neither case, however, is there any sense in asking which causes which. The co-generative logic allows us to give a renewed sense to each, namely, here, the sense of an everyday and exercisable praxis.

An everyday practice

An understanding of the dimension of everyday praxis in the transcendental *épaché* implies describing three complementary facets of this concrete act. In a recent work written jointly with Franciso Varela and Pierre Vermersch (Depraz *et al*. 1999, 2003), a dynamic description was proposed for the movement of the reduction.[3]

The different stages of this transcendental pragmatic of the reductive movement are:

1. A phase of the *suspension* of prejudices, which transforms the type of attention that the subject pays to his or her own lived experience, and which represents a rupture with the natural attitude.
2. A phase of *conversion of attention* from 'the exterior' to 'the interior', which has the structure of the reflexive conversion.
3. A phase of *letting-go* or *reception* of experience.

The term *épaché* refers collectively to these three organically interlinked phases, for the simple reason that phases 2 and 3 always presuppose that phase 1 is reactivated and undergoes continuing activation. Let us note that the 'suspending movement' of phase 1 is also at work, each time with a differentiated quality, at each stage of the structuring of the reflecting act.

---

[3]The description presented here is synthesized from Depraz *et al*. (1999*a*, *b*, 2001). For further details of this analysis of the *praxis* of the reduction, see Depraz *et al*. (2003).

The initial (suspending) phase involves three distinct modes of activation:

- an external existential event capable of playing the role of activating the suspending attitude, for example the encounter with the death of another or aesthetic surprise;
- the mediation of others — this could be decisive, if there is an injunction to accomplish the movement, or even a less directive attitude (as when someone plays the role of a model);
- self-directed injunctions — as far as individual training is concerned, these are presupposed, and, in any event, long cycles of training are required and an apprenticeship to the point of stabilization.

These three modes of cultivation are not mutually exclusive, but work together, the one in relation to the other; they are so many motivations, worldly, intersubjective, or even individual. All three, presenting differently in different individuals — and indeed in the same individual over the period of his or her development — come together to make possible, then to maintain, the possibility of phases 2 and 3. It is worthwhile, therefore, to maintain the suspending disposition even as one's attention becomes converted (phase 2) or the attitude of reception is deployed (phase 3).

To speak of the *initial* phase in connection with the suspension immediately suggests a remark: this 'initialization' has already taken place and, at the same time, it is produced each time as if in a new manner. We find ourselves here in the provisional circle of having to describe an act just as we are performing it. The question of initialization is masked in its radical character through an already-established beginning that serves to describe the same conduct.

The two later phases are complementary and presuppose, as I have said, the initial phase as well as its active maintenance. They correspond with two fundamental changes in the orientation of the cognitive activity: the first comes out of a change of *direction* of attention, the one that lets go of the spectacle of the world in order to return to the interior world. In other words, perception is substituted for the most part for an *apperceptive act*. There is here a massive obstacle to change, namely, the necessity of being diverted from habitual cognitive activity towards the external world. The second fundamental change consists of passing from a movement, still voluntary, to an attentional switch from the exterior toward the interior, toward simple receptivity and listening. In other words, from phase 2 to 3, one passes from a 'going to search' to a 'letting come', a letting 'reveal itself'. The principal obstacle to this third phase rests in the necessity of crossing an *empty time*, a time of silence, an absence of holding on to immediately available givens and things of which one is already conscious.

We have here two reversals of the most habitual cognitive functioning. Of these, the first is the condition of the second. This, in turn, signifies that the second cannot arise if the first has not already taken place. Thus, the two reversals are:

- a reversal of the *direction* of the attention from the exterior to the interior (phase 2)
- a change in the *quality* of the attention, which passes from going-to-search to letting-come (phase 3).

The first reversal remains governed by the distinction between the interior and the exterior; it is moved by a certain dual doubling and carries an undeniable content of voluntary activity. The second, by contrast, is characterized by a passive disposition of receptive waiting. This allows any residual duality of the first reversal to be avoided.

Such a description of the practical everyday transcendental *époché* leads us to look again at the schizophrenic *époché*. Does not the alteration of the self that is evident at the onset of an episode of schizophrenia precisely match up with the three phases of the *époché* described above?

Phase 1. First, there is the interruption of the continuity of the everyday course of actions and thoughts. This corresponds with the very structure of suspension, with the opening of an abyss. More specifically, it reflects the mode of release of the existential event, in the manner of an external motivation.

Phase 2. The interruption of actions and thoughts in turn reveals a duality between the exterior and the interior, which the verb *schizein* (to split) translates well. This provides a concrete instantiation of reflection as a dual doubling structure. There is also an inflexion of this dual doubling, a withdrawal to the interior world because of the difficulty of confronting external reality. This inflection corresponds in structure with the reflexive conversion, i.e. the redirection of attention from the exterior to the interior. In schizophrenia, withdrawal toward the interior — a version of autism — is first suffered as the result of a change of attention. None the less, structurally we have here a homologue of the conversion of attention in phase 2 of the *époché*.

Phase 3. Finally, there is the paradoxical behaviour of the person with schizophrenia, the ambivalence of his or her thoughts, which can lead to several related phenomena. For instance, there may be hyperreceptivity, an attitude of hyperlucidity inverting the loss of contact with the exterior, or the withdrawal of the self in a perspicacious detachment, a lucid disengagement. This is very close to the receptive attitude, of waiting and of letting-come, which corresponds to the third phase of the revisited transcendental *époché*.

Given these similarities, the schizophrenic *époché* offers a valuable experiential or empirical milestone for apprehending more concretely the praxis of the *époché* and its possible achievement through training. In brief, the experience of a person with schizophrenia teaches us through his or her own capacity to suspend, to change the direction of our attention to one of letting-come. But what degree of schizophrenia is necessary actually to practise the *époché*, to exercise it? What is the 'wise folly' required here?[4]

A practice to cultivate: exercising the *époché*

Discussion of the transcendental *époché* in the practical terms of training implies a thoroughgoing challenge to the initial distinction between standard-experience and limit-experience. Correspondingly, it challenges the discontinuity between normal experience and pathological experience.

However, these discontinuities — those of the phenomenologists and the clinicians — have always been considered naive in oriental cultures, be these Buddhist or Taoist meditators, or practising physicians (these are often the same). Meditation practices, as exemplified by the work of Yuasa (1987) and Yanaguchi (1997)[5], show that there is a continuous gradation between everyday experience and types of elaborated experience. If there is a gradation, it is because one can, through training and interior labour or effort, cultivate an attention to oneself that is the first step toward the *recapturing of a finer quality of lived experience*. Access to this finer level of internal experience is thus given neither immediately nor in advance, but presupposes an apprenticeship. Indeed, there are cycles of apprenticeship, in every case requiring a longer period of time than the simple access to the perception of an apple blossom or the familiar situation of a meal taken with the family. It is worth noting, however, that these apparently daily experiences can themselves be recaptured at a level of granularity that requires no less labour or training than experiences which at first glance seem more difficult to access, for instance the possibility of capturing an emotion of fear at the very moment it emerges, or of accessing the memory of an instant as it appears.

If training can be used in connection with very simple emotional or retentive experiences as well as in regard to more delicate situations of loss of sense, this again shows that there is no rupture between the everyday and the exceptional, between the familiar and the liminal. This is the case, paradigmatically, with the transcendental *époché*, which, instead of limit-state or speculation, is thus made practical in an everyday way. But it is also the case for the schizophrenic *époché*, its existential analogon. For this now no longer appears, as it did in the first section, as a pathological liminal experience, inaccessible to anyone from the perspective of standard normality. Thus we have here an everyday schizophrenic *époché* (which suggests that the normal subject can equally undergo training to achieve a comparable experience) and, at the same time, an incarnate transcendental *époché*.

---

[4]Compare in connection with the wise folly of the Epistles of St Paul, and Trungpa (1995).
[5]I rely for all of this point on these two remarkable books (Yuasa 1987, Yamaguchi 1997).

The importance of the embodied nature of this experience cannot be overstated. The everydayness of the schizophrenic *époché*, the concrete exercise of the transcendental *époché*: these two practices, linked by their co-generativity, acquire a renewed significance from the possibility of what in phenomenology is called corporeity (or bodiliness). Training in connection with the *époché* includes a bodily labour. What Yuasa and Yamaguchi teach in their work on meditation is precisely a remarkable focus on corporeity; that aspect which Husserl called *Leib*, they call the 'subtle body'; and this is in opposition to the 'gross body', which is the aspect of bodily experience that Husserl called *Körper*. To practise the *époché* is to be attentive to the changes in our bodies, to the forces that cross the subtle body, because it is here that a finer and more incarnate consciousness of movements of suspension, of conversion of the attention, and of letting-come — the three phases of the *époché* — can all be found. The schizophrenic *époché* examined in its everydayness thus makes us conscious of the weight of our bodiliness, and of the difficulties of liberating ourselves from the *Körper* in the direction of the *Leib*.

Conclusion

What are the limits of the phenomenological description of trancendental experience? Could one describe the *époché* completely? Is its practice an asset in view of its complete description? The limits of description are the very limits of corporeity. The more one makes the effort to become attentive to the subtle bodily movements (that is, at one and the same time bodily and conscious), the more one gives oneself the resources to progress in descriptive fineness and completeness. In this process, the schizophrenic *époché* helps us to push back the limits of the description of the transcendental *époché*: it makes us attentive to ourselves, via the other, in our difficult embodiment.

References

Blankenburg, W. (1971*a*). *Der Verlust der natuerlichen Selbstverstaendlichkeit*. Stuttgart: Enke.

Blankenburg, W. (1971*b*). *La Perte de l'Evidence Naturelle*. Paris: Presses Universitaires de France.

Depraz, N. (2001*a*). Lucidité du corps. De l'empirisme transcendantal en phénoménologie. Dordrecht: Kluwer.

Depraz, N. (2001*b*). De l'empirisme transcendantal: entre Husserl et Derrida. In: *Actes du Colloque J. Derrida, Juin 1999*. Paris: Alber.

Depraz, N., Varela, F., and Vermersch, P. (1999). The gesture of awareness. In: *Phenomenal Approaches to Consciousness* (ed. M. Velmans). Amsterdam: John Benjamins.

Depraz, N., Varela, F., and Vermersch, P. (2000). [French paper] *Etudes Phénoméno-logiques.*

Depraz, N., Varela, F., and Vermersch, P. (2003). *On Becoming Aware: The Pragmatics of Experiencing.* Amsterdam: Benjamins Press.

Fink, E. (1974) *De la Phénoménologie.* Paris: Minuit.

Goddard, J.-Ch. (1999). *Le Transcendental et le Spéculatif dans l'Idéalisme Allemand.* Paris: Vrin.

Kimura, B. (1986). *'Réflection et Soi chez les Schizophrènes'* en Ecrits de Psychopathologie Phénoménologique. Paris: Presses Universitaires de France.

Landgrebe, L. (1982). *Faktizität und Individuation.* Hamburg: Meiner.

Merleau-Ponty, M. (1945). *Phénoménologie de la Perception.* Paris : Gallimard (*The Phenomenology of Perception* (trans. C. Smith), London: Routledge & Kegan Paul, 1962).

Naudin, J. (1997). *Phénoménologie et Psychiatrie, Les Voix et la Chose.* Toulouse: Presses Universitaires du Mirail.

Parnas, J. (2000). The self and intentionality in the pre-psychotic stages of schizophrenia. A phenomenological study. In: *Exploring the Self. Philosophical and Psychopathological Perspectives in Self-Experience* (ed. D. Zahavi), pp. 115–47. Amsterdam: John Benjamins.

Sass, L. A. (2001). Schizophrenia, self-experience, and so-called 'negative-symptoms'. In: *Exploring the Self* (ed. D. Zahavi), pp. 149–84. Amsterdam: John Benjamins.

Schütz, A. (1962). *Collected Papers I.* The Hague: M. Nijhoff.

Schütz, A. (1964). *Collected Papers II.* The Hague: M. Nijhoff.

Schütz, A. (1966). *Collected Papers III.* The Hague: M. Nijhoff.

Schütz, A. (1996). *Collected Papers IV.* Dordrecht: Klüwer.

Stanghellini, G. (1997). For an anthropology of vulnerability. *Psychopathology,* **30:** 1–11.

Stanghellini, G. (2000). Vulnerability to schizophrenia and lack of common sense. *Schizophrenia Bulletin,* **26**(4): 775–87.

Trungpa, C. (1995). *Bardo. Au Dela de la Folie.* Paris: Seuil.

Yamaguchi, I. (1997). *Ki also leibhaftige Vernunft, Beitrag zur interkulturellen Phànomenologie de Leiblichkeit.* Munich: Fink.

Yuasa, Y. (1987). *The Body. Toward an Eastern Mind–Body Theory.* New York: State University of New York Press.

13 How can the phenomenological–anthropological approach contribute to diagnosis and classification in psychiatry?

Alfred Kraus

Introduction

In an Indian tale three blind men were asked to identify what they touched when an elephant was presented to them. The first one, touching the legs said: 'I am touching pillars'. The second, touching the ears, identified them as fans. And the third, touching the back, said: 'This is a bed'. None of them identified the elephant, even if all the identified elements were considered together.

This is analogous to the situation with our modern glossary diagnostics and corresponding classifications. Traditionally, in medicine, there have always been two kinds of diagnostic process: one directed to the whole patient, the other to the symptoms and signs of the presupposed disease. Whole-person diagnostics, however, even if still used implicitly to some extent in practice, is now formally proscribed, at any rate for research. We are required to make a definite diagnosis based on given inclusion and exclusion criteria, even if the diagnosis gained in this way contradicts our practical experience. We are obliged to apply non-specific, even ambiguous, criteria, and to establish diagnoses based on these criteria in the absence of an immediate intuitive grasping of the experience of the whole person. The disorders defined in our classifications, similarly, are no more than summaries of groups of criteria that often have no understandable interconnections and, as such, are not determined by whole diagnostic entities. Again, we are not allowed to pre-suppose such whole entities. We have, so to say, to close our eyes, and — as in our Indian tale — this carries the risk of drawing conclusions that, from a traditional clinical point of view, are false.

It is the task of phenomenological–anthropological psychiatry (P-A psychiatry) to make a holistic diagnosis, oriented to the person of the patient, scientifically sound by reflecting upon its elements and by translating these into scientific terms, drawing particularly on philosophical phenomenology and anthropology.

In this chapter I will compare phenomenological-anthropological diagnostics (P-A diagnostics), as developed within P-A psychiatry, with symptomatological–criteriological diagnostics (S-C diagnostics), as developed in our official classifications, such as the ICD and DSM. The two approaches, I believe, are complementary and should supplement each other. Later in the chapter, I illustrate the strengths of the P-A approach with three examples: melancholia, hypomania, and hysterical personality disorder. First, we must consider what is understood by the terms 'phenomenological' and 'anthropological', and hence by P-A psychiatry.

What is phenomenological–anthropological psychiatry?

Phenomenological psychiatry is characterized by a central concern with phenomena. Some authors, outside the P-A tradition, equate phenomena with symptoms, but they are crucially different (Rovaletti 2000). Thus, the term 'phenomenon' is limited to that which, in our lived experience, is revealed or disclosed by itself without any theoretical presuppositions. The term 'symptom', by contrast, is related to a medical concept of disease. By definition, a symptom points to a disease that, as such, does not necessarily show or disclose itself to us in direct experience. Fever is a case in point. Fever is a symptom that points to any of a large number of hidden diseases.

Under the heading of P-A psychiatry (see also Krau 2001) we sum up a number of approaches with a different philosophical background, all of which are concerned, in one way or another, with clinical phenomena, some of them with an anthropological orientation. At the clinical level these approaches are not always sharply distinguished, but I will outline them briefly before turning to their role in psychiatric classification and diagnosis. (For further reading, see the list at the end of the chapter.)

At least three classical types of phenomenology can be differentiated (Blankenburg 1980; Parnas and Zahavi 2002). The first is *eidetic phenomenology*, which points to the logos, or essence, of phenomena (Blankenburg 1991). An essence is an invariant feature of something given in experience (e.g. describing the invariant features of all trees instead of the contingent features of a particular tree). An eidetic or essence-based phenomenology seeks to characterize such general essences. It is thus the science of the logos (or essence) of phenomena, concerned not with facts (as in empirical science) but with essences.

For psychiatry, however, phenomenology has become important not only as an eidetic science, but also as a *phenomenology of constitution*[1]. Here, the

---

[1]Sometimes called 'transcendental phenomenology'.

empirical objects or essences as such are not of interest. Rather, what is of interest is how phenomena are constituted, that is, apprehended or understood by the observer. But 'to apprehend' and 'to understand' are intentional acts. Hence, whereas in empirical sciences one starts with the presumption of observer independence from phenomena, in the phenomenology of constitution the phenomenon is seen as a correlate of the observer's constituting intentional act. That means that every meaningful being is bound to a constituting act: the phenomenon is structured by so-called transcendental subjectivity. Phenomenology of constitution thus seeks to understand how phenomena are constituted and how the observer's conscious intentionality is related both to the 'objectivity' of the world and to phenomena.

It is important to note in passing that, despite his importance in the development of modern descriptive psychopathology, Karl Jaspers' (1965) understanding of phenomenology and of phenomena is quite different from that of the phenomenology of constitution. For Jaspers, 'phenomenon' is almost interchangeable with the concept of 'subjective symptom'. His psychopathology is methodologically based on the intuitive understanding (*anschauliche Vergegenwärtigung*) of the other person's mental life by empathic understanding.

Under the heading of existential-hermeneutic approaches we list different daseinanalytic and existence-analytic approaches. Not all have an anthropological orientation. Here 'anthropological' and 'anthropology' have a special meaning, which is different from that in biological and cultural anthropology. 'Anthropological' here conveys not only a humanistic orientation. It implies also a methodological focus on the essence of human existence as expressed in the individuality, subjectivity, freedom, and historicity of individual people. Phenomenological–anthropological psychiatry thus attempts not only to understand psychopathological phenomena by comparing them with normal psychological phenomena (e.g. understanding social phobia through normal shame), it also seeks to conceive of psychiatric disturbances, such as schizophrenia and mania, as modifications of what are called essential structures of our 'being-in-the-world'. Such essential structures include intersubjectivity, temporality, spaciality, embodiment, and self-awareness.

In the frame of Daseinanalysis the introduction of anthropological 'dimensions'[2] by Binswanger (1956), has been particularly fruitful for both psychopathology and classification in psychiatry. Binswanger (1956) developed this concept in his book *Drei Formen missglückten Daseins* ('Three forms of miscarried Dasein'), with examples such as eccentricity and 'high flowness'. Following Blankenburg (1982), who contributed much to the further development of this approach, Daseinanalysis is oriented to the structure of an individual's mode of 'incarnation' — its self-constitution or

---

[2]The term used by Binswanger (1956) is usually translated as 'proportions'.

self-realization. As with Heidegger's (1962) concept of Dasein, the starting point of the Daseinanalytical approach is not a personality with individual qualities set within an independent environment, but the 'being-in-the-world', i.e. the set of *relationships* to self, to others, and to the world. Binswanger's 'Daseinsanalyse', however, is different from Heidegger's 'Daseinsanalytic' (1962), in so far as it brings the ontologically determined 'existentials' of Heidegger into the frame of concrete human existence. As an empirical method it is metaontic, as Needleman (1963) has written.

Other anthropological proportions are, for example, future- and past-relatedness, self-realization and world-realization, authenticity and inauthenticity, individuation and community-relationship, and, as we shall see in the third clinical example below, under- or non-identification and over-identification. It is important to note that these dimensions, even if sometimes running contrary to one another, build up a dialectical relationship that can be distributed between extremes in a scalor way. This is fruitful for psychopathology, because it means that the abnormal is not measured by only one norm, be it a real or ideal norm or a mean. Rather, the 'abnormal' as well as the 'normal' are located on one or more scales along which deviations can always occur in at least two directions between extremes. Thus, there are no absolute norms, positively discriminating the normal from the abnormal. Instead, dimensions of deviation are taken into consideration that need other criteria in order to be called 'pathological'.

Problems of description and classification

The significance of the P-A approach for diagnosis and classification can be appreciated best by comparing it with traditional diagnosis. Thus, in traditional diagnosis, even in psychiatry, the complaints of patients tend to be fitted to medical terminology (as, for example, in speaking of being depressed or having hallucinations). But this is not necessarily what the patient feels or experiences. What the patient's experience primarily comprises are phenomena of a certain relationship to one-self, to others, and to the world. What is 'given', that is to say, is a particular kind of 'being-in-the-world' which is *experienced* by the patient and *observed* by the diagnostician. Only secondarily on the basis of the medical model of disease does the diagnostician discern symptoms based on his or her observations.

In discerning symptoms, however, in traditional diagnosis, we are already prejudiced against what we are told by the patient or what we observe by the assumption of an underlying dysfunction to which the symptoms can be traced back. This assumption predetermines the way we describe the symptoms, for instance speaking of *disorders* or *disturbances* of thinking, of perception, of drive, and so on. This in turn not only reduces the richness of the multiple meanings of the original phenomena to simple 'dysfunctions', it can even distort the description of symptoms. Often we are uncertain about the kind of dysfunction involved: we are unsure whether to speak of an affective or a mood disorder, for example. Such terms may have a heuristic value, but they often presuppose what has still to be proven by research. In this vein, van Praag (2000) even recommended that psychiatric diagnosis should be 'functionalized' to facilitate biological and pharmaceutical research. He proposed that symptoms should be ranked according to their relationship to the pathophysiological substratum underlining a particular condition. Symptoms would thus be organized in vertical hierarchies according to their diagnostic 'valence' (or significance) rather than in their current largely horizontal groupings.

In reducing phenomena to symptoms, and even more in reducing them to criteria (giving them exact definitions), there is always the danger, which was well recognized by Jaspers (1965), of making the phenomena more distinct or 'pseudo-precise' than they really are. This is particularly true for psychotic symptoms. For example, is it justified to define the hearing of voices in schizophrenia as disturbances of perception if the person concerned hears the voices, not as coming from outside, but in their head or in some other part of their body? Another example, discussed below, is mood disturbance in people with melancholia.

Modern psychiatric classification, as it is represented in the glossaries of diagnostic classifications such as ICD and DSM, is characterized by two main developments. The first is the use of criteria instead of symptoms, the second the use of categories of disturbances, or 'disorders', instead of diseases (Kraus 1994; Sadler 1992). This is an important advance because in psychiatry, apart from cerebral organic diseases such as dementia, the notion of a symptom as relating to a well-defined underlying disease entity has become more and more questionable. In psychiatry, in consequence, the symptom as a sign of a specific disease entity has less value than in somatic medicine. In psychiatry, moreover, the symptom is often less specific and less precise. It cannot be 'isolated' from other aspects of the patient's experience as clearly as it can as in somatic medicine. Kurt Schneider (1967), therefore, argued that we should speak in psychiatry of characteristic traits (*Merkmale*) rather than of symptoms. Modern glossary diagnostics follow Schneider in speaking of criteria instead of symptoms. Thus, whereas in somatic medicine symptoms are used to characterize a given disease, leading to a definite explanation of the underlying dysfunction, criteria are used in psychiatry only to differentiate between diagnoses. If a certain number of criteria are met, and exclusion criteria not given, a particular disorder must be diagnosed.

However, this approach to diagnosis — important as it has been in detaching psychiatry from a naive medical model — has been achieved at the cost of trading validity for reliability (Spitzer and Degwitz 1986). Consistently with the concern to differentiate between disorders, criteria have been selected in order to be as reliable as possible. Because all symptoms cannot be equally well defined, the symptoms included in our glossaries have been selected for definability rather than for their centrality to the essence of the psychopathological entity (e.g. leaving out schizophrenic autism). The concern with exact definition favours, in particular, observable symptoms against phenomena of inner experience and sensations (as in psychotic experience). This entails not only an impoverishment in the range of descriptions of mental illness, but also of the richness and multiple meanings of the descriptive terms employed. The result is that neither the criteria used nor the diagnostic entities they define get close to the essence of the phenomena with which they are concerned. In focusing only on the limiting boundaries of diagnostic entities, our classifications tend to become over-inclusive, for example lumping together melancholic (endogenous) and reactive as well as neurotic forms of depression under the same category of 'depressive episode', the latter being differentiated mainly by degrees of severity. Because genetic, biological, and psychosocial factors, as well as responses to treatment, allegedly show little variation between these kinds of depression, quantitative differences were assumed to be more important for diagnosis than qualitative–phenomenal differences. The consequence has been that modern glossaries do not allow the possibility of expressing the clinical intuition of a change in the patient as a person and of his or her 'being-in-the-world'. Yet such intuitions could be cruial to more precise characterization of the clinically relevant features of the patient's experience. Monti and Stanghellini (1996) have compared the use of phenomenonology in this way with the sharpening of a psychopathological razor.

Schneider (1967) went so far as to question whether, in the case of endogenous psychoses, we are justified in speaking of a diagnosis at all. In the absence of biological markers and of identifiable causes, he said, we can take into account only psychological facts. For this reason he spoke of a 'differential typology' instead of a 'differential diagnosis'. Modern glossaries have followed him in this respect only in so far as they no longer claim to present a nosological but only a diagnostic system, even if many terms in the glossaries retain a nosological resonance (Tatossian 1996). Certainly Schneider (1967), in his proposal for a differential typology, had Max Weber's ideal types in mind. Jaspers (1965) differentiated diseases in the sense of a genus that can be related to an organic cause like paralysis from disorders such as endogenous psychosis, which he regarded as ideal types. Recently, Schwartz and Wiggins (1987) in the USA, Frommer (1996) in Germany, and Tatossian (1996) in France, have shown the importance of the concept of ideal types for diagnosis in psychiatry.

Yet another proposal for a typological system of classification in psychiatry builds on Wittgenstein's (1961) concept of family resemblances (Cantor *et al.* 1980; Blashfield *et al.* 1989). Without going into details, this approach is based on the observation that people with schizophrenia, for example, resemble one another, even though they have not a single symptom in common. All these typological approaches share the idea that the entities defined in psychiatric classification are prototypical concepts.

One of the advantages of a prototypical model of classification is that, unlike a deterministic, categorical system, no specific number of criteria is necessary and sufficient to assign a real case to a given category. A category is defined by certain traits coming together more often in that category than in others. Hence, all that can be said is that the more traits that are present in a given case, the closer the case corresponds to the prototype, and hence the more that case is typical of the category in question.

Phenomenonological–anthropological psychiatry has developed a further typological concept that has a notable affinity with the concepts mentioned above. As a typology of essences, it is derived from Husserl's '*Wesenschau*' (intuition of essences) and is strongly influenced by existential philosophy, particularly by the philosophy of Heidegger, Sartre, and Merleau-Ponty. In clinical applications we speak of phenomenological types or, if existential aspects are concerned, of existential types (Kraus 1991). The approach involves working out invariant features by imaginative variation.

Although differing in detail, each of these P-A approaches involves a more person-centred or holistic approach to diagnosis than the medical symptom-based approach. This is well illustrated by the existential approach just outlined (I come to some clinical examples in the next section). Thus, in this approach we seek to understand the general structure of the phenomena of a given disturbance in terms of the particular individual's 'being-in-the-world', that is the patient's relationship to him- or herself, to others, and to the world. Particular weight is laid upon the patient's actual experiences. Whereas S-C diagnosis is oriented to the morbus, this approach is oriented to the person. We try to understand the disturbance within the context of the whole person. As illustrated in the next section, we try to understand a disturbance of thought or of mood in schizophrenia and mania by an alteration of the whole 'being-in-the-world' of the person concerned.

An important question is the extent to which phenomenological or existential types overlap with our traditional entities of disease, or indeed underpin them, or may even help to define new ones. Many of our traditional entities are not founded on 'facts', but to a large extent on eidetic or constructive entities. Thus, the borders of these entities are often the 'borders of ideas'. It is not, however, only the way we establish our diagnostic entities, but also diagnosis itself that is called into question in psychiatry from these considerations. One can put in question whether even illness has the same meaning in psychiatry as in somatic medicine as Häfner (1983) seems to assume. An important argument for illness being different, not only in personality disorders but also in disorders such as endogenous psychosis, is that illness in psychiatry cannot be separated from the person to the patient. As we will see in the next section, this is true not only in respect of the consequences of the disorder for the patient, but also in its origin. One does not 'have' schizophrenia in the same way as one 'has' a somatic disease, because it is always also a kind of being.

To avoid speaking of 'schizophrenics' or 'hysterics, as, for instance, DSM-IV does, might have not only a scientific but also a humanistic rationale. However, excluding the subject as an agent in this way, in the context of his or her illness, can also be seen as a scientific prejudice, in that it neglects the most important human aspect of these disturbances as a kind of being. Mental illness is further discriminated from somatic in that its assessment implies value judgements to a much greater degree. As Fulford (1989) has shown, this is because psychiatry is concerned with aspects of human experience and behaviour in which values are highly and legitimately diverse. In Fulford's work, this is the basis of a quantitative rather than qualitative difference between mental illness and somatic illness. But it shows, again, the importance of the individual in psychiatry, of particular persons in specific cultural and social contexts, and in particular relations with others. Fulford shows how, contrary to a naive medical model, a number of mental disorders are actually defined by reference to social evaluative norms, by the expectations of society, by what is acceptable, age-appropriate, and so on.

Clinical examples

The following clinical examples illustrate how P-A methods relating to the 'being-in-the-world' of the person make it possible to derive more specific descriptions of phenomena relevant to psychopathology, and hence how phenomenological types can contribute to establishing diagnostic entities. This will lead, in the final section of the chapter, to a more detailed comparison between P-A and S-C diagnosis.

Melancholic depression

My first example is the diagnosis and classification of depression. The contemporary unitary model of depression in ICD-10 makes no division between melancholic, reactive, and psychogenic categories. This model thus assumes that the *quality* of depressive mood is identical in each of these groups. Even in other categories, such as schizophrenia and epilepsy, depressed mood is assumed to have the same quality. Quantitative differences in mood, according to the ICD-10 lexicon, are all that matters diagnostically. Indeed 'depressed mood' itself is quantitatively defined in ICD as 'lowered mood'. Depressed mood, following the glossary guidelines, is qualitatively identical even with sadness, yet this is inconsistent with the clinical experience of many psychiatrists who distinguish melancholic mood from normal sadness. Analogous to the so-called praecox feeling in schizophrenia there is a 'feeling of melancholia' (*Melancholiegefühl*). Earlier classifications, such as the DSM-III, spoke of a distinct *quality* of melancholic depression (although without elaborating on it). Patients themselves often differentiate their depression from ordinary feelings of sadness.

Some of the most common elements of the distinct quality of melancholic mood are listed in Table 13.1. The distinct quality is based in part on the ineffable character of the experience: patients cannot give a reason for their feelings, unlike in the case of ordinary sadness. They will say that there is a blunting, a loss of liveliness and vigour, and an alien quality that cannot be shaken off. The mood has an unremitting or overwhelming quality: it feels as though it is being forced upon the patient, who cannot distance himself from it or set it aside. He may also say it closes off access to 'himself', that he cannot be himself in this kind of mood. Indeed, he would rather like to be sad but cannot feel any emotions; he has no feelings at all. This is also the case with happy or pleasant occasions. The patient feels indifferent not only to his immediate surroundings but also to his family; and such indifference is itself a source of suffering. Even the perception of the world is less intense, plastic, or lively. Many patients will say that they feel their melancholic mood in a bodily way as a common weakness, often also in localized bodily feelings. It is a feeling of being enclosed in oneself. Every action is so demanding and exhausting. One cannot differentiate this inhibition from one's altered mood. The clinician, consistently with these descriptions given by the patient, will observe a certain numbness and rigidity, an invariability in the patient's mood. The patient often shows no facial movement or weeping as would be expected in other states of sadness, such as mourning. There may also be an inability to generate emotions and cognitions in opposition to the melancholic mood — what I have called 'intolerance of ambiguity' (Kraus 1988).

All these phenomena are not usually found in other kinds of depression or in sadness. Their presence does not necessarily mean a high severity of being depressed, as the ICD-10 glossary assumes. There are also melancholic states of

Table 13.1 The qualities of melancholic mood

The melancholic experiences the altered mood as forced upon him or her.
The patient has no access to it.
Inability to 'be' him or herself in the depressed mood.
A feeling of bluntness and liveliness, and of strangeness.
Being depressed is without reason.
The patient has no influence on the mood.
The patient cannot differentiate it from a common inhibition.
It is to a large extent invariable.
The patient is unable to develop emotions and cognitions opposite to the melancholic mood (intolerance of ambiguity).
The patient cannot achieve a distance from it.
Inability to behave sadly (cannot weep, facial expression is without emotion, etc.).
The melancholic mood is experienced in a bodily way as a common weakness, etc., but also in localized bodily feelings.

low severity. At its core, the melancholic mood alteration is — paradoxically formulated — rather a lack of mood. Normally there is a feeling of oneself in every kind of mood, but the melancholic patient, by contrast, usually reports a strangeness, a lack of capacity to be himself in this kind of mood. The core of melancholia, then, involves what in phenomenology is called a loss of ipseity, a kind of depersonalization, distinct from the concept of depressed mood. We speak of a melancholic depersonalization (Kraus 2002). This does not exclude a depressed mood from also being present. However, depressed mood is not what is specific to melancholia and what differentiates it from other states of depression.

I have argued elsewhere (Kraus 2002) that a kind of depersonalization is the structural characteristic also of other phenomena of melancholia, such as disturbance of drive, melancholic delusion, etc. I cannot go into details here, but if a kind of depersonalization does prove to be a common characteristic of all melancholic phenomena, this would unify all these phenomena within a certain phenomenological type. Such a type would be a distinct diagnostic entity in the sense of P-A diagnostics.

Mania

In mania as well as in depressive states, we find in the glossary to ICD a number of criteria that are not integrated with one another. Each of these criteria, moreover, may be satisfied by many normal individuals as well as by individuals in other diagnostic categories. Take, for example, the criterion 'loss of usual social inhibitions'. What the trained phenomenological diagnostician perceives in the manic patient is not only her (disinhibited) behaviour as such, but also the fact that the behaviour emerges from a different kind of relationship to herself and others. The manic patient fails to acknowledge her real role as well as the roles of others in a given situation.

Binswanger (1960) described this as an inability of the patient with mania to 'appresent' (Binswanger's term) herself, and others, as a partner, a mother, a patient, and so on. In the light of modern role-theory we can say that there is a loss of reciprocity in social roles. This reciprocity is evident e.g. in me speaking to you and in you hearing me, or, in driving, between road-users. In every social situation we develop an objective identity that is legitimated by its reciprocity with the social roles of others and by the fulfilment of the respective role-expectancies of our role-partners. But the patient with mania experiences this reciprocity as a restriction of her identity. In order to expand her identity, she rejects every determination by her real social roles, negating these in favour of a harmonizing 'oneness' of ego and world. This is very different from other kinds of loss of distance in everyday life in that, because of her altered way of 'being-in-the-world', the patient with mania cannot behave in any other way.

This change of being and consequent loss of freedom is 'co-experienced' — *'miterfahren'*, as Jaspers (1965) says — if we qualify a lack or loss of distance, which as such is non-specific, specifically as a manic behaviour. This holistic experience of a different constitution of the 'being-in-the-world' of the patient with mania allows a diagnosis to be made not from outside, but from the side of the patient, from the side of his or her self-realization. This makes it possible also to understand in part the patient's loss of social inhibition and thus to develop a better therapeutic relationship.

Hysterical or histrionic personality disorder

My third example shows how phenomenological types can be established as diagnostic entities (Kraus 1996). ICD-10 and DSM-IV employ the term 'histrionic'. For reasons mentioned above we use the traditional terms of 'hysterical' and 'hysteria'. The less specific term, histrionic, associates theatrical behaviour with a disturbance.

ICD-10 lists six criteria for this disorder (a–f):

a) self-dramatization, theatricality, exaggerated expression of emotion;

b) suggestivity;

c) shallow and labile affectivity;

d) continual seeking for excitement and activities in which the patient is the centre of attention, etc.;

e) inappropriate seductivity in appearance or behaviour;

f) over-concern with physical attractiveness.

As with depression and mania, the number of criteria is arbitrary and there is no interconnection between them. In contrast to this criteriological approach to diagnosis, P-A diagnosis refers a single phenomenon to the uniformity of a certain 'being-in-the-world'. The structure of this particular kind of being is a failure by the patient to identify with his or her actual being (Kraus 1996). This failure of identification may be misunderstood because the psychoanalytical literature maintains that people with hysterical characters show a strong tendency to identifications with others (e.g. Fenichel 1945; Schilder 1939). But these identifications with others, expressed through easily interchangeable roles, are possible only because the hysterical character is not, or is only partly, identified with him- or herself. Eidelberg (1938) called this pseudo-identification. The specific effect of countertransference (described by Hoffman 1979), the impression of being fragmented, fragile, and contradictory, is based on this failure of identification. This structure of 'non-identification' unifies all single phenomena, the behaviours, feelings, and emotional expressions listed in ICD and DSM criteria; it gives them more specificity and makes them understandable as the expression of a certain type of being-in-the-world.

The phenomenological structure of non-identification in people with hysteria is best described by Jaspers. Referring to the 'hysterical personality', he wrote: 'Instead of being content with its talents and possibilities . . . [*it has*] . . . the need to appear to itself and to others as being more than it is, to experience more than it is capable of experiencing (Jaspers 1965, p. 370). That means the person is not what he is pretending to be. The hysterical person looks at himself as he has manipulated others to see him; he deceives himself and others by pretending feelings he actually does not have. Exclusively determined by wishes and needs, he lives in a dominating future with little anchor in the past and present.

This phenomenological account differs in two respects from the account of hysterical personality in ICD-10. First, the ICD-10 describes the histrionic personality mainly in terms of behaviours opposed to an outside world. Phenomenological description, by contrast, adds the relationship of the person to himself, not only in the sense of a centricity to self, of self-indulgence and so on, but of self-*deception*, what J. P. Sartre (1943) called '*mauvaise foi*' — bad faith. The second difference is about integration and wholeness. Each ICD criterion of histrionic personality disorder can also be found in normal people: for instance, the criterion (e), of inappropriate seductivity in appearance or behaviour, or (f) over-concern with physical attractiveness. All of these criteria can also be found in other disturbances, such as mania. In the latter case this can lead to the diagnosis of an additional personality disorder. In phenomenological diagnosis the structural characteristic of non-identification is common to all the phenomena of the hysterical personality. Therefore, the lack of this structural characteristic would preclude characterizing an isolated behaviour as hysterical; in the case of a mania, it would suggest rather a pseudo-hysterical manic symptom.

Phenomenological and criteriological approaches to diagnosis also provide different understandings of the relationship between hysterical personality disorder and conversion and dissociative disorders (e.g. a 'paralysed' arm with no neurological cause). ICD-10 identifies dissociation and conversion already as such as hysterical disorders, distinguishing them sharply from histrionic personality disorder. P-A diagnosis suggests that in certain cases conversion and dissociation may be an expression of the hysterical personality's non-identification, namely, in this case, treating his or her own body like a quasi-object, the body of someone else. However, mechanisms of dissociation and conversion may, under traumatic circumstances, be possible in everyone, even in animals as an acute reaction, and need not be combined with a lasting self-deception (Kretschmer 1974). Such mechanisms are thus not uniquely hysterical in origin. In hysterical personalities we always find dissociation within the frame of a non-relationship with themselves, in so far as the person concerned denies real problems and difficulties, being also dissociated from his real emotional, cognitive, and volitional states. Self-deception is thus essential to specifically hysterical dissociation. Correspondingly, the diagnosis of hysterical personality disorder and hysterical symptoms, or its replacement with other terms, cannot avoid taking into consideration the changed relation of the individual to him or herself. The true pathological element in hysteria as well as in Mania and in melancholia is not the behaviour as such, but the restricted capacity of behaving in another way, which is founded in a changed way of being, a changed relationship to one's own being. This changed 'being-in-the-world' is worked out in so-called phenomenological or existential types (Kraus 1991). It presupposes an existential understanding of human identity as a dialectical relationship between non-identity and identity. This dialectic of giving up identifications but also of identifying anew through the facticity of one's real being is given up in hysteria. This non-identification in hysteria can be opposed to other existential types, for example to the over-identification with one's being found in melancholia (Kraus 1991).

With the establishment of phenomenological or existential types, an anthropological understanding of these disturbances is to some extent possible, relating it to the general conditions of our 'being-in-the-world'. In this way, psychiatric classification can be founded, in part, on philosophical anthropology.

Overview and conclusions

In this chapter I have outlined some of the main differences between phenomenological–anthropological (P-A) and symptomatological–criteriological (S-C) diagnosis. These are summarized in Table 13.2. Thus, P-A diagnosis is oriented to the eidos of the phenomena, to the person, to his or her life world, and to the subjective experience of disturbance. Hence, in P-A diagnosis, the disturbance has the status of 'being', whereas in S-C diagnosis the disturbance has the status of 'having'. In S-C diagnostics, furthermore, the distinct and complex phenomena of a disturbance are reduced to easily definable and (fairly) reliable criteria, defined by inclusion and exclusion criteria, which have no interrelationship of meaning. Objectifiable behavioural aspects, therefore, are in the foreground. The model of disturbance or disease is that of somatic medicine. In P-A diagnostics, by contrast, the phenomena describe particular modes of experience and behaviour, which are understood in a unified way as expressions of specific phenomenological or existential types of relationship of the patient to him or herself, to others, and to the world.

The acquisition of all this information about the patient as a person, and about the life-world, requires a very different patient–diagnostician relationship. In S-C diagnosis the patient is mainly a supplier of data, which the diagnostician has to relate to the pre-given prescriptions of the glossary in order to make a diagnosis. To carry out this objectifying function, then, the S-C diagnostician needs to have a certain distance from the patient. In P-A diagnostics, by contrast, the diagnostician has a more engaged function,

Table 13.2 Summary of differences between P-A and S-C diagnosis

Phenomenological–anthropological	Symptomatological–criteriological
Holistic; oriented to the life-world 'logos' of the phenomenon	Reductive
Being ill as a subjective experience (illness, *mal*, *affection*, *Kranksein*); category of being	Disease (medical model of body medicine) (disturbance, *maladie*, *Krankheit*); category of having
Psychopathological: entity as an ideal phenomenological or existential type	Psychopathological: entity as a generic concept
Oriented to the person as a subject, to the history of the individual — *maladie de la personne* (Lacan); *Lebensgeschichte* (Binswanger)	Oriented to the 'morbus', to the function of the body — *maladie de la fonction* (Lacan); *Lebensfunktion* (Binswanger)
Phenomenon: reveals itself without theoretical presupposition; certain kinds of experience and behaviour as expression of a certain relationship to one's self to the world and to others	Symptoms as the result of some dysfunction; inclusive and exclusive criteria; related to a medical concept of disease
Single phenomenon: points directly to the whole diagnostic entity; is determined qualitatively by the whole; has a special quality in different disturbances	Single criterion: has a decisive importance only in correlation with other criteria; can be the same element in different disturbance entities
Internal connection of single phenomena; diagnostic entity as an integral whole	No internal connection of the criteria; diagnostic entity as a serial summing up formula
Weight lies on form	Weight lies on content
Weight lies on validity	Weight lies on reliability
Exchange of profound experience is possible	Exchange of profound experience is not possible
Experiencing subject is in the centre; subjective experience is a criterion of verification	Subjectivity is excluded; subjective experience is not a criterion of verification
Experience: of something new; can cross expectancies; has an open end	Experience: controllable; repeatable; expectancies are confirmed or not
Patient is an active partner in diagnostic process, capable of orienting, theorizing, and interpreting; shows him or herself from the side of freedom and relation to the future	Patient is a supplier of data; is mainly an object of investigation
Investigator is to a large extent dependent on the cooperation of the patient	Investigator is more independent of the patient

helping the patient to describe his disturbance as precisely as possible, but also to understand and interpret it to a certain degree. This is possible only if the diagnostician has a close relationship to the patient. Similarly, in S-C diagnostics the diagnostician has to assess in a straight-line way whether the patient does or does not have certain symptoms which satisfy or not certain criteria, in order to verify or falsify a diagnosis, whereas in P-A diagnostics the diagnostician has to carry out the movement of a 'hermeneutic circle'. This is an interactive process, through which the meaning of a patient's experience of disorder is progressively explored by proceeding from a particular experience to an evolving holistic understanding and then back again to the single phenomenon.

What, then, do we gain from P-A diagnosis? The examples outlined above suggest that, at the level of diagnosis itself, P-A diagnosis provides a fuller and more specific description of the phenomena of mental disorder; thus, in the first example, P-A diagnosis helped to identify the features that differentiate melancholia from other forms of depression and from normal sadness. In P-A diagnosis, then, the emphasis is on validity, whereas in S-C diagnosis it is on reliability. The phenomenological or existential types described above for mania and hysterical personality disorder, furthermore, suggest unifying structures underlying the otherwise unrelated symptoms or criteria by which these disorders are defined in ICD and DSM. These structures — or 'psychopathological organizers' as Monti and Stanghellini (1996) call them — may indeed be central to distinguishing pathological from normal forms of these symptoms.

The very different relationship between patient and diagnostician required by P-A diagnosis may be important also for psychotherapy and rehabilitation. In both of these areas it is important that the patient is seen not merely as a bearer of symptoms, as the object or victim of an illness, but also (as in phenomenological diagnostics) as somebody who is capable of initiating behaviour, of action, of reflection, and so on. The guidelines and norms of rehabilitation and psychotherapy thus connect directly with the diagnostic process itself. Similarly, because forensic psychiatry has mainly to do with the *incapacity* to behave in accordance with social norms, P-A diagnosis is also of significance for this field. Tatossian (1996) was right in saying that operational criteria are not sufficient when it comes to assessing the capacity of a patient to act freely.

Finally, fruitful connections with empirical research are also possible, as Sadler (1992) and Mundt and Spitzer (1997) demonstrated. In this respect, Fulford's (1989) demonstration of the role of value judgements in the meanings even of such 'scientific' concepts as disease and dysfunction offers a clear link between analytical philosophy and phenomenological anthropology. Value judgements are particularly important in P-A diagnostics, but it is a particular endeavour of P-A psychiatry to keep these under control by clarifying the relevant anthropological presuppositions. Even if phenomenological or existential types as such are not identic with real or natural entities of diseases related to certain causes, they can pave the way for finding these in a similar way as K. Jaspers (1965) showed with his ideal-types.

Far from being antithetical then, as many on both sides have believed, P-A and S-C diagnosis offer complementary approaches to diagnosis and classification in psychiatry. The current dominance of the S-C approach makes it all the more important that we develop rigorous methods for the P-A characterization of mental distress and disorder as meaningful experiences of individual human beings.

Further Reading

Overviews in English of the significance of the P-A approach for psychiatry in general are given by Blankenburg (1980) and Kraus (2001), and specifically for diagnosis and classification by Kraus (1994), Mishara (1994), and Parnas and Zahavi (2002).

References

Binswanger, L. (1956). *Drei Formen missglückten Daseins*. Tübingen: Niemeyer.

Binswanger, L. (1960). *Melancholie und Manie*. Pfullingen: Neske.

Blankenburg, W. (1980). Anthropologisch orientierte psychiatrie. pp. 182–97. In: Ergebrine für die Medizin. Z. Psychiatrie Die Psychologie des 20. Jahrhunder, vol. X (ed. U. Peters). Zurich: Kindler.

Blankenburg, W. (1982). A dialectical conception of anthropological proportion. In: *Phenomenology and Psychiatry* (ed. A. J. J. De Koning and F. A. Jenner), pp. 35–50. London: Academic Press.

Blankenburg, W. (1991). Phänomenologie als Grundlagendisziplin der Psychiatrie. *Fundamenta Psychiatrica*, **5**: 92–101.

Blashfield, R. K., Sprock, J., Haymaker, D., and Hodgin, J. (1989). The family resemblance hypothesis applied to psychiatric classification. *Journal of Nervous and Mental Disease*, **177**: 492–7.

Cantor, N., Smith, E., French, R., and Mezzich, J. (1980). Psychiatric diagnosis as prototype categorization. *Journal of Abnormal and Social Psychology*, **89**: 181–93.

Eidelberg, L. (1938). Pseudo-identification. *International Journal of Psychoanalysis*, **19**: 321–30.

Fenichel, O. (1945). *The Psychoanalytic Theory of Neurosis*. New York: W. W. Norton.

Frommer, J. (1996). Charakterisierung der eigenen Persönlichkeit und subjektive Krankheitsvorstellungen: Ihre Bedeutung für die klinische Diagnostik. In: *Psychopathologische Methoden und psychiatrische Forschung*. (ed. H. Sass.) Jena Stuttgart: G. Fischer.

Fulford, K. W. M. (1989). *Moral Theory and Medical Practice*. Cambridge: Cambridge University Press.

Häfner, H. (1983). Allgemeine und spezielle Krankheitsbegriffe in der Psychiatrie. *Nervenarzt*, **54**: 231–8.

Heidegger, M. (1962). *Being and Time* (trans. J. MacQarrie and E. Robinson). New York: Harper & Row.

Hoffmann, S. O. (1979). *Charakter und Neurose*. Frankfurt: Suhrkamp.

Jaspers, K. (1965). *Allgemeine Psychopathologie*. Berlin: Springer.

Kraus, A. (1988). Ambiguitätsintoleranz als Persönlichkeitsvariable und Strukturmerkmal der Krankheitsphänomene Manisch-Depressiver. pp. 140–9. In: *Persönlichkeit und Psychose* (ed. W. Janzarik). Stuttgart: Enke.

Kraus, A. (1991). Methodological problems with the classification of personality disorders: the significance of existential types. *Journal of Personality Disorders*, **5**: 82–92.

Kraus, A. (1996). Identitätsbildung Melancholischer und Hysterischer. In: *Hysterie Heute* (ed. G. H. Seidler), pp. 103–10. Stuttgart: Ferdinand.

Kraus, A. (1994). Phenomenological and criteriological diagnosis. Different or complementary? In: *Philosophical Perspectives on Psychiatric Diagnostic Classification* (ed. J. Z. Sadler, O. P. Wiggins, and M. A. Schwartz), pp.148–60. Baltimore: John Hopkins University Press.

Kraus, A. (2001). Phenomenological–anthropological psychiatry. In: *Contemporary Psychiatry Vol. 1: Foundations of Psychiatry* (ed. F. Henn, N. Sartorius, H. Helmchen, and H. Lauter), pp. 340–55. Berkin: Springer.

Kraus, A. (2002). Melancholie: eine Art von Depersonalisation? In: Affect und Affektive Störing (ed. Th. Fuchs). Paderborn: Schöring.

Kretschmer, E. (1974). *Hysterie, Reflex und Instinkt*. Stuttgart: Thieme.

Mishara, A. (1994). A phenomenological critique of commonsensical assumptions in DSM III-R: the avoidance of the patient's subjectivity. In: *Philosophical Perspectives on Psychiatric Diagnostic Classification* (ed. J. Z. Sadler, O. P. Wiggins, and M. A. Schwartz), pp. 129–47. London: John Hopkins University Press.

Monti, E. P. and Stanghellini, G. (1996). Psychopathology: an edgeless razor? *Comprehensive Psychiatry*, **3**: 196–204.

Mundt, C. and Spitzer, M. (1997). Psychologie heute. In: *Pychiatrie der Gegenwart, 4. Auflage, Band 1: Psychopathologie* (ed. H. Helmchen, F. Henn, H. Lauter, and N. Sartorius). Berlin: Springer.

Needleman, J. (1963). *Being-In-The-World. Selected Papers of Ludwig Binswanger*. New York: Harper & Row.

Parnas, J. and Zahavi, D. (2002). The role of phenomenology in psychiatric diagnosis and classification. In: *Psychiatric Diagnosis and Classification* (ed. C. M. Mai, W. Gaebel, J. J. López, and N. Sartorius). Chichester, UK: J. Wiley.

Rovaletti, M. L. (2000). The phenomenological perspective in the clinic: from symptom to phenomena. *Comprendre III*.

Sadler, J. Z. (1992). Eidetic and empirical research. A hermeneutic complementarity. In: *Phenomenology, Language and Schizophrenia*. New York: Springer.

Sartre, J. P. (1943). *L'être et le Néant*. Paris: Gallimard.

Schilder, P. (1939). The concept of hysteria. *American Journal of Psychiatry*, **95**: 1389–413.

Schneider, K. (1967). *Klinische Psychopathologie*. Stuttgart: Thieme.

Schwartz, M. A. and Wiggins, O. P. (1987). Diagnosis and ideal types: a contribution to psychiatric classification. *Comprehensive Psychiatry*, **28**(4): 277–91.

Spitzer, M. and Degwitz, R. (1986). Zur diagnose des DSM-III. *Nervenarzt*, **57**: 698–704.

Tatossian, A. (1996). Troubles affectivs et schizophrenie: aspects coneptuels synopse. Numeró Special.

van Praag, H. M. (2000). Functionalization of psychiatric diagnosis or providing biological psychiatry research with a stable foundation. *Temas*, **58**: 79–97.

Wittgenstein, L. (1961). *Tractatus Logico-philosophicus*. London: Routledge & Kegan Paul.

14 Incomprehensibility

Markus Heinimaa

Introduction

This chapter is from a series of studies in the philosophy of psychiatry that investigate the logic of some central psychiatric concepts, such as 'psychosis' (Heinimaa 2000*a*), 'delusion' (Heinimaa, in press), 'understanding', and 'person' (Heinimaa 2000*b*). The key theme to emerge from these studies is the centrality of the grammar of 'understanding' and concepts related to its absence or demise (e.g. 'incomprehensibility') in describing the philosophical grammar of these concepts. In what follows, and for the purpose of having a clearer picture of the grammar of 'understanding', we look at the concepts indicating radical failures of understanding and study the logic of 'incomprehensibility' in the light of the illumination provided by Lars Hertzberg, Cora Diamond, Ludwig Wittgenstein, and Peter Winch. Some implications of the logical distinctions made to understanding psychiatric conceptualisations are drawn.

Concern about 'incomprehensibility' is not entirely absent from the psychiatric literature. Karl Jaspers' work (1959) is notorious in making the clinical distinction between the understandable delusions of affective psychoses and the 'essentially incomprehensible' delusions of schizophrenia to a central nosological element; for Jaspers, this is the distinction between essentially incomprehensible disease processes as against understandable psychological reactions and development (Blankenburg 1984). The influence of this delineation was strong in pre-war German psychiatric literature. Notwithstanding occasional attempts to raise the issue (Oppenheimer 1974), the recent period of Anglo-American dominance in psychiatric thinking has mostly neglected the whole issue (Corin and Lauzon 1992) — if not proposing its deliberate suppression (Jenner *et al.* 1986; Roberts 1992). Nevertheless, the intrinsic presence of this concept remains ubiquitous in psychiatric discourse and psychiatric classifications; DSM-IV (*Diagnostic and Statistical Manual of Mental Disorders*, 4th edition), for instance, draws heavily on 'incomprehensibility' when describing the diagnosis of schizophrenia (American Psychiatric Association 1994, p. 276).

Psychiatric concepts and incomprehensibility

What is the content of the claim that psychiatric conceptions are internally connected to 'incomprehensibility'? The concept is most clearly evident with bizarre delusional psychopathology. It is seen, for example, in the following description of a patient who, while staying in the clinic for months, never once looked up but all the time kept his eyes turned down and commented on this himself (Callieri 1960, p. 254):

> Früher streckte mein Auge sich vorwärts und ich sah die Realität ver-schwommen, verdunkelt, verfinstert. Dann waren es für mich Anstrengung und Mühe, die Umwelt genauer zu sehen; aber ich sah alles wie eine Fläche, wie ein Gemälde: das Auge wünschte nicht mehr dort hinten in die Tiefe zu sehen. Nun ist das Auge gesunken, ist niedergegangen, hat für sich Raum und Platz *unten* gewonnen und hat sich dem Niederen angepaßt . . . immer besser paßtes sich an, immer bequemer, immer tiefer; es schaut klar im Niederen, ganz unklar aber in der Höhe. Die Höhe ist ihm verhindert. Ich bin jedoch überzeugt, daßes unaufhörlich kämpft, und ich meine, daßes ihm nach und nach gelingen wird, sich aufzurichten . . .[1]

The patient describes how 'the eye' (not 'his eye', emphasizing the exteriority of the eye to his person) earlier used to reach forward and found reality vague, obscured, and darkened, difficult to perceive clearly, with flat appearance like a painting. And he explains that 'the eye' did not wish to see into this depth, that 'the eye' has sunk, it has gone down, and has found place and space for itself from underneath, and it has adjusted to below, being more and more comfortable with this. He also remarks that he is certain that 'the eye' is fighting relentlessly to look up and will in the end succeed in this.

Assessing this clinical note, we are struck not only by the peculiarity of the description of this 'eye-as-a-separate-person', but also by the quality of self-evident factuality in the patient's description of his circumstances. The otherness of 'the eye', and his struggle with it, is difficult to fathom and some-what eerie. It seems clear that we would be at quite a loss in describing our impressions of this patient if we did not have concepts such as 'strange, odd, bizarre, and incomprehensible' at our disposal.

In studying the role of incomprehensibility in psychiatric discourse, concepts such as 'madness' and 'psychosis' are the most obvious candidates

---

[1] Earlier my eye stretched itself forwards and I saw reality blurred, obscured, and darkened. Then to me, it was exertion and effort to see the environment more exactly, but I saw everything like a flat area, like a painting: the eye no longer wished to look further into the depth. Now the eye has sunken, it has gone down, and has won for itself place and space from *underneath*, and it has adjusted to below . . . better and better it adapts itself, ever more comfortable, ever deeper; it sees clearly down there, very unclearly, however, into the height. The height is kept from it. However, I am convinced that it fights relentlessly, and I think that it will, succeed in straightening itself little by little. (Callieri 1960, p. 254, trans. M.H.).

on which to focus. With 'madness', the conceptual connection seems unproblematic enough. It can also be shown that the connections between 'madness' and 'psychosis' are not only historical but conceptual. In an earlier paper (Heinimaa 2000a), I discussed the question 'What is psychosis?' from the conceptual point of view. Taking into account both the historical development of 'psychosis' and the definitions given to it in modern psychiatric nosology (DSM-III-R, DSM-IV, International Classification of Diseases (ICD) 10), the close connections between the grammar of psychosis and the grammars of 'understanding' and 'person' become evident.

According to the analysis presented in Heinimaa (2000a), psychosis is connected with the factual reporting of incomprehensibility (i.e. stating as a generally valid fact that a patient and/or his or her expression are incomprehensible, not understandable), and the uses of the concept 'psychosis' mark the very limits of a person's intelligibility to others as an understandable person.

Recently, there has been a tendency towards narrower and disorder-specific definitions of psychosis (DSM-IV gives five different syndrome-dependent definitions of psychotic symptoms); nevertheless, the concrete descriptions and guidelines on how to use the concept have to rely on 'incomprehensibility' to be practically applicable (Fulford 1989; Rudnick 1997).

The concept of delusion is also an important tool in the vocabulary of psychiatry. Not only 'bizarre delusion', as above, but also 'delusion' itself is a concept whose grammar is beyond adequate description, if we refrain from referring to the 'incomprehensibility' of certain linguistic moves or acts (David 1999, Heinimaa in press). Empirical psychiatric research has addressed the problems inherent in including the presence of 'bizarre delusions' as a strong criterion of the diagnosis of schizophrenia. In particular, the criterion has been shown to have poor inter-rater reliability (Flaum *et al.* 1991) and the option of dropping it altogether has been put forward (Goldman *et al.* 1992). No further general discussion on the logic of this criterion has nevertheless ensued.

Louise Silvern, in her paper, 'A hermeneutic account of psychology' (Silvern 1990), points out how, besides psychosis, other psychiatric illness concepts (e.g. 'neurosis') may involve changes in psychological functioning that are conceived as incomprehensible. Likewise, according to Jaspers, in every neurosis there is a point at which the person in good health no longer understands the patient and is accustomed to consider the patient, if not 'mad', at least with certain qualifications as basically 'mentally disturbed' (Jenner *et al.* 1986). Also, whenever the limits between 'normal psychological reactions' and pathological phenomena are discussed, the writers in one or other way seem to be obliged to discuss the limits of understanding involved in the pathological phenomena (see, for instance, Kopelman (1994) on drawing the boundary between grief reactions and depression).

German Berrios (1991), in his critical account of Jasper's influence on psychiatry, contests the significance of 'incomprehensibility' as, according to him, this is subject to the state of art of psychological theory and thus a contingent condition of psychiatric morbidity (p. 10):

> It is clear, that the assessment of comprehensibility depends on the state of progress of psychological theory: delusions incomprehensible today may not be so tomorrow

Berrios' dismissal, however, does not seem pertinent in this context: His criticism concerns the theoretical significance of 'incomprehensibility', that is, its significance for the theory of psychopathology, which according to him might be subject to changes in psychological theory ('might' — even this contention has to be made with some reservations), but not its philosophical significance (which field of questioning is not limited to what is 'psychological').

Gadamer (1993), on the other hand, in his paper 'Hermeneutik und Psychiatrie', acknowledges the question as a substantial one, but warns of the extremely thin ice on which we are walking when discussing psychiatric phenomena in these terms (pp. 207–9):

> ... in der Erfahrung des Berufslebens, begegnet dem Psychiater solche Unverständlichkeit und Unheimlichkeit, die ihm Wahnsinn als seelische und geistige Erkrankung bedeutet ... Ist es noch verständlich oder ist es unverständlich, wenn Nietzsche as 'Dionysos oer der Gekreuzigte' unterzeichnet hat? Der Begriff der Verständlichkeit erweist sich als äusserst vage.[2]

According to Gadamer, a psychiatrist meets in his work with incomprehensibility and uncanniness that means to him madness as a mental or spiritual illness. Gadamer also points out how concepts as rigid as incomprehensibility, even when concerning a person who escapes all attempts at understanding, are close to unacceptable in connection with human life.

In summary, we see that the concept of incomprehensibility lies like a hidden thread in the linen of psychiatric discourse, cutting across nosological categories and becoming ever more clearly significant the closer we move towards concrete psychiatric discourse.

The meaning of 'incomprehensibility'

Given the conceptual connections between 'incomprehensibility' and psychiatric concepts, what are the consequences of this logical point? I

---

[2] '... in the experiences of professional life, the psychiatrist meets with such unintelligibility and uncanniness, that means to him insanity as a mental and spiritual disease. Is it yet understandable, or is it incomprehensible, when Nietzsche signed [letters] as "Dionysos or the crucified"? The concept of understandability proves to be extremely vague.' (Gadamer 1993, pp. 207–9, trans. M.H.).

tackle this question by asking about the meaning of the concept. A natural strategy is to discuss the logical features of this concept by comparing it with 'understanding'.

The connections between 'understanding' and 'incomprehensibility' are not as straightforward as one might think. Lars Hertzberg, a Finnish philosopher with a long-term interest in Wittgenstein's philosophy and conceptual issues in the human sciences, has discussed the logic of understanding in his paper 'Förståelsen och dess gränser' (Hertzberg 1995) ('Understanding and its limits'). He points out that there are (at least) three different kinds of failures of understanding:

1. Misunderstanding: 'He misunderstands the instructions.'
2. Not-understanding: 'He fails to understand the instructions, however much he ever tries.'
3. Incomprehension: 'He finds the instructions are incomprehensible.'

We can further characterize these cases in terms of the kind of understanding involved, as follows:

(1) misunderstanding as a form of understanding;

(2) not-understanding as a privation of understanding;

(3) incomprehensibility as an understanding that there is nothing to understand.

The first case appears to be of little concern to us: misunderstanding can be interpreted as a variant (although incorrect) understanding and it is thus on the same logical level as 'understanding' itself. The distinction between cases 2 and 3, and their logical features, is less clear, and the third case is of specific interest here: is it reasonable to conceive of 'incomprehensibility' in terms of a specific form of 'understanding'?

In psychiatric work it is a common experience that there are cases where we experience a shift from conceiving things in terms of 'not-understanding' to 'understanding'. Often we are also prone to experience that not-understanding had to do with certain features of our interaction, certain 'obstacles' to understanding, which then cleared away — possibly due to systematic efforts to obtain a clearer idea of things concerned, or due to better communication with the patient. After the fact, we may interpret that the non-understanding was a case of misunderstanding: maybe we missed some vital information or misinterpreted it for a while. And we may also be prone to take this as a paradigm for dealing with all cases of not-understanding.

Hayward and Taylor (1956) exemplify this clinical experience in the following extract from a rich account of the experiences of a patient with schizophrenia and a therapist in the course of intensive psychotherapy (p. 222):

> In the past there has been a tendency to dismiss the patient as using 'neologisms' or 'bizarre gestures' or the like. Actually, if the therapist will take the time to listen to the patient, or observe him minutely, over a prolonged period, he will begin to see 'method in the madness'.

Hayward and Taylor point out that dismissive attitudes towards patients' expressions and an unwillingness to give prolonged attention to patients' expressions or behaviour are clinical obstacles to more accurate understanding of their communications. Their account also implies that one could speak of a kind of misunderstanding here, although a rather complex one, relating to a lack of attention and willingness really to hear a patient's point in her communications.

However, these conclusions cannot do away with the fact that we were obliged to use the concept of not-understanding to make our point, to open ourselves to the question of understandability. Recognizing a 'problem for understanding' requires that we use 'not-understanding' in some circumstances. And here the ambiguity of not-understanding emerges: what do we do when we say that the patient's speech is incomprehensible? Is this an expression for the lack of determination of meaning (case 2) or are we expressing a somehow definite understanding of not-understanding (case 3)?

An example of case 2, lack of determination of meaning, is found in the following clinical note, in which Hayward and Taylor (1956) describe the kind of 'suspension of comprehension' that the therapist may experience when dealing with the communications of a patient (p. 226):

> It cannot be emphasised too much how difficult it is to be aware of many of these problems when working with a patient who gives little or no verbal explanation. Rather the therapist has to resign himself to feeling like a person travelling backward. He can see a good deal of where he has been but it is often impossible to see where he is or where he is going.

In Hayward and Taylor's account, the therapist 'has to resign himself' to temporary lack of comprehension; 'incomprehensibility' might be used in this case in the sense of 'lacking determination of meaning'. In practice, the therapist probably wavers between judging the communications she is involved in as being *somehow* understandable, as being incomprehensible but potentially comprehensible, and as being simply incomprehensible — but possibly it is just this wavering that might be expressed in using 'incomprehensibility' in this sense.

For a clinical example of case 3, of not-understanding as a definite understanding, consider Jaspers' original description of the distinction between understandable forms of psychopathology and essentially incomprehensible schizophrenic pathology (Jaspers 1959, p. 483):

> Das [einfühlbar, verständlich] pathologische Seelenleben . . . können wir anschaulich erfassen als Steigerung oder Herabsetzung uns bekannter Phänomene und als Auftreten solcher Phänomene ohne die normalen Gründe und Motive. Das [auf eigene Weise unverständlich, im wahren Sinne ver-

rückt, schizophren] pathologische Seelenleben . . . erfassen wir auf diese Weise unzureichend. Es treten hier vielmehr Veränderungen allgemeinster Art auf, die wir nicht anschaulich miterleben können, die wir jedoch von außen irgendwie fassbar zu machen suchen.[3]

Here, Jaspers makes the distinction between emotionally approachable and understandable pathology, in which morbid psychical changes can be clearly comprehended as exaggeration or diminution of familiar phenomena or as their appearance without normal reasons or motives, and peculiarly incomprehensible, in real sense 'insane' schizophrenic pathology, in which this kind of understanding is not sufficient. He continues that here changes of a very general nature appear, which cannot be empathized with, but which we nevertheless try to make comprehensible from the outside. The implications of Jaspers' account are clear: he states as an empirical fact that some psychiatric phenomena are basically incomprehensible and can be approached only from the outside. Thus the 'un-understandability' of relevant clinical phenomena is a definite understanding of their incomprehensibility.

Having demonstrated the clinical relevance of this distinction, the meaning of this ambiguity is discussed below in the illuminations given by the writings of Cora Diamond, Ludwig Wittgenstein and Peter Winch.

Diamond on nonsense

First, to elucidate this inherent ambiguity of 'incomprehensibility', we use as our guide Diamond's well-known paper, 'What nonsense might be' (Diamond 1986). The reasoning in this paper is particularly helpful to discussions of 'incomprehensibility' (see also Hertzberg 2001). Diamond starts her discussion with two examples of nonsense sentences:

1. Caesar is a prime number.
2. Scott kept a runcible in Abbottshire.

Diamond distinguishes between a natural view, according to which these sentences are nonsense for different reasons (in (1) there is a mistake in categories, i.e. the sentence contains contradictory meanings, and (2) contains a nonsense word, i.e. the sentence is lacking in meaning), and what he calls the

---

[3]Pathological psychic life of the first kind [meaningful, allowing empathy] we can comprehend vividly enough as an exaggeration or diminution of known phenomena and as an appearance of such phenomena without the usual causes or motives. Pathological psychic life of the second kind [in its particular way ununderstandable, 'mad' in the literal sense, schizophrenic psychic life] we cannot adequately comprehend in this way. Instead we find changes of the most general kind for which we have no empathy but which in some way we try to make comprehensible from an external point of view. (Jaspers, 1962, p. 577).

Frege–Wittgenstein view, in whch these examples are given a similar verdict: they are both nonsensical because the expression as a whole is not given meaning.

According to Diamond, the natural or 'positive' conception of nonsense, namely, the idea that the sentence is nonsense because of the categories of the expressions in it, is implicitly the idea of their forming a sentence that does say something — something that holders of the natural view regard as an impossibility and which they deny is really sayable at all. This is the incoherence of the natural view, as, from the Frege–Wittgenstein perspective, there is no basis whatsoever in making this kind of distinction.

The Frege–Wittgenstein or 'negative' conception of nonsense would be that in these 'strings of words' no determination of meaning has been given — that they have the form of words that appear to be expressing something, or to be trying to express something, but they are empty of meaning and hence we cannot say what they mean. According to Diamond (1986, pp. 133–4):

> For Wittgenstein there is no kind of nonsense which is nonsense on account
> of what the terms composing it mean

This distinction can be applied to the grammar of incomprehensibility. Thus, we notice that saying 'He finds the instructions are incomprehensible' (case 3 in previous section) implies that an understanding has been expressed, namely the understanding that the instructions are incomprehensible, incoherent, faulty, etc. It implies that something substantial has been said about these instructions and the description 'positive conception of incomprehensibility' can be applied to it.

On the other hand, when uttering 'He fails to understand the instructions, however much he ever tries' (case 2), no positive assumptions as to the presence of incomprehensible phenomena are made, and one could say that this expression does not say anything about incomprehensibility prevailing, but only shows that where we expect comprehensibility we do not meet with this. This implies that nothing whatsoever of substance has been said about these instructions and the description 'negative conception of incomprehensibility' is an apt one.

Although consistent, this is all very obscure. Can this distinction be given a more concrete or tangible account? Can it be made more immediately meaningful? To clarify this, I look more closely at Wittgenstein on nonsense in *Philosophical Investigations*.

What do we do with 'incomprehensibility'?

When a question about the meaning of a concept troubles us, Wittgenstein's suggestion is to take heed of the way we use the concept in our everyday life, to search for examples of how we are prone to use the concept. But what does Wittgenstein himself do with the concept of 'nonsense', which is a ubiquitous turn of argument in his writings. Wittgenstein himself explains the role of 'nonsense' in philosophical discussions as follows (1953, §500):

> When a sentence is called senseless, it is not as it were its sense that it is senseless. But a combination of words is being excluded from the language, withdrawn from circulation.

This section in *Philosophical Investigations* stems from an earlier, more extended, version published in *Philosophical Grammar* (Wittgenstein 1974, p. 130), in which the context of this comment is more openly apparent (Diamond 1986):

> How strange that one should be able to say that such and such a state of affairs is inconceivable! If we regard thought as essentially an accompaniment going with an expression, the words in the statement that specify the inconceivable state of affairs must be unaccompanied. So what sort of sense is it to have? Unless it says these words are senseless. But it isn't as it were their sense that is senseless; they are excluded form our language like some arbitrary noise, and the reason for their explicit exclusion can only be that we are tempted to confuse them with a sentence of our language.

Wittgenstein's main point seems to be that when saying that something is nonsense we are not doing very much — we are only leaving some expressions out of consideration, and these expressions do not count for us in any positive sense.

What do we do with 'incomprehensibility' in more ordinary contexts of life? Someone might comment on the text in a poem, 'Hell, this text is quite incomprehensible', and put it away. The same might happen when listening to an unfamiliar piece of music.

We can take also an even more concrete example. Think of assembling a ready-made chair from written instructions, where one of the assembly phases is totally missing but this is not indicated. We may recognize the lack and say that these instructions are deficient. We may in some cases also say that these instructions are incomprehensible, as a kind of shorthand for recognizing their incompleteness. (Or we may find it incomprehensible that such a mistake has taken place at all.) But there are also cases where we may only say (in exasperation) that these instructions are incomprehensible, put them away, and try to proceed with the assembly by ourselves.

So, it seems, 'incomprehensibility' marks where we stop trafficking with things or persons as we had been trafficking with them before.

The important point is to notice that 'incomprehensibility' is not a contentual expression: it does not *refer* to either 'meaninglessness' or to 'the non-existence of meaning'. It just points out where the limits of comprehension lie in giving itself to our use as this limit. And this is the main point of calling this 'negative conception of incomprehensibility': it is negative in terms of lacking any substantial reference.

This also means that the concept of incomprehensibility does not tell us anything about the conditions of its manifestation. It only shows us that what we have pursued with understanding is not available. We thus have to try to find understanding in a novel way. This may involve explanation, interpretation, etc.

Winch on 'Ceasing to exist'

In trying to describe this elusive conceptual point, I add to these examples Peter Winch's illuminating discussion of what the notion of dismissing a referential (i.e. positive) conception of incomprehensibility amounts to, in his paper 'Ceasing to exist'.

One of the examples that Winch discusses comes from Isaac Bashevits Singer's short story called 'Stories from behind the stove', part of which recounts an incident in which an old peasant suddenly vanishes without trace or explanation of any kind. The point of the discussion is to make us recognize that the purported explanation of this happening by Zalman the glazier ('People do vanish') is not an explanation at all but 'just an expression of despair at the prospect of finding an explanation' (Winch 1987, p. 85). Singer (1970) reads as follows:

'People do vanish', he said. 'Not everyone is like the Prophet Elijah, who was taken to heaven in a fiery chariot. In the village of Palkes, not far from Radoshitz, a peasant was ploughing with an ox. Behind him walked his son, sowing barley form a bag. The boy looked up and the ox was there but his father had gone. He began to call, to scream, but there was no answer. His father had disappeared in the middle of the field. He was never heard from again.'

'Perhaps there was a hole in the earth and he fell in?' Levi Yotzchoch suggested.

'There was no hole to be seen — and if there had been a hole, why didn't the ox fall in first? He was in the lead.'

'Do you mean that the demons carried him away?'

'I don't know.'

'Perhaps he ran away with some woman,' Meir the eunuch suggested.

'Nonsense, an old man of seventy — maybe more. A peasant does not run away from his earth, his hut. If he wants a woman, he goes with her into the granary.'

'In that case, the Evil Ones took him,' Levi Yitzchoch said judiciously.

'Why just him?' Zalman the glazier asked. 'A quiet man, Wojciech Kucek — that was his name. Before the Feasts of the Tabernacle, he used to bring branches for covering the Sukhoth. My own father bought from him. These things happen . . .'

According to Winch (1987, p. 104), in this story:

> ... the various positive accounts which are suggested by members of Zalman's audience ... of the mysterious disappearances are quickly dispatched. But the arguments by which they are dispatched cannot be said to point in the direction of the storyteller's account since, as I just said, he gives no account ... His words do not locate any definite point in the stream of life. So it is not so much that that what is said conflicts with our understanding of things ... It just fails to connect with it.

In the same vein I'd like to express my point like this: saying that something is incomprehensible is not an explanation at all, but just an expression of despair when our ordinary ways of comprehending people and situations elude us. It is not an alternative explanation to what is taking place but belongs to a different logical space than any explanation or understanding we may come up with. That is, 'incomprehensibility' is not a form of understanding at all but marks the limits of the understanding we are in.

Applying these insights into the clinical examples described earlier in this chapter, we notice first that the difficulties in expressing the 'resignative' aspects of psychotherapy may in some cases be can be brought more clearly to focus when we recognize that saying we are confronted with the 'incomprehensible' is just an expression of legitimate despair at not knowing where we stand in relation to the patient. Second, regarding Jaspers' comment in the section on the meaning of 'incomprehensibility', it seems clear that incomprehensibility cannot have the kind of factual role as a basic psychopathological concept envisaged by Jaspers.

Further suggestions

I will conclude by making three suggestions concerning the clinical implications of this conclusion.

First, think of the concept of 'psychosis'. As pointed out earlier, besides being conventionally understood as a referential expression (picking up a clinical syndrome or state), the uses of the concept also mark the very limits of a person's intelligibility to others. As I see it, this dual structure or inherent ambiguity of 'psychosis' can be described in terms of the positive and negative readings of 'incomprehensibility'. We can use 'psychosis' as a clinical concept with a certain degree of reliability, but when confronted with the task of giving a comprehensive, positive account of its content (i.e. describing 'psychosis' as a referential expression and consequently assuming a stable reference for it), our task inevitably fails and we are forced to propose exceedingly narrow explications of psychosis (such as DSM-IV definitions of psychosis) to fill the gap between its real clinical uses and assumed scientific status. On the other hand, applying the negative conception of incomprehensibility consistently to the concept of psychosis leads us to the conclusion that the concept 'psychosis' cannot in principle be severed from the clinical contexts of its use, and only by appreciating this are we able to make sense of our ways of using it in the clinical environment.

Second, these deep conceptual obscurities concerning the concept of psychosis are even more urgent when we move from 'full-blown' psychotic states to syndrome entities where overt psychoticism has a more marginal, but nevertheless real, clinical role. For instance, recently extensive interest has emerged in the prodromal symptoms and features of psychosis and the possibilities of early detection and intervention of schizophrenia and other psychoses (McGlashan and Johannessen 1996). It seems clear that having a good grasp of the logical features of 'psychosis' is essential for coping with both clinical and ethical issues related to concepts such as 'attenuated psychotic symptoms' or 'at-risk mental state' (Heinimaa 1999; Schaffner and McGorry 2001).

Third, relating to the clinical significance of having 'incomprehensibility' and related concepts (e.g. 'impossibility') at our disposal, I would like to propose the following clinical example, which comes from clinical work, namely supervision in connection with ordinary psychiatric treatment.

A resident discusses a patient contact, which he has experienced as an especially burdening one. The patient's life history appears to him astoundingly sordid. The resident asks: 'What can I do with this patient? It seems quite inconceivable, impossible, that someone's life could be like this!' The supervisor's impression is that the resident responds to this agonizing life story with bewilderment, looking for 'instant solutions' to cope with the overwhelming anxiety. (Like 'Nobody's life can be like this. It must be she/he is exaggerating, or this is a depressive symptom, or . . .'). The supervisor describes her observations on the case, and repeats and legitimizes the supervisee's experience of an 'impossible' life story. She suggests that the thing to do at this moment is not to escape the 'impossible', but to let the impossible show itself as it is, that is, as impossible.

The supervisee found this to be helpful. But the point of this story is that the concept of 'impossible' gives us a tool to endure and cope with extraordinary phenomena, and this does not necessitate our having a theory of 'impossibility' and its references at our disposal to legitimise the use of this concept in psychiatric work. We do not need to 'know' what 'incomprehensibility' or 'impossibility' refer to in order to be able to use them in a fruitful way in clinical encounters.

References

American Psychiatric Association (1994). *Diagnostic and Statistical Manual of Mental Disorders: DSM-IV*. 4th ed. Washington, DC: American Psychiatric Association.

Berrios, G. E. (1991). Delusions as 'wrong beliefs': a conceptual history. *British Journal of Psychiatry*, **159**(Suppl. 14): 6–13.

Blankenburg, W. (1984). Unausgeschöpftes in der Psychopathologie von Karl Jaspers. *Nervenartz*, **55**: 447–60.

Callieri, B. (1960). über das Phänomen der 'Persönlichung' des Auges. *Nervenartz*, **31**: 253–6.

Corin, E. and Lauzon, G. (1992). Positive withdrawal and the quest for meaning: the reconstruction of experience among schizophreniacs. *Psychiatry*, **55**: 266–78.

David, A. S. (1999). On the impossibility of defining delusions. *Philosophy, Psychiatry, Psychology*, **6**: 17–20.

Diamond, C. (1986). What nonsense might be. In: *Ludwig Wittgenstein: Critical Assessments*. Vol. 2: *From* Philosophical Investigations *to* On Certainty: *Wittgenstein's Later Philosophy* (ed. S. Shanker), pp. 125–41. Surry Hills, Australia: Croom Helm.

Flaum, M., Arndt, S., and Andreasen, N. C. (1991). The reliability of 'bizarre' delusions. *Comprehensive Psychiatry*, **32**: 59–65.

Fulford, K. W. M. (1989). *Moral Theory and Medical Practice*. Cambridge: Cambridge University Press.

Gadamer, H.-G. (1993). *über die Verborgenheit der Gesundheit*. Frankfurt: Suhrkamp.

Goldman, D., Hien, D. A., Haas, G. L., Sweeney, J. A., and Frances, A. J. (1992). Bizarre delusions and DSM-III-R schizophrenia. *American Journal of Psychiatry*, **149**: 494–9.

Hayward, M. L. and Taylor, J. E. (1956) A schizophrenic patients describes the action of intensive psychotherapy. *The Psychiatric Quarterly*, **30**: 211–48.

Heinimaa, M. (1999), Conceptual problems of early intervention in schizophrenia. *Hong Kong Journal of Psychiatry*, **9**: 20–4.

Heinimaa, M. (2000a). On the grammar of psychosis. *Medicine, Health Care and Philosophy*, **3**: 39–46.

Heinimaa, M. (2000b). Ambiguities in the psychiatric use of the concepts of the person: an analysis. *Philosophy, Psychiatry, Psychology*, **7**: 125–36.

Heinimaa, M. (in press). Incomprehensibility: the role of the concept in DSM-IV definition of schizophrenic delusions. Medicine, Health Care and Philosophy.

Hertzberg, L. (1995). Förståelsen och dess gränser. *Glänta*, **1–2**: 107–12.

Hertzberg, L. (2001). The sense is where you find it. pp. 90–103. In: *Wittgenstein in America* (ed. T. G. McCarthy and S. C. Stidd). Oxford: Clarendon Press.

Jaspers, K. (1959). *Allgemeine Psychopathologie*. 8th ed. Berlin: Springer.

Jaspers, K. (1962). *General Psychopathology*, translated by J. Hoening and M. W. Hamilton. Manchester: Manchester University Press.

Jenner, F. A., Monteiro, A. C., and Vlissides, D. (1986). The negative effects on psychiatry of Karl Jaspers' development of Verstehen. *Journal of the British Society for Phenomenology*, **17**: 52–71.

Kopelman, L. M. (1994). Normal grief: good or bad? Health of disease. *Philosophy, Psychiatry, Psychology*, **1**: 209–20.

McGlashan, T. H. and Johannessen, J. O. (1996). Early detection and intervention in schizophrenia: rationale. *Schizophrenia Bulletin*, **22**: 201–22.

Oppenheimer, H. (1974). Comprehensible and incomprehensible phenomena in psychopathology: a comparison of the psychology of Sigmund Freud and Karl Jaspers. *Comprehensive Psychiatry*, **15**: 503–10.

Roberts, G. (1992). The origin of delusions. *British Journal of Psychiatry*, **161**: 298–308.

Rudnick, A. (1997). On the notion of psychosis: the DSM-IV in perspective. *Psychopathology*, **30**: 298–302.

Schaffner, K. F. and McGorry, P. D. (2001). Preventing severe mental illnesses — new prospects and ethical challenges. *Schizophrenia Research*, **51**: 3–15.

Silvern, L. E. (1990). A hermeneutic account of clinical psychology: strengths and limits. *Philosophical Psychology*, **3**: 5–27.

Singer, I. B. (1970). Stories from behind the stove. In: *A Friend of Kafka*, pp. 61–74. Harmondsworth: Penguin Books.

Winch, P. (1987). *Trying to Make Sense*. Oxford: Blackwell.

Wittgenstein, L. (1953). *Philosophical Investigations*. Oxford: Basil Blackwell.

Wittgenstein, L. (1974). *Philosophical Grammar* (ed. R. Rhees). Berkeley: University of California Press.

Section 6   A New Kind of Science

15 Anxiety — animal reactions and the embodiment of meaning

Gerrit Glas

Introduction: nature and narrative in clinical anxiety and anxiety research

Psychiatric and psychotherapeutic literature on anxiety seems to suggest that there are, broadly speaking, two main types of anxiety. There is on the one hand the medical literature, in which anxiety is described as a dysfunctional alarm response that is elicited by biological, cognitive, and learning mechanisms. Although multifactorial in its origin, this alarm response itself is a primarily *biological* reaction, which is built into the hardware of the brain. There is on the other hand a large, older, body of literature that describes anxiety as an *existential* phenomenon, expressing the meaning of universal facts of life such as, for instance, the threat of absurdity, isolation, and/or imminent non-being. So, there are two discourses on anxiety, one emphasizing that anxiety is part of the natural human endowment (but elicited by the wrong cues), the other highlighting that all forms of anxiety, even pathological ones, in some way reflect omnipresent human conflicts and challenges.

Most striking in this context is the complete disregard in each of these approaches for the other approach. Existential and/or psychotherapeutic literature almost completely neglects the biological aspects of anxiety. Modern pharmacological and neuroendocrine studies on anxiety, on the other hand, show only a superficial interest in the typical human aspects of anxiety. This state of affairs suggests that the relationship between 'nature' and 'narrative' is not only at the heart of psychiatry's understanding of anxiety, but is also deeply problematic.

My problem is, in short, whether these two discourses on anxiety should be kept apart or whether they can in some way be integrated. Should the clearly biological underpinnings of the emotion of anxiety, and in particular pathological forms of anxiety, be seen as completely distinct from the deeply human, existential meanings of this emotion, or should both be considered as two aspects, or manifestations, of the same phenomenon? Is there just one anxiety or are there two? And, if there exist two or even more anxieties, how are they related? More specifically, could it be that there are many anxieties with existential meaning that builds on differentiations in their biological (and other) roots?

These questions provide the broad outline. Within that outline, there are sub-questions, such as: do recent clinical and neuroscientific findings challenge long-standing notions about anxiety, or about emotion in general, or about brain processes, or about the relationship between subjective experience and more or less objective behaviours? Could it be that the anthropological approach to psychopathology offers an important alternative for the almost inevitable 'either–or' (biological or psychological) of the majority of theoretical accounts of anxiety. Is there a concept of anxiety in which even the most elementary forms of anxiety in some way express typical human meanings of anxiety?

Many of these questions will be left aside or briefly touched on only in this chapter. In the first part I give a short introduction into the clinical and scientific aspects of pathological forms of anxiety. Then I offer a succinct overview of different forms of basic, or existential, anxiety. In the final two sections I enter the philosophical discussion that arises when the biological and existential vocabularies are brought together.

Clinical and scientific issues in the study of anxiety

From a broad historical perspective, it seems that there are at least three trad-itions in the study of anxiety (see Glas 1994). First, and foremost, there is the *medical* tradition, which from Antiquity until now dominated the theoretical literature on anxiety and which, at least in the past 150 years, favours a bio-logical approach to anxiety. According to this approach, anxiety is rooted in a dysbalance of a physiological or endocrine equilibrium. Subjective feelings of fear and/or anxiety are the epiphenomena of this dysbalance.

Second, the concept of anxiety as *inner threat* must be distinguished. Well known as this is in the present time, one can hardly imagine the revolutionary significance of this concept when it emerged in the late nineteenth- and early twentieth-century psychoanalytical literature. Contemporary defenders of this view can be found in psychotherapeutic circles and in some branches of cognitive psychology. They do not deny that fear and anxiety can be related to events in the outside world, but they maintain that in addition there is an inner drama that contributes to the rise of anxiety. People fear, for instance, to be out of control and/or vulnerable.

Finally there is the *existential* concept of anxiety, a concept that dates back to philosophers such as Pascal (1980) and Kierkegaard (1844/1980) and that, via existential phenomenology, inspires the work of anthropological psych-iatrists and existential psychotherapists in our time (Goldstein 1940; Yalom 1980). According to this concept, the feeling of anxiety is seen as the expression of a frustrated urge for self-realization or as the expression of the imminent annihilation of personal identity and psychic integrity.

In the introduction above, I placed the inner threat and existential concepts of anxiety together. From what has been said here, one may grasp that there are also important differences between the subjective–psychoanalytic and the existential–anthropological approach. The latter concentrates primarily on existence as such, which is broader and, depending on one's point of view, also more fundamental than the restriction to inner experience.

From a *clinical* point of view, the experience of anxiety is often a double- or multi-layered one. On the surface, there exists a concrete fear, or a number of fear symptoms, that conform(s) to the criteria of one of the DSM-IV anxiety disorders. These symptoms are of three kinds: behavioural, physiological, and mental. Their explanation is also considered to be threefold: behavioural, (neuro)physiological, and cognitive. Learning theorists try to explain the oversensitivity to particular situations. They describe types of conditioning and the routines that animals and persons use to avoid the cues that elicit fear behaviour. Neurophysiological and neuroendocrine explanatory models (animal and human) describe correlations between overt behaviour and changes in the balance between neurotransmitter systems and the underlying brain circuitry. Psychopharmacologists study the way in which pharmacological agents influence mood, affect, and behaviour as a result of their effects on brain subsystems. Cognitive theorists describe how emotional information is processed and how this information processing affects the way the person interprets the world. All this knowledge — behavioural, (neuro)physiological, and cognitive — forms a body of knowledge. This body of knowledge is general by nature: it aims at general constellations of clinical phenomena. This general knowledge is collected in textbooks, learned by trainees, and then, again, applied to the individual patient. Trainees are educated to unravel the idiosyncratic story of the patient and to detect the general aspect, i.e. those symptoms and signs that are accounted for by the body of knowledge just mentioned.

At a deeper level, however, there are aspects of the phenomenon of anxiety that cannot be accounted for by such an objectifying approach. By listening to the patient one can often find a vital, sensation-like, experience that is much more difficult to describe because it lacks a definite object (see Glas 1997). I quote the account of an anonymous surgeon in *The Lancet* of 1952 (pp. 83–4):

> It is as difficult to describe to others what an acute anxiety state feels like as to convey to the inexperienced the feeling of falling in love. Perhaps the most characteristic impression is the constant state of causeless and apparently meaningless alarm. You feel as if you were on the battlefield or had stumbled against a wild animal in the dark, and all the time you are conversing with your fellows in normal peaceful surroundings and performing duties you have done for years. With this your head feels vague and immense and stuffed with cottonwool; it is difficult, and trying, to concentrate; and, most frightening of all, the quality of your sensory appreciation of the universe undergoes an essential change [cited by Landis 1964, pp. 241–2]

It is my impression that this more basic or fundamental anxiety is often related to pervasive and global feelings of unconnectedness, powerlessness, absurdity, and/or doubt. Anxiety is, in these cases, not primarily the *consciousness of* being unconnected, out of control, and unable to make choices. It is rather *the ways in which* this powerlessness, unconnectedness, and lack of control are *embodied* and *lived*. Understanding anxiety from an anthropological perspective means that one understands the crucial importance of this conceptual shift — the shift from anxiety of 'something' to anxiety as an elementary expression of an underlying central thme in a person's life.

In contemporary *scientific* research the biological approach to anxiety prevails. It is now widely accepted — I follow here LeDoux (1996) — that there are at least two fear-mediating neuronal systems; one involving the amygdala and the other the hippocampal system. The term *amygdala* refers to two small nuclei at each side of the limbic system of the brain. These nuclei are now considered to play an important role in the regulation of conditioned fear responses, i.e. in acquired reactions to fear-provoking stimuli that are often not consciously perceived. Reactions to these fear-provoking stimuli consist of changes in bodily posture and an increase in muscle tension, blood pressure, attention, and the excretion of stress hormones. The operations of the amygdala are supposed to proceed without accompanying consciousness, although there are neuronal connections between the amygdala and the neocortex. Furthermore, it is assumed that the amygdala has the capacity of 'implicit emotional memory'. It forms the 'quick and dirty' part of the alarm system, in the sense that it gives rise to a processing system that reacts quickly and is broadly tuned to a wide variety of fear stimuli. These stimuli remain unnoticed, in many cases.

The other, *hippocampal* fear-mediating, system has the capacity of 'explicit emotional memory', indicating that its remembrances are conscious and 'narrowly tuned' to a limited set of fear-provoking cues. When the hippocampus is involved in the processing of fear, confrontation with signals of threat evokes a cognitive, more complex and slower, fear response, and in most cases the subject is aware of the source of threat.

The important thing to notice here is that both systems function *in parallel*: they are not completely separate, or linear (i.e. in a time sequence), or operating in a strictly hierarchical way. Parallel functioning means that both systems are activated together when confronted with a stimulus that is related to stimuli that were present during the initial trauma. I quote LeDoux (1996, p. 202):

> Through the hippocampal system you will remember who you were with and what you were doing during the trauma, and will also remember, as a cold fact, that the situation was awful. Through the amygdala system the stimuli will cause your muscles to tense up, your blood pressure and heart rate to change, and hormones to be released, among other bodily and brain responses. Because these systems are activated by the same stimuli and are functioning at the same time, the two kinds of memories seem to be part of one unified memory function.

Both systems, together, maintain a delicate balance, the one system releasing the output of the thalamus, the other inhibiting it. LeDoux is inclined to the view of William James, according to which the emotional quality of memories is accounted for by the feedback of peripheral bodily sensation. The neurologist Damasio (1994; see also 1999) has argued for a similar, more refined, mechanism, consisting of the activity of so-called 'as-if' loops in which it is not only the actual but also the imagined bodily feedback that influences a person's feelings and decisions. In this case, it is the representation of all kinds of bodily responses to imagined actions that serves as a signal, indicating the adaptive value of future action, the expected degree of satisfaction of oneself or others, and even the moral significance of one's endeavours. Damasio, in fact, seems to return to an Aristotelian position, in which emotion serves as a disposition that enables the person to find a position in the middle, between the extremes of too much and too little of a certain behaviour. The capacity to find such an equilibrium is itself an instance of morality; it is the expression of a moral virtue.

A typology of fundamental anxieties

In this section I present a short overview of a number of existential or, as I prefer to call them, basic or fundamental anxieties (for a more elaborate account see Glas 2001). This concentration on fundamental anxieties is not meant to detract from the importance of the anxieties that are well known from psychoanalytical and cognitive literature. However, as it is my aim to illustrate how the biological approach to anxiety converges with broader clinical approaches, these basic anxieties seem even more suitable than the psychoanalytical and cognitive approaches, which describe more or less 'regional' configurations of anxiety. The basic anxieties, as we conceive them, refer to behaviours and feelings that are expressed by and refer to the person in his or her totality, whereas the psychoanalytical and cognitive anxieties refer to conflicts and issues that are bound to more or less specific situations.

The basic anxieties are often more at the background, but are none the less of crucial importance in understanding the patient. Table 15.1 presents seven basic anxieties: pervasive feelings with an underlying theme, a theme that refers to a structural dimension of human existence.

Anxiety related to loss of structure

Anxiety related to *loss of structure* (chaos), then, refers to the inability of maintaining a relationship to oneself and/or the world. Psychotic anxieties are often characterized by loss of structure. From the perspective developed here, psychotic anxiety is not merely a reflection of a disturbance in thinking or

Table 15.1 Typology of basic anxieties: their themes and underlying structure

Type	Theme	Structure
Anxiety related to loss of structure	Chaos	I-self relationship
Anxiety related to existence as such	Facticity	Capacity to shape one's existence
Anxiety related to lack of safety	Vulnerability	Physical protection
Anxiety related to unconnectedness	Isolation	Affective connectedness
Anxiety related to doubt and inability to choose	Irrevocability	Historicity; capacity to will
Anxiety related to meaninglessness	Absurdity	Mastery; capacity to entrust
Anxiety related to death	Non-existence	Openness; capacity to transcend

perception, because it is the relationship to the world and to oneself as such that is threatened. The person lives in an unfamiliar, uncanny, and depersonalized world. There is not a perceptual disturbance as a result of which the person has unfamiliar feelings and sensations, which in their turn cause anxiety. The subjective quality of these anxieties suggests that there exists a much more immediate relationship, in the sense that anxiety is the very expression or manifestation of a change in position toward oneself and the world. In short, the anxiety is *itself* the manifestation of a state of chaos and disruption, rather than an anxiety *of* chaos, such as in fear of loosing control.

A woman aged 68 with long-standing obsessive–compulsive disorder and a history of anorexia nervosa in her youth has obsessions with a psychotic quality. She says: 'When I look around, especially when I am at home and the sun shines through the windows, then I see all the swarming particles of dust, moving in the air, forth and back in the draught. It is overwhelming. Maybe, I am contaminated. But that is not the central issue. I cannot say what really frightens me. Perhaps, it is because I cannot control them. I simply cannot get rid of them. I am paralysed and feel strange, as if I am surrounded by a thick, trembling, and yet invisible substance. Sometimes, when this occurs and when I am anxious, I hear voices. Sometimes, I can simply not perceive the objects around me, as if they have faded away and been replaced by the dust. My perception is changed, then, and I cannot think clearly anymore.

Anxiety related to existence as such

Anxieties related to *existence as such*, represent a horror — or even nausea — of the brute fact of one's existence, or a disgust with the world. Sometimes this horror, or disgust, is directly primarily to one's body, for instance in case of anorexia nervosa. The theme of these anxieties is the facticity of life (its matter-of-factness). What occurs in one's life does not offer any promise. Everything seems to be neutral. What exists is not genuine, not alive; life feels like inert matter. Nothing responds; one's inner experience feels frozen. The structural condition to which this anxiety refers is the *capacity to shape one's existence* in spite of the unpredictability of human existence.

Anxiety related to lack of safety

Anxiety related to the theme of *lack of safety* depends primarily on the (non)existence of physical safety. The person experiences the world as insecure and inhospitable. The vulnerability of human existence manifests itself here in a more specific feeling of disruption that results from lack of *physical* protection. One may think, here, of the intense terror and desperation after physical or technological disasters. This anxiety points to physical protection or the availability of an ecological niche as a structural condition without which human beings cannot flourish.

The patient is aged 34, an unmarried woman with a part-time job as a remedial teacher. She has had a phobia of electricity, lightning, thunderstorms, and loud noises since she was 11 years old. At that age, she witnessed a short-circuit of the light in a globe in her bedroom and panicked. A few days later, she panicked again after being confronted with a loud noise in the playground at school. The ensuing phobic reactions worsened over the years, leaving her an invalid, with many somatic complaints, a slipped disc in her back (partly) because of strong and long-standing muscle tension, and almost unmanageable anticipatory anxiety when the use of electrical equipment can no longer be avoided and/or thunderstorms are announced on the weather forecast. She describes this anxiety as a blockade, originating in her head; or as a tension or inner pressure leading to paralysis. She also calls it a warning signal that she may not be able to manage the situation. Lifting her arm or her hand to switch on the light or an electrical device then becomes an enormous task.

Panic is a kind of explosion, a sudden discharge of pressure. Just like the pressure in the atmosphere explodes as a thunderstorm, she says, so the trembling, the pounding of her heart, and the feeling of going mad are a kind of explosion. During the night she listens in complete darkness to all the little noises in her house and in the street, the ticking of the clock, the noises of the central heating, and so on. When the anxiety increases, these sounds fade away, what remains is complete silence, which is experienced as a pressure, and as pain, everywhere pain, paralysing and alarming at the same time. Sounds that penetrate this silence are felt as bouts of pain.

The anxiety presents itself here in a physical way and refers primarily to lack of physical protection. However, the case also illustrates that the basic anxieties may overlap. Apart from anxiety related to lack of physical protection, this patient is also at the edge of chaos (lack of structure) and is affectively unconnected. A person can suffer from more than one fundamental anxiety.

Anxiety related to unconnectedness

Anxiety that centres around the theme of *unconnectedness or isolation* is perhaps the pre-eminent existential or basic anxiety. This anxiety resembles separation anxiety — which is, of course, well known from psychoanalysis — but it differs from separation anxiety in that the emphasis here is on the incapacity to connect as such, rather than on past or anticipated events of separation. What prevails is a tormenting feeling of distance, the awareness of an unbridgeable gap. This feeling can amount to the awareness that one lives in a vacuum and is about to suffocate, or that one lives in an unreal world in which things not are what they seem to be and in which attempts to connect fail as if there were a glassy wall between the person and the surrounding world. The structural condition to which this anxiety refers is the condition of *affective connectedness*.

Anxiety related to doubt and inability to choose

Anxiety related to the theme of *doubt and inability to make choices* refers to the structural dimension of time and the anthropological category of the will. Doubt and inability to make choices are major symptoms of obsessive–compulsive disorder. From an anthropological point of view, obsessive-compulsives have difficulties in coping with the irrevocability of decision-making. Indecision may give the impression of openness; in fact, however, it is an avoidance of genuine openness, in the sense that it does not allow decisions to become concrete and, because of that, does not lead to engagement and commitment when these are required. This is the kind of anxiety Kierkegaard is referring to when he speaks of the human person in a state of mental vertigo at the abyss of freedom. This anxiety is experienced as 'unbearable lightness', as a kind of weightlessness that avoids responsibility, in contrast to the heaviness that is inherent to the first three basic anxieties (related to the themes of destruction of the I–self relationship, of facticity, and of physical protection).

A 34-year-old woman with a long history of social phobia, and many unsuccessful attempts of behavioural therapy by experienced therapists, reports that her hands and her head tremble all the time, when she visits a public place or goes to birthday parties and other meetings. Work has never been an option. She lives alone. On closer inspection, it appears that treatment resistance is not so much a result of the severity of the symptoms of her social phobia, as much as a sign indicating that she has difficulties with life itself. In a fundamental way, the woman has yet to 'decide' really to live, i.e. to engage herself in a life in which she uses her capacities and relates in a more active way to her background and upbringing. Her emptiness betrays an avoidance of making decisions at all. Her disease (i.e. her trembling) gives her an illusory sense of control in a situation that is marked by lack of control and lack of willpower. Shaking is safer than engaging. She seems to be open, but this openness is only superficial. Beneath the surface there is an endless postponement of even trivial decisions and an avoidance of engagement.

Anxiety related to meaninglessness

Anxiety related to *meaninglessness* is perhaps the most well known anxiety, as well as a major theme in existentialist and post-modern prose. Anxiety borders, here, on perplexity. Its theme is the absurdity of human existence, with perhaps a dual aspect of uncontrollability of being forgotten or lost in a cosmic sense. The structural condition that is supposed to conquer these anxieties is the *capacity to entrust oneself to others* and/or to a *transcendent reality*.

Anxiety related to death

Anxiety related to *death*, finally, brings us to the theme of non-existence. Death anxiety is by no means an easy construct. It should certainly not be restricted to the fact of one's (own) death in the future, or to the process of dying. Death anxiety also refers to the anxiety that exists when a person relates to his or her own finitude and mortality as such. Anxiety, conceived in this way, is closely connected with life itself: it is a living of the 'possibility of one's own impossibility to exist' (this formulation echoes Heidegger's in *Sein und Zeit*). Death anxiety refers, here, to the category of possibility as a lived and full reality, and not to possibility as an empty and merely logical or statistical possibility. To live the reality of possibility presumes the capacity to transcend one's own limited perspective.

Towards an integrated view of anxiety

We have now explored some of the biological and existential aspects of the phenomenon of anxiety. Both come together in the clinical situation. Of course, a lot has had to be omitted, for instance the enormous body of literature on the psychodynamic and cognitive aspects of anxiety. However, we do not really need these other perspectives to bring us to the right position to highlight some of the underlying conceptual issues. I will limit myself to one issue. This issue concerns the question whether there are conceptual barriers opposing the idea that there are biological precursors of the basic anxieties.

I cannot go deeply into the empirical part of this question, mainly because, to my knowledge, there exists no research on the neurobiological correlates of the basic anxieties. Let me just remark that concepts such as 're-entry' and 'global mapping', as they are developed by neuroscientists such as Edelman, Tononi, and others, suggest the possibility of gaining some insight into the biological underpinnings of activities like projecting oneself into the future, acquiring a sense of basic trust, learning of past experiences, and so on. These concepts suggest that in areas such as the association areas of the brain past experiences and factors influencing these experiences are represented, compared, and subjected to a kind of inner enactment. Along this line it could be imagined that global pictures of the world, linked with values, emotions, and the concept of the self, give rise to or (at least) contribute to the experiences of the basic anxieties we have discussed (see Edelman 1992, p. 170; Hundert 1989, Chapter 8).

Let us, however, concentrate on the conceptual part of our question, by assuming that there are indeed biological 'precursors' of the basic anxieties. What could this mean? More precisely, what configuration of concepts and explanatory models would contribute most to a position in which different levels of conceptualization are neither kept completely separate, nor simply reduced to one another (the existential to the biological or the biological to the existential)?

What is needed first is, I would suggest, a firm opposition to any temptation whatsoever to reify subsystems of the brain (see Edelman and Tononi 2000, pp. 143–4). Subsystems, such as the hippocampus or the thalamus, cannot function in isolation. Of course, the majority of scientists agree with this, just as everybody agrees with the idea that the brain itself cannot function in isolation. However, rejection of reification means much more. It also implies an awareness of the more subtle temptations that are inherent in psychiatric language and in suggestive graphic representations, such as magnetic resonance (MR) images and schemes in books. Psychiatric language is often simplifying. Pictures and schemes in books draw arrows between hypothetical entities represented as coloured boxes, suggesting a direction of causality of activities in and between these boxes. The boxes refer to particular brain subsystems; the arrows suggest the direction of causality. The suggestive power of these simplifying schemes and formulations may give rise to the impression of independence of the subsystems.

When reification is successfully resisted, one is ready to face another difficult problem: the question of how the process of differentiation of the various subtypes of basic anxiety should be conceptualized, taking into account the biological underpinnings of even the most refined of these anxieties. Is the scientist caught in a dilemma between either a bottom-up or a top-down approach, or could one think here of a combination of the two? From a hierarchical point of view the differentiation and opening up of the biological basis of the fundamental anxieties occurs more or less top-down. Higher-order processes regulate the differentiation of biological processes and make them suitable for their function within more refined emotional processes. Parallel models, on the other hand, avoid making a choice between top-down and bottom-up approaches. Reductionist models, finally, favour a bottom-up approach: higher-order process may be reduced, causally and/or conceptually, to lower-order processes.

The least one can say is that there are empirical reasons to question a purely reductionist approach. In a simplified model of brain functioning, one could, for instance, say that specificity and differentiation increase with the level in the hierarchy. At the lowest level, the reactions of the animal (or person) show a fixed pattern. The behavioural repertoire at this level is limited — compare, for instance, the four basic alarm responses of Isaac Marks (freezing, flight, defensive attack, and submission; Marks 1987). Higher-level behaviour builds on lower-level functioning in the sense that it moulds and refines this behaviour. From a reductionist point of view, one could now suggest that it does not matter whether there exists an overprediction or an underprediction of danger: both are mismatches and, because they are mismatches, they cause fear (see Gray 1982). Interestingly enough, however, at higher system levels the difference between overprediction and underprediction does matter and in fact may give rise to different kinds of fear; for instance *worry* in case of overprediction of fear and *anxious surprise* when there is an underprediction of fear (see Rachman and Lopatka 1986*a,b*). Worry is an anticipatory, forward-looking emotion, whereas anxious surprise is a backward-looking feeling.

This is an example that pleads against a reductionist approach. Reductionist accounts cannot do justice to differentiations at the higher system levels that are important for the existence of phenomena at that level.

Perhaps one could proceed by assuming that the choice between parallel and hierarchical models, and, more precisely, the assignment of a locus of control in the process of differentiation, depends on the context in which a particular process is studied. Even on a very elementary level, one could imagine that the anxieties we have discussed are manifestations in the domain of feeling and behaviour, of differentiation and refinement at higher system levels, levels at which the integration of the different aspects of human functioning in broader contexts belongs to the tasks of the person. The fundamental anxieties could then be conceptualized as different manifestations of a refined, almost intuitive, kind of orienting oneself in the world in a wider sense. The feeling mode, then, refers not only to the level of bodily survival (as is the case in the so-called orienting reflex or Marks' acute alarm responses), but also to many other areas that are vital for human existence, including the psychic, social, and spiritual realms. The structural dimensions to which the themes of the basic anxieties refer could then be conceptualized as analogies of other structural modes *within* the psychic or feeling mode.

Dooyeweerd's ontology and the conceptual analysis of brain functioning

The ontology to which I implicitly refer above was originally developed by the Dutch philosopher Herman Dooyeweerd (1953–1958) and has subsequently been modernized (Clouser 1991, 1996; Hart 1984), applied, and refined in fields such as physics (Stafleu 1987), biology (Zylstra 1996), technology (Schuurman 1980), information theory and social systems theory (Basden 2000; de Raadt 1991), economy (Goudzwaard 1979), and medicine (Hoogland and Jochemsen 2000; Jochemsen & Glas 1997) and neuroscience (Glas 2002). In the Dooyeweerdian ontology there are three fundamental distinctions:

- the distinction between modes (or functions) and entities
- the distinction between the law-side and the subject-side of both modes and entities
- the distinction between active (subjective) and passive (objective) functioning within a particular mode.

Modes refer to the ways in which entities function. Any entity functions actively in more than one mode; the entity of a tree, for instance, functions in a biotic, a physical, and a geometrical mode. The tree functions, in other words, according to biotic, physical, and geometrical laws or law-like regularities. Modes refer primarily to this law(like)-side of the way things (entities) function. However, modes also have a subject-side: the way things are is, in other words, also 'subject', i.e. subjected to these laws and/or regularities.

Entities, like modes, have both a law-side and a subject-side. The identity of an entity is, on the one hand, dependent on its membership of a particular class of things (law-side) and, on the other hand, strictly individual (subject-side).

Finally, things may behave as subjects or as objects in a particular mode. Their functioning conforms to subject- and object-functions respectively. A tree, for instance, may become the object of juridical, economic, and/or aesthetic appreciation. It then functions in the corresponding modes, i.e. as a legal object (when a person has an argument with a neighbour whose tree overarches the person's yard), as an economic object (when one buys a tree), or as an aesthetic object (when one admires its beauty). Modes in which an entity becomes the object of an activity of another entity or person are modes in which that entity functions passively. It functions according to the corresponding object-function. So, in the aesthetic appreciation of the tree, the tree functions as an aesthetic object, in the sense that the aesthetic mode of the tree is opened up. This view, therefore, regards aesthetic perception as not merely a subjective phenomenon in the mind of the perceiver, but primarily as a relational phenomenon in which the aesthetic mind of the perceiver opens up, or discloses, aesthetic qualities of the perceived object, qualities that are not merely added or attributed to the object but belong to that particular object in an intrinsic way (for a similar account, see Scheler 1916).

These Dooyeweerdian distinctions help to make clear what is required to resist deep-rooted tendencies to identify the brain as a *concrete*, morphologically discernable *entity*, with the results of scientific research into the *biotic* (and other) *functions* of the brain. This identification, as discussed above, implies reification. From a modal (or functional) point of view neuroscientists study the brain (or parts of it) as an 'organ' in which certain functions obey particular biotic (and other) regularities and laws. However, what occurs when this modal point of view is identified with the brain as a tangible and visible entity is that two conceptual gaps are neglected: the gap between entity in a law-like/structural and entity in an subject-side/individual sense, and the gap between the modal (functional) and the entity point of view.

Modern neuroimaging techniques are especially interesting in this respect, because they are highly suggestive of the tangibility of what in fact belongs to the structural (law-side) features of brain functioning. Looking at the different colourings of the MRI scans of panicking patients and normal controls, one may be tempted to say: 'We now see what panic disorder *is*'. However, utterances like these overlook the conceptual distinction between what is structural (law-side) and what is individual (subject-side). Panic disorder is a term that refers to a taxonomy that defines typical features of a class of phenomena. One can never 'see' panic disorder, like one sees a tree or any other visible entity. Panic disorder is a diagnosis constructed upon a set of observations, defined in a particular classification system. Even if this set of observations contains particular features of a MRI scan (which, in the future, could be the case), this would not allow one to say that what one sees 'is' panic disorder, because panic disorder is a term that refers primarily to the law-side of reality. Strictly speaking, one can only say that what one observes conforms to (particular) criteria of panic disorder.

The other conceptual distinction that is easily overlooked, the one between the modal and the entity point of view, is more difficult to apply in medicine, because medicine's key concepts often refer to entities such as panic disorder (or any other disease or physiological subsystem) and not to modes of functioning. However, in a more sophisticated approach it is easy to discern that even in applied sciences, such as medicine and technology, one cannot avoid the modal point of view, because entity concepts, such as the concept of class in biological taxonomies, are almost always originally conceived from a particular scientific perspective in which, more or less implicitly, one particular modal point of view is used. The concept of class, for instance, is primarily a biological concept, although attempts have been made — until now unsuccessfully — to reduce it to numerical regularities.

So, scientists should resist the force of suggestive shortcuts. Scientifically speaking, even the term 'brain' is an unqualified word that refers primarily to ordinary experience. When concepts derived from ordinary language are transposed to a scientific level they may become carriers of other, different, meanings, some of which have clearly substantialist connotations.

In response to all-too-easy identifications between entities of everyday experience and concepts referring to entities that are produced by the scientific mind, I would like to argue for a view in which the brain as a concrete, visible, part of the human body is seen as responding to, and operating within, a number of part-structures, and in which these part-structures, seen from their law-side, are seen as functioning within the structural whole of the human body.

Stated briefly, there are three ways to resist the all-too-easy identification (hypostazation) of the brain as a concrete 'organ' with what neuroscientific investigators say about the brain.

(1) The *modal* point of view should be sharply distinguished from the *entity* point of view. In other words, the functioning of the brain according to the laws and regularities of a particular modal aspect should be distinguished from the functioning of the brain as an entity. The modal term denotes a particular aspect of the functioning of the brain, whereas the entitary term refers to the brain as a thing-like structure(s) or to thing-like structures of parts of the brain. Of course, both the expression 'modal function' and the expression 'entity' are used in an abstract sense here. What one actually investigates are always (except in certain post-mortem cases) brain processes — molecular, neurochemical, and neuroendocrine processes. In the laboratory one never encounters brains as such, but brains involved in all kinds of processes. This brings us to the second distinction.

(2) What has just been said seems trivial — maybe it really is. However, the term 'process' may obscure the important difference between what is *law-like* about a particular brain process and the process itself, as a sequence of *concrete* events. Propositions about the lawfulness of the brain process are of a different order, compared with propositions describing sequences of events. I emphasize this, because there is a rather strong tendency in philosophy of science to blur this distinction. The explanation of a particular state of affairs is, then, limited to the description of the causal history of that state of affaires, whereas laws are viewed as laws of the *models* that provide the conceptual framework for these descriptions, and not as laws governing *real* processes. According to this approach, laws are merely instrumental (Cartwright 1991; van Fraassen 1989).

(3) Finally, reification, or hypostazation, is also precluded if the notion of interwovenness of part-structures is taken into account. We might begin with a distinction between four of these structures: a physical, a biotic, a psychical, and an act-structure. These part-structures obey their own internal structural principles, each of them having their own qualifying (modal) function, whereas all are encompassed within the structural whole of the human body. 'Body' should be taken here to denote the human person in a full sense, including the functioning of the person in social, economic, legal, aesthetic, moral, and

religious relations. These ways of functioning are all corporeal, according to Dooyeweerd, in the sense that they are nothing apart from human corporeality.

When this view is taken seriously, it implies that each part of the human body, the brain included, at the same time functions in all part-structures and in the body as a structural whole. This means that the brain functions not only within the physical and biotic part-structure, but also in the psychical part-structure and in the act-structure.

Does this mean that the brain 'feels', 'thinks', or 'loves'? No, it does not, because being a subject (or agent) differs from 'functioning within a particular modal aspect' and from 'functioning within a particular part-structure'. There is no homunculus hidden between the convolutions of the brain, nor a ghost in the machine. However, this does not coerce us to the alternative of considering the brain as 'merely' a biological organ, or as a computer or biochip.

Does this mean that the brain itself, as part of the human body, functions in an active sense within modes 'higher' than the biotic mode? Or, are these higher-than-biotic functions opened only in a passive sense? Again, I think we should try to avoid the either/or. I am not an advocate of stretching language to the extent that one maintains that brains *as such*, as entitary structures functioning within the biotic part-structure, actively function within the psychical (or social, moral, etc.) mode. To maintain this would be to transform the ordinary meaning of the term brain into a metaphor denoting a mixed psycho-physical entity without clear conceptual boundaries.

However, the brain is more than passive substrate. The least that can be said from the perspective developed here is that the biotic part-structure is encapsulated within the psychical part-structure in a 'foundational' sense. The term foundational means here, roughly speaking, that psychic functioning is co-determined by biotic functioning, whereas biotic functioning is opened up by psychic functioning. To be more precise: in so far as the brain functions in accordance with the law-like regularities of the biotic part-structure, 'higher' than biotic object-functions are opened up, in such a way that the brain as a biological entity fits with the functioning of those parts of body that conform to the regularities of the psychic part-structure and the act-structure. To reiterate, object-functions are those functions or modes in which a particular entity, such as the brain, functions as an object, i.e. needs another entity or person to develop aspects or functions of itself, which without this interaction would remain 'closed'. Because of this structural interwovenness, 'higher'-than-biotic modes of functioning are opened up *within* the biotic substructure (which itself is an entitary structure). The psychical part-structure is, in its turn, in a foundational sense bound within the act-structure (and the physical within the biotic).

In short, the functions of the brain, as a biotic part-structure, are opened up in the direction of the psychical and higher functions, and, at the same time, do not loose their internal biotic destination. This opening up of object-functions (i.e. functions of a substructure that are developed when this structure becomes the object of the activity of another, 'higher', structure) implies that there is an increasing tendency toward functional specialization and a growing potential for variation (see Hundert 1989, Chapter 8). Therefore, it is in an *indirect* sense that one might say that the brain functions within the psychical part-structure and the act-structure.

Practically and theoretically this means that the relevant context expands the 'higher' the part-structure one studies. The brain viewed from the perspective of the body as a psychical structure is engaged in all kinds of psychical processes. At the level of the psychical part-structure, the brain cannot be studied in isolation, for we enter here into the domain of temperament, emotion, and sensory perception. Traits and functions within this domain are dependent on processes in both the central and the peripheral nervous system (cf. the regulation of the sympathetic and parasympathetic tonus); and on changes in endocrine and immune functioning in virtually all parts of the body. Brain functioning in a psychical sense is integrated in the functioning of the body as a whole. Therefore, saying that the brain sees, smells, or feels is an abstraction (because the brain is only part of the body). Saying that seeing, hearing, and feeling are brain functions is also an abstraction. It is conceptually more accurate to say that seeing, hearing, and feeling are activities of the human person, which — as processes — can be studied from the perspective of the psychical part-structure that, in its turn, is founded in a biotic part-structure. One could add, here, that there is an irreversible order in this foundational relationship between the biotic and psychical part-structure. The irreversibility, or asymmetry, consists of the fact that without the biotic (and physical) part-structure the psychical part-structure does not exist, whereas the biotic part-structure may exist (and be conceptualized) without presuming the higher part-structures.

Conclusion

In this chapter the question was raised whether pathological forms of human anxiety are simply remnants of some archaic animal reaction or must be seen as totally distinct from animal physiology, for instance as bearers of existential meaning. I explored a third position, which suggests that in the human world animal reactions can be opened up to social, moral, and even existential meanings.

It was suggested that this position is compatible with recent work of neurologists and neuroscientists such as LeDoux, Edelman, and Damasio. Given the relative lack of empirical research on anxiety as an existential phenomenon, it is important to concentrate also on the conceptual issues that are involved. Putting the mind back in the brain is one important step. Opening up the brain in such a way that brain functioning obeys psychological regularities and is responsive to social norms and moral values is another.

Our discussion amounted to the question of how the process of differentiation, from the biological precursors to the fundamental anxieties, takes place. What are the driving forces behind it? Can these driving forces be identified? In the hierarchical approach, we suggested, these driving forces are conceptualized as acting top-down. Reductionist explanations will favour a bottom-up approach. Parallellists tend to hold back their answer, because any answer will oblige them to take either a hierarchical or a reductionist position. The systems perspective that has been developed here on the basis of Dooyeweerd's ontology departs from the premise that our notion of development presupposes a widening context in which the process of differentiation takes place: the higher the modes that are actively or passively opened up, the wider the context that is implied. In the interaction with this context, both bottom-up and top-down regulations may occur.

Of course, many questions remain to be answered. To pursue these questions would extend the boundaries of this chapter. If anything emerges from the above account, it is that anxiety is a rich and intriguing emotion. Its complexity gives an idea of the many dimensions along which human existence unfolds.

References

Basden, A. (2000). The Dooyeweerd pages. Online Available at: http://www.basden.u-net.com/Dooy/

Cartwright, N. (1991). The reality of causes in a world of instrumental laws. In: *The Philosophy of Science* (ed. R. Boyd, P. Gasper, and J. D. Trout), pp. 379–86. Cambridge: MIT Press.

Clouser, R. A. (1991). *The Myth of Religious Neutrality. An Essay on the Hidden Role of Religious Belief in Theories*. London: University of Notre Dame Press.

Clouser, R. A. (1996). A sketch of Dooyeweerd's philosophy of science. In: *Facets of Faith and Science, Vol. II.* (ed. J. M. van der Meer), pp. 81–97. Lanham: University Press of America.

Damasio, A. R. (1994). *Descartes' Error. Emotion, Reason, and the Human Brain*. New York: Avon Books.

Damasio, A. R. (1999). *The Feeling of What Happens. Body, Emotion and the Making of Consciousness*. London: Vintage, Random House.

De Raadt, J. D. R. (1991). *Information and Managerial Wisdom*. Idaho: Paradigm.

Dooyeweerd, H. (1953–1958). *A New Critique of Theoretical Thought*, Vols I–IV (especially Vol. III). Amsterdam, Paris, Philadelphia: Presbyterian and Reformed Publishing Company.

Edelman, G. (1992). *Bright Air, Brilliant Fire. On the Matter of the Mind*. London: Penguin Books.

Edelman, G. and Tononi, G. (2000). *A Universe of Consciousness. How Matter Becomes Imagination*. New York: Basic Books.

Glas, G. (1994). A conceptual history of anxiety and depression. In: *Handbook on Anxiety and Depression* (ed. J. A. den Boer and A. Sitsen), pp. 1–44. New York: Marcel Dekker.

Glas, G. (1997). The subjective dimension of anxiety: a neglected area in modern approaches to anxiety? In: *Clinical Management of Anxiety; Theory and Practical Applications* (ed. J. A. den Boer, E. Murphy, and H. G. M. Westenberg), pp. 43–62. New York: Marcel Dekker.

Glas, G. (2001). *Angst — Beleving, Structuur, Macht.* Amsterdam: Boom.

Glas, G. (2002). Churchland, Kandel and Dooyeweerd on the Reducibility of Mind States. *Philosophia Reformata*, **67**: 148–72.

Goldstein, K. (1940). *Human Nature in the light of Psychopathology.* New York: Schocken Books.

Goudzwaard, B. (1979). *Capitalism and Progress: A Diagnosis of Western Society* (ed. and trans. J. Van Nuis Zylstra). Toronto: Wedge.

Gray, J. A. (1982). *The Neuropsychology of Anxiety. An Enquiry into the Functions of the Septo-hippocampal System.* Oxford: Oxford University Press.

Hart, H. (1984). *Understanding Our World. An Integral Ontology.* Lanham: University Press of America.

Hoogland, J. and Jochemsen, H. (2000). Professional autonomy and the normative structure of medical practice. *Theoretical Medicine*, **21**(5): 457–75.

Hundert, E. M. (1989). *Philosophy, Psychiatry, Neuroscience. Three Approaches to the Mind. A Synthetic Analysis of the Varieties of Human Experience.* Oxford: Clarendon Press.

Jochemsen H. and Glas, G. (1997). *Verantwoord Medisch Handelen.* Amsterdam: Buijten & Schipperheijn.

Kierkegaard, S. (1980). *The Concept of Anxiety. A Simple Psychologically Orienting Deliberation on the Dogmatic Issue of Heriditary Sin.* (ed. and trans. R. Thomte in collaboration with A. B. Anderson). Princeton, New Jersey: Princeton University Press (original in Danish, 1844).

Landis, C. (1964). *Varieties of Psychopathological Experience* (ed. F. A. Mettler). New York: Holt, Rinehart & Winston.

LeDoux, J. (1996). *The Emotional Brain. The Mysterious Underpinnings of Emotional Life.* New York: Touchstone/Simon & Schuster.

Marks, I. M. (1987). *Fears, Rituals, and Phobias: Panic, Anxiety, and their Disorders.* New York: Oxford University Press.

Pascal, B. (1980). *Pensées* (ed. Lafuma). Paris: Editions du Seuil.

Rachman, S. and Lopatka, C. (1986*a*). Match and mismatch in the prediction of fear — I. *Behavior Research and Therapy*, **24**: 387–93.

Rachman, S. and Lopatka, C. (1986*b*). Match and mismatch of fear in Gray's theory — II. *Behavior Research and Therapy*, **24**: 395–401.

Scheler, M. (1916). *Der Formalismus in der Ethik und die materiale Wertethik. Neuer Versuch der Grundlegung eines ethischen Personalismus.* Berne: Francke.

Schuurman, E. (1980). *Technology and the Future: A Philosophical Challenge.* Toronto: Wedge Publishing Foundation.

Stafleu, M. D. (1987). *Theories at Work. On the Structure and Functioning of Theories in Science, in Particular During the Copernican Revolution.* Lanham, New York: University Press of America.

Van Fraassen, B. (1989). *Law and Symmetry.* Oxford: Clarendon Press.

Yalom, I. (1980). *Existential Psychotherapy*. New York: Basic Books.

Zylstra, U. (1996). The influence of evolutionary biology on hierarchical theory in biology, with special reference to the problem of individuality. In: *Facets of Faith and Science*. Vol. 2 (ed. J. M. van der Meer), pp. 287–99. Lanham: University Press of America.

16 Linguistic markers of recovery: semantic and syntactic changes in the use of first person pronouns in the course of psychotherapy

Werdie (C. W.) van Staden and Christa Krüger

Introduction

The semantic (meaning-driven), but not the syntactic (grammatical), use of first-person pronouns changes with recovery (i.e. with good outcome) in the course of psychotherapy. This was the core finding in a study that combined philosophical and empirical methods to examine the use of first-person pronouns during recovery (Van Staden 1999*a*). As we describe in this chapter, philosophical methods were crucial to distinguish the relevant semantic use of first-person pronouns from their syntactic use. Empirical methods were then employed to test whether semantic and/or syntactic usage changed during recovery in a sample of actual patients.

A natural way to study first-person pronoun usage in relation to recovery would be simply to count and compare in positivist fashion the various first-person pronouns used by patients before and after recovery, for instance at the commencement and termination of psychotherapy. This would be relatively easy to do. However, apart from Spence's work (Spence *et al.* 1994, Spence 1995) of the analyst–analysand relationship, empirical studies of this kind have not been reported. This is perhaps doubly surprising, given the importance of concepts such as self and ego (the natural expression of which are by means of first-person pronouns) in psychoanalytical and psychotherapeutic theory (Glover 1988).

This positivist approach of simply counting pronouns, however, measures only syntactic usage rather than the meanings carried by the personal pronoun in a given context (i.e. their semantic usage). Hence one reason for the absence of reported studies in the literature could be, simply, that syntactic usage fails to show any changes in psychotherapy – it is notoriously difficult to publish studies with negative findings!

In the study described in this chapter, therefore, we extended our approach to include semantic usage. Semantic variables are considerably more difficult to define in ways that are suitable for empirical study, in particular permitting reliable identification sentence by sentence. The semantic variables employed in the present study were derived by one of us from a study of Frege's semantic theory and the logic of relations (Van Staden 1999*a*, Van Staden, in press). This philosophical work (as, for example, in Frege 1966, Lemmon 1996) provided the theoretical backbone for the examination of sentences as expressions of (1) relations and (2) the semantic positions that are inherent to relations. The particular interest here, of course, is those relations that are expressed by patients in illness and recovery. This link with illness and recovery is discussed further below. First, though, the empirical questions are: (1) whether semantic variables derived in this way could be reliably identified, and (2) whether they did indeed change in the course of successful psychotherapy.

The details of the empirical study have been reported elsewhere (Van Staden 1999*a*). In this chapter we outline the main features of the study and then discuss the theoretical and practical significance of our key finding: that semantic, but not syntactic, usage of personal pronouns changed during the course of successful psychotherapy.

Empirical study of first-person pronoun usage

In the empirical study we examined a series of verbatim transcripts of psychotherapy sessions. Essentially, we compared a group of patients with a good outcome (i.e. recovered) with a group of patients with a poor outcome (non-recovered). The transcripts in question were part of an archive, now based at the University of Ulm in Germany, and derived from a major study of psychotherapy carried out originally at Pennsylvania State University, USA, in the 1970s (the Penn Study; see Luborsky *et al.* 1988).

The Penn Study transcripts offered a number of advantages for the empirical study, and also some disadvantages. First, they were complete and unedited, so that we had direct access to the words and phrases actually used. Second, the Penn investigations had carried out a comprehensive outcome rating experience, including both clinically objective and self-report measures (Luborsky *et al.* 1988). From this, as described in detail in Van Staden 1999*a*, we were able to derive two groups: ten patients with the best and ten with the worst outcome. As the basis of our comparative study, this key procedure was thus based on completely independent ratings.

Linguistic Variables

Syntactic usage of first-person pronouns is defined by the declension — whether 'I' or 'me', 'we' or 'us'. A variant of syntactic usage is pragmatic usage. As defined by early twentieth-century pragmatists, this is similar to syntactic usage but fixes the implied tense: 'I' always symbolizes the 'present self' and 'me' always symbolizes the 'past self' (Mead 1934; Wiley 1994). However, for the purposes of the empirical study described here, pragmatic usage is not distinguished from syntactic. Thus, for syntactic usage, the variables were 'I', 'me', 'we', and 'us', as well as 'implied I' and 'implied me' for instance in 'I ate my food and (I) talked to her' and 'she said (to me) . . .'.

For semantic use, the variables were the semantic positions that were expressed by the first-person pronouns: 'alpha position' and 'omega position', as well as 'unclear position' for instances where a semantic position was not expressed clearly. These are positions in relations, as defined in the linguistic theory noted above. Their nature and significance is described in more detail later in this chapter.

Empirical Methods

The empirical paradigm was designed for statistical comparison of change between the commencement and termination of psychotherapy in groups of patients with the best and the worst outcome. The groups were compared for change in the frequencies of the respective variables pertaining to syntactic usage, pragmatic usage, and semantic usage of first-person pronouns. The independent samples t test and the Mann–Whitney U test (MWU) were used for this comparison.

As noted above, 10 patients with the best and 10 with the worst outcome were selected from the transcripts of patients who had undergone psychotherapy in the Penn Study (there were 73 patients in all). These groups showed no significant differences in age, sex, marital status, religion, or diagnosis. The patients were treated once or twice a week by 18 psychodynamically oriented therapists for a minimum of 8 to a maximum of 264 sessions, with a median of 32 sessions during a median of 34 weeks.

Transcripts of two commencement and two termination sessions were analysed for each patient, amounting to the examination of 80 sessions. The presence or absence of the variables at each verb phrase was recorded in binary codes, and then entered into a statistical software program from which were determined the frequencies of the variables, their change between commencement and termination sessions, and the statistical comparisons.

The reliability of the recordings was assessed by sampling 100 successive verb phrases from a random psychotherapy transcript and subjecting them to an analysis by five final-year medical students. The students received a 15-minute training session for the identification and recording of the variables. The mean concordance rate between the study recordings and the student recordings was 94% (standard deviation 1.85; range 92–97%). The Kendall coefficient of concordance among the recordings of the students was 0.0011, which is highly satisfactory.

Results

Syntactic variables

There were no significant differences between the best and worst outcome groups in the change of syntactic usage of first-person pronouns. This is illustrated for the frequency of use of 'I' in Fig. 16.1. Thus, the frequency of 'I' changed very little between the start and finish of psychotherapy for both patient groups; best-outcome patients had a mean increase of 0.33(SD 9.11)%, and worst-outcome patients had a mean increase of 0.50(SD 6.63)%. Statistical comparison of changes in the usage of 'I' between patients with the best and worst outcomes confirmed that they were not significantly different ($t = 0.049$, 16.15 d.f., $P = 0.962$).

Similarly, no significant differences were found between the two groups of patients in terms of change in the usage of 'me' ($t = 0.099$, 15.27 d.f., $P = 0.339$), 'implied I' ($U = 35.0$, $P = 0.257$), or 'implied me' ($U = 38.0$, $P = 0.364$). The frequency of 'we', in contrast to 'I', showed a mean increase for both patient groups between commencement and termination, but because of the large variance among patients this difference was not statistically significant ($U = 23.0$, $P = 0.131$). The pronoun 'us' was used too infrequently to allow meaningful statistical comparison.

Semantic variables

In contrast with the syntactic and pragmatic variables, the outcome groups differed significantly in the change of semantic variables. As illustrated in

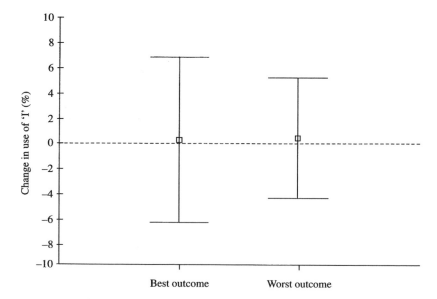

Fig. 16.1 Changes in the frequency of use of 'I' during therapy in 10 patients with the best outcome and in 10 with the worst outcome. Values are mean with 95% confidence intervals. $P = 0.962$

Figs 16.2 and 16.3, the best-outcome group showed an increase in alpha positions (mean increase of 7.14(SD 7.38)%) and a decrease in omega positions (mean decrease of 17.79(SD 19.95)%), whereas the worst-outcome group

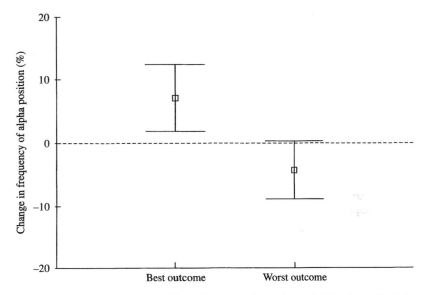

Fig. 16.2 Changes in the frequency of the alpha position during therapy in 10 patients with the best outcome and in 10 with the worst outcome. Values are mean with 95% confidence intervals. $P = 0.002$

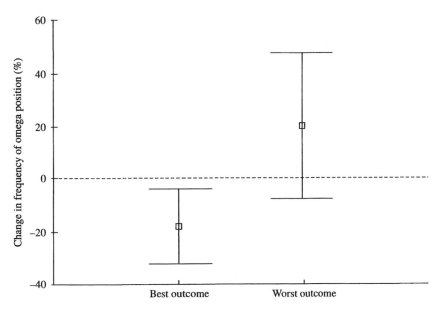

Fig. 16.3 Changes in frequency of the omega position during therapy in 10 patients with the best outcome and in 10 with the worst outcome. Values are mean with 95% confidence intervals. $P = 0.028$

showed the inverse, i.e. a decrease in alpha positions (mean decrease of 4.40(SD 6.46)%) and an increase in omega positions (mean increase of 20.18(SD 38.74)%). These changes are highly statistically significant (alpha position: $t = -3.72$, 17.69 d.f., $P = 0.002$, mean difference -11.54, 95% confidence interval -5.06 to -18.07; omega position: $U = 21.0$, $P = 0.028$). For the 'unclear' position, no significant differences were found between the patient groups ($U = 42.0$, $P = 0.545$).

Theoretical significance of the changes in semantic usage

Derivation of the semantic variables

The semantic variables employed in this study were derived from the semantic theory of Gottlob Frege, which in turn is based on his philosophy of mathematics and the logic of relations (Frege 1966; Lemmon 1996). According to this theory, sentences are taken to be expressions of relations and the semantic positions that are inherent to relations. The alpha semantic position in a relation is occupied by what in linguistic theory is called the *owner* of that particular relation. Correspondingly, the omega semantic position in a relation is occupied by the *accidental* to that particular relation.

These positions are fairly easy to identify. For example, say we have a relation, an action in this case, between x and y, where x feeds y. Whose action is this? The owner of this action is x. Thus, x occupies the alpha position in this relation. Who is the accidental to this action (if no other relations that may bear on this particular action are taken into account)? The accidental to this action is y. Thus, y occupies the omega position. For those relations that are actions, the alpha position is commonly known as the position of the 'agent'.

The distinction between the semantic positions thus may seem like a distinction known commonly as that of 'agency'. However, the distinction extends more broadly, because all relations are not actions. Some relations are, for example, states or attitudes. For these, the same questions can be asked to identify the semantic positions. For example, when x knows y, or x needs y, x is the owner of the knowledge or the need. x occupies the alpha position. The omega position is occupied by the accidental to this knowledge or this need (provided that other relations bearing respectively on these particular states are not taken into account). Similarly, when x is against y, x is owner of this attitude and y is the accidental to it. x occupies the alpha position and y the omega position.

Note that these semantic positions should not be mistaken for grammatical positions, but are positions irrespective of their being expressed in language. For example, 'I stroked the dog' is the verbal or written expression of a particular relation that pertained between 'I', the speaker in this case, and the dog.

This action happened irrespective of whether it was expressed in language. The speaker occupied the alpha position in this relation ('stroking') irrespective of whether it was expressed. It just happens to be that in English' and many other languages, first-person pronouns are used to express the semantic positions of the speaker in relations as he or she experiences them. In fact, a language has in some instances more than one way of expressing the same semantic position. For example, the speaker and the dog still occupy the alpha and the omega positions respectively when the relation used in the above example is expressed by 'The dog was stroked by me'.

Change in semantic positions with recovery

Occupancy of semantic positions as expressed by first-person pronoun usage was found to change with recovery in the course of psychotherapy. It changed in that alpha positions were taken up and omega positions were relinquished.

This finding is congruent with work on the concepts of illness and recovery. The combination, moreover, of this finding and work on the concepts of illness generally, as well as in psychotherapy, suggests that these changes in semantic usage of first-person pronouns are markers of recovery in general. The reason is that the concepts of illness and recovery in general imply these changes in the semantic positions.

Holmes and Lindley (1989) conceive of recovery in psychotherapy as the gaining of personal autonomy, which entails agency and/or liberty. Theories of illness also suggest that recovery entails gaining agency (Fulford 1989), gaining liberty to perform actions, gaining capacity for action (Flew 1973), gaining the ability to do things (Nordenfelt 1987, 1994; Whitbeck 1981), the cessation of disability or impairment in functioning (American Psychiatric Association 1994, p. xxi), and gaining understanding or rationality (in case of recovery from mental difficulties) (Gardner 1993).

In so far as an individual procures agency in his or her gaining of autonomy during recovery, this individual gains capacity for action. This gain is evidenced in an individual's execution of an action that was previously beyond their capacity. Thus, the procurement of agency goes hand in hand with the capacity (or ability) to execute an action that was previously beyond an individual's capacity (or ability). The more agency is procured, the more actions that were previously beyond the individual's capacity (or ability) can now be performed, and *vice versa*.

In so far as actions *are* performed as a result of the procurement of an increased capacity or ability for action, occupancy of the alpha position is taken up because, as we saw above, the owner of an action occupies the alpha position. In other words, the procurement of agency or, equivalently, the procurement of the capacity or ability for action entails an increased capacity or ability to occupy the alpha position. In so far as the increased capacity or ability for actions proceeds to actions, occupancy of the alpha position is taken up.

An individual's procurement of liberty may involve, first, the procurement of liberty to execute actions. The more liberty an individual has to execute actions, the more actions may follow. In case more actions follow, more frequent occupancy of the alpha position follows. Second, an individual's procurement of liberty may involve the procurement of liberty from restrictive actions (by others or things) upon this individual (Holmes and Lindley 1989). As we saw above, the semantic position of an individual upon whom an action is executed is the omega position. The more an individual procures liberty from actions upon him or her in his or her experiences, the less frequently he or she occupies the omega position.

'Recovery' as reflected in one's experiences, may extend beyond actions to non-actions. It may extend to rationality, for example. Action is a necessary condition for rationality, to the extent that reasoning and thinking, for example, are actions (Lindley 1986). However, rationality also has non-actions as necessary conditions to it, for example the *states* of knowing and understanding, which are not actions. We do not 'do' them, yet they are necessary conditions for rationality. The procurement of knowledge, understanding, and rationality (as in psychotherapy or cognitive therapy, for example) implies that a patient takes up occupancy of the alpha position, as such a patient would become the owner of this knowledge or this understanding (as it is reflected in the expressions 'I know . . .' and 'I understand . . .').

Thus, prima facie, concepts of illness and recovery imply changes in the semantic positions as found in the empirical study. So, a meaning-driven enquiry into these concepts as well as the empirical investigation suggest the same finding. Neither method produced this finding, however, in isolation from the other, even though they are from disparate origins (natural sciences and conceptual enquiries).

Brief methodological annotations about nature and meaning

The core finding presented here resulted from a strong synergy between methods from the natural sciences (i.e. an empirical quantitative investigation) and meaning-driven methods (i.e. philosophical analysis). A strong synergy can be claimed because the methodological contributions from both natural and meaning-driven domains cross-fertilized one another to exceed — as synergy is defined (Sykes 1983) — the sum of the individual contributions.

Methods from the natural sciences were used to examine the natural ways in which first-person pronouns had been used grammatically, but these methods were equally suited to examine meaning-driven usage of first-person pronouns, once the meaning-driven variables had been defined.

Meaning-driven variables, in turn, had been defined by philosophical, or meaning-driven, methods. Meaning-driven methods, furthermore, highlighted the potential extent or generalizability of the core finding. That is, shifts in the semantic positions may be relevant to recovery in general.

Provided, then, that changes in semantic usage of first-person pronouns are markers of recovery in general, the core finding of the empirical study may be applicable in practice not only to psychotherapy, but also to recovery in general.

Potential practical applications

The empirical study and the previous section have been concerned with changes in the semantic positions when recovery was something given. A converse approach could be taken in applying the core finding practically. That is, changes in the semantic positions as expressed in first-person pronoun usage may serve as an indication of recovery.

Applications in clinical assessment

The clinical assessment of semantic positions during or after treatment could complement standard ways of assessing progress and outcome. The focus might be on semantic positions in certain *target relations* that are characteristic of a specific disorder, similar to the standard monitoring of *target symptoms*. Alternatively, semantic positions could be assessed for *all* expressed relations (as has been done in the empirical study described), similar to assessing recovery by means of existing *global* measures of outcome (Phelan *et al.* 1996) such as 'quality of life' questionnaires (Lehman 1996) and assessments of 'functioning' (American Psychiatric Association 1994, pp. 30–2).

Such assessment would add value to standard ways of assessing progress and outcome in that, unlike the standard clinical assessments and measures of outcome, it does not require the patient or the clinician to *reflect on* the outcome as such. Rather, it reveals progress and outcome as reflected *within* the patient's account. Thus, as an independent measure, an assessment of the semantic positions would overcome the potential bias or mistaken representation of outcome, which is incurred when a patient or a clinician has to *reflect on* progress or outcome. As a linguistic measure, furthermore, it could provide a method for tracking progress in the course of treatment, allowing the therapist to avoid blind alleys, and to build on themes that are proving helpful.

Applications in treatments

Tracking the semantic positions may aid the clinician's understanding of a patient's experiences of illness, and thereby facilitate a more empathic doctor–patient relationship (Kaplan *et al.* 1994). This relationship in turn may enhance recovery, especially for patients who suffer from psychiatric disorders.

Understanding a patient better by tracking his or her semantic positions may be deployed more directly in psychotherapy in order to enhance recovery (Van Staden 1999b). By means of understanding the similarity of a patient's semantic positions in various relations, the patient (and therapist) may attain the prerequisites for recovery in psychodynamic therapy (i.e. understanding and insight). For example, a patient may come to understand that he or she is often in a position of being ridiculed (which is an omega position) in relations with people of the opposite sex. Alternatively, in cognitive behavioural therapy (Beck 1976; Hawton *et al.* 1996) a therapist may suggest a change in the occupancy of semantic positions. Thereby, a patient may contemplate and learn to occupy desirable semantic positions in certain situations (Van Staden 1999b).

It is worth noting, finally, that other linguistic variables, besides semantic usage of the first-person pronoun, may be relevant to the theory and practice of psychotherapy. Thus the empirical study described above included, *inter alia*, the use of the negative. This showed no change with recovery in the course of psychotherapy. So far as it goes, then, this is evidence against the traditional view of overcoming denial as being a component of recovery. Of course, not all denial is expressed by negatives, nor are all negatives expressions of denial, although they are at least suggestive. The same is found for verbs that express obligation (e.g. 'I ought to . . .'). These also showed no change, which, again so far as it goes, is contrary to the expectations of rational emotive therapy, a key feature of which is to encourage patients to recognize, and then give up, restrictive feelings of obligation (Ellis 1996).

In all these cases, then, aspects of patient's semantic usage would inform the therapist about his or her initial semantic positions and about change thereof. However, much further research is required to establish the validity, reliability, and practical viability of these applications. Even more, replication studies in specific diagnostic groups and other forms of treatment are required. These could provide sound empirical substantiation for the meaning-driven claim that these changes in the semantic positions are necessary features of recovery in general.

References

American Psychiatric Association (1994). *Diagnostic and Statistical Manual of Mental Disorders (DSM-IV)*. 4th ed. Washington, D.C.: American Psychiatric Association.

Beck, A. T. (1976). *Cognitive Therapy and the Emotional Disorders*. New York: International Universities Press.

Ellis, A. (1996). Rational-emotive therapy. In: *Current Psychotherapies*. 4th ed. (ed. R. J. Corsini), pp. 197–238. Itasca, Illinois: F. E. Peacock.

Flew, A. (1973). *Crime or Disease?* New York: Barnes & Noble.

Frege, G. (1966). *Translations from the Philosophical Writings of Gottlob Frege*. (trans. P. Geach and M. Black). Oxford: Basil Blackwell.

Fulford, K. W. M. (1989). *Moral Theory and Medical Practice*. Cambridge: Cambridge University Press.

Gardner, S. (1993). *Irrationality and the Philosophy of Psychoanalysis*. Cambridge: Cambridge University Press.

Glover, J. (1988). *'I': The Philosophy and Psychology of Personal Identity*. London: The Penguin Press.

Hawton, K., Salkovskis, P. M., Kirk, J., *et al.* (ed.) (1996). *Cognitive Behavioural Therapy for Psychiatric Problems*. Oxford: Oxford University Press.

Holmes, J. and Lindley, R. (1989). *The Values of Psychotherapy*. Oxford: Oxford University Press.

Kaplan, H. I., Sadock, B. J., and Grebb, J. A. (1994). *Synopsis of Psychiatry*. Ch. 1. Baltimore, Maryland: Williams & Willkins.

Lehman, A. F. (1996). Measures of quality of life among persons with severe and persistent mental disorders. In: *Mental Health Outcome Measures* (ed. G. Thornicroft and M. Tansella), pp. 75–92. Berlin: Springer.

Lemmon, E. J. (1996). *Beginning Logic*. 2nd ed, pp. 179–87. London: Chapman & Hall Medical.

Lindley, R. (1986). *Autonomy*. New York: MacMillan.

Luborsky, L., Crits-Christoph, P., Mintz, J., *et al.* (1988). *Who Will Benefit From Psychotherapy: Predicting Therapeutic Outcomes*. New York: Basic Books.

Mead, G. H. (1934). *Mind, Self, and Society*. London: University of Chicago Press.

Nordenfelt, L. (1987). *On the Nature of Health: An Action–Theoretic Approach*. Dordrecht, Holland: D. Reidel.

Nordenfelt, L. (1994). Mild mania and a theory of heath: a response to 'Mild Mania and Well-Being'. *Philosophy, Psychiatry, and Psychology*, **1**(3): 179–84.

Phelan, M., Wykes, T., and Goldman, H. (1996). Global function scales. In: *Mental Health Outcome Measures* (ed. G. Thornicroft and M. Tansella), pp. 15–26. Berlin: Springer.

Spence, D. P. (1995). When do interpretations make a difference? A partial answer to Fliess's Achensee question. *Journal of the American Psychoanalytic Association*. **43**: 689–712.

Spence, D. P., Mayes, L. C. and Dahl, H. (1994). Monitoring the analytic surface. *Journal of the American Psychoanalytic Association*. **42**: 43–6.

Sykes, J. B. (ed.) (1983). *The Concise Oxford Dictionary*. Oxford: Clarendon Press.

Van Staden, C. W. (1999a). *Linguistic changes during recovery: a philosophical and empirical study of first person pronoun usage and the semantic positions of patients as expressed in psychotherapy and mental illness*. MD thesis, University of Warwick, UK.

Van Staden, C. W. (1999b). 'I' or 'me': the logic of human relations. In: *Heart & Soul: The Therapeutic Face of Philosophy*. (ed. C. Mace), pp. 87–103. London: Routledge.

Van Staden, C. W. (in press) Linguistic markers of recovery: theoretical underpinnings of first person pronoun usage and semantic positions of patients. *Philosophy, Psychiatry, and Psychology*.

Whitbeck, C. (1981). A theory of health. In: *Concepts of Health and Disease* (ed. A. L. Caplan, H. T. Engelhardt, J. J., McCartney). Reading, Massachusetts: Addison Wesley.

Wiley, N. (1994). *The Semiotic Self*. Padstow, UK: Polity Press.

Section 7   Future Possible?

17 Magic, science, and the equality of human wits

Paolo Rossi

The secret knowledge

Becoming a magician — either in the sphere of natural magic or in that of demonic magic — is not the same as becoming an accountant, a professor of biology, or a theoretical physicist, for a very simple reason. In the universe of magic, science and truth have a fundamental characteristic: they are not accessible to all people, neither in fact nor in principle.

The term *initiation*, has always been used and is still used (not by chance) in reference to magic. In order to know the truths of magic and to practise magic, a person must embrace a principle greater than human nature, and must assume a role that is qualitatively different from that which people have by nature. A nature that is in some way divine must be superimposed on the person's original nature. St Thomas's definition of grace — *quaedam similitudo divinitatis participata in homine* (Tommaso d'Aquino 1984, p. 105) — could, if removed from its context, be inserted in many natural magic texts. As D. P. Walker has written, magic is always on the point of turning into art, science, applied psychology and, mainly, religion (Walker 1958).

Magical techniques are, together, a way to operate on the world and a process of religious regeneration. Magic is also salvation. The domination of nature presupposes the achievement of individual perfection, and the process that permits the achievement of perfection coincides with that which leads to the domination of nature (Eliade 1956). Not everyone can achieve perfection. Consequently, not everyone can know the world and operate on it. The ascetic discipline, withdrawal from the world, and the capacity to raise oneself to a level unattainable by other people, are some of the elements that constitute a magical type of knowledge.

This mode of thinking gives rise to several closely bound themes which reappear in innumerable texts, and are taken up and repeated by several authors. These are: (1) the secret and reserved character of knowledge, the divulging of which would have ill-omened consequences; (2) the extreme difficulty and complication of procedures and rituals that permit one to approach the truth; (3) the distinction between the narrow group of sages or 'true people' and the *promiscuum hominum genus* or the mass of the profane; (4) the extraordinary character of the personality of the magician who can accomplish impressive feats and who has reached a level of knowledge that sets him or her apart.

Corpus hermeticum

The 14 treatises of the *Corpus hermeticum*, which Marsilio Ficino translated from the Greek between 1463 and 1464, were circulated widely as a manuscript, and 16 editions were printed between 1471 and the end of the fourteenth century. These texts date to the second century AD, but throughout the sixteenth century were attributed to the legendary Hermes Trismegistus, a contemporary of Moses and indirect teacher of Pythagoras and Plato. They form the basis of the great rebirth of magic in the fifteenth and sixteenth centuries, and operated strongly on the culture of the ages of Ficino and Kepler. The text of the *Picatrix latinus* was also widely read in the fifteenth and sixteenth centuries in a Latin version derived from the Arabic through a lost Spanish version. The Arabic text probably dates to the eleventh century, but it is an essential treatise for understanding the philosophical and artistic culture of the Renaissance (Garin 1976).

Ad laudem et gloriam altissimi et omnipotentis Dei, cuius est revelare suis praedestinatis secreta scientiarum: the theme of secrecy appears in the first lines of the *Picatrix* and reappears time and time again. The 'secret' that the book intends partially to reveal cannot be acquired if knowledge is not acquired first. The secret cannot be possessed except by the sage and by the person who studies science in an orderly way. Science is divided into two parts: one is manifest, the other hidden. The hidden part is deep, but those who explore it will attain what they desire and will be able to draw from it what they want. The words that refer to the ordering of the world are the same ones that Adam received from God, and they can be understood only by those sages who dedicate themselves constantly to the sciences and who have understood the essence of the Being by drawing on the truth. It is, in any case, a *magna profunditas* (great profundity) of things 'difficult for the intellect', a science *nimis profunda* (too deep) (Perrone Compagni 1975, pp. 290, 301, 330). The suggestions presented in magical texts are, by nature, far from beastly persons (*a bestialibus hominibus sunt natura remoti*). Only very few sages are able to understand the secrets written by other sages in their books using an occult language. Persons who do not exert themselves in science are defective, persons of weak opinion. Consequently, he must be called man only because he has the form and figure of man: *homo appellari non debet nisi nomine, forma et figura hominis* (Perrone Compagni 1975, p. 296).

The material and the essential man

In the hermetic–magical tradition, the themes of a distinction between two types of person, and the themes of secrecy and difficulty, seem to be inextricably bound up with one another (Nock and Feftugière 1945–1954):

> Is the intellect, Trismegistus, not of the same quality in all men?

> Not all men, Asclepius, reach real knowledge . . . The intimate union of sensation and intellect is proper to man. But not every man possesses intellect. There are in fact two types of men: the material and the essential man (*Corpus Hermeticum*; I, p. 98; II, p. 303)

Around 1330, Bono da Ferrara wrote that the art of alchemy is extremely difficult because of equivocations, allegory, and metaphor. The *oratio* of alchemical philosopher is written 'in alien and enigmatic terms, with extraneous and impossible figures'. The philosophers speak a language that only they know. This allows them to understand one another and to exclude all others (*loquela extranea ab omnibus aliis et nota solis eis*) (Bonus 1602, pp. 123, 132, 398):

> I pray and beseech all those who understand these things and in whose hands this precious gem will arrive, to communicate it to men who dedicate themselves to these problems, who ardently desire this art and who are learned in natural principles. They must instead hide it from the profane and from children, for they are undeserving.

The authority of rank, the merit of sainthood and of doctrine, and the dignity of nature are elements that constitute the figure of the sage for Cornelio Agrippa, who writes two centuries later. Agrippa presents the secrecy of truth, and the processes that permit a person to attain it, as closely linked to the distinction between the divine and mortal beings (Agrippa 1967, p. 25):

> Secrets must be communicated verbally only, through a small group of sages and the sacred arcana must be guarded by a small number of elects . . . Every experiment of magic abhors the public, wants to be hidden, grows stronger in silence and is destroyed when revealed.

This arcanum, writes Paracelsus in a text of 1584, had already been considered occult by the ancient Fathers, so as not to be reached by the hands of the undeserving. We beseech, in imitation of those Fathers, 'to deal with and conserve this divine mystery in secret' (Paracelsus, 1584, p. 27). Sublimated mercury, the great German physician affirms in another text, becomes gold, silver, copper, and iron; it appears malleable like wax, liquifies in the sun like snow and, finally, returns to its primitive state. This is a secret that must be kept well hidden and must not be revealed to those who are unworthy of it (Paracelsus 1584, p. 79):

> A goose will prefer a turnip to a gem; therefore the common people are not
> worthy of knowing this secret, and God has expressly forbidden throwing
> pearls before swine.

We have placed very few examples before the eyes of the reader,
Giovambattista Della Porta writes in *Magia naturalis*, but these and what can
be derived from them must be kept with a faithful heart, so that they are not
degraded by reaching the hands of profane persons who belong to the herd
(*ne passim per manus ignari et gregarii hominis pervenientia vilescant*)
(Della Porta 1607, p. 544).

Even Robert Fludd, in the seventeenth century, referred to the herd of the
profane, in one of his many answers to Johannes Kepler, who had accused him
of 'dabbling in tenebrous enigmas'.

For *all* the exponents of magic and alchemistic culture, the texts of ancient
wisdom take the form of sacred texts, which include secrets that only a few
people can decipher. The truth is hidden in the past and in the profound. It
must be searched for and individuated beyond the expedients that were wisely
used to hide it from the unworthy. As when dealing with the sacred texts, it is
necessary continuously to go *beyond the letter*, in search of a message that
is more and more hidden. That message expresses a truth, which is always
the same. History is only apparently varied. It contains a single, immutable,
sapientia (Fludd 1659, pp. 41–2):

> When Aristotle wrote of the *prima materia*, Plato of the *hyle*, Hermes of the
> *umbra orrenda*, Pythagoras of the *symbolical unity* and Hippocrates of the
> *deformed chaos*, they were all writing in reality of the *darkness* or *dark abyss*
> of Moses.

There is an impassable difference between regenerated persons and those
who have only human form and figure. This theme had crossed both the *pious*
and *psychiatric* currents of Renaissance magic, as well as those currents
linked to demonic and necromantic magic. However, in the years in which
Robert Fludd wrote, the theme of the distinction between sages and common
people had undergone an extremely harsh criticism.

The 'moderns' against magic

Only if you have not underestimated the historical significance of magic,
alchemy, and astrology in the Renaissance and in seventeenth-century culture,
only if you clearly know how slight was the armour with which many philosophers advanced to attack the prevailing magical view of nature, can you realize
the meaning of and reasons for the numerous polemic and extremist statements
presented by many contemporaries of Bacon, Descartes, and Mersenne.

Doctrines concerning the sources and processes of knowledge, on the
nature of human beings, and on the roads to the truths, multiply and are

expressed with a disconcerting radicality. They are born within different perspectives, with different presuppositions at their core. Sometimes they even have very different meanings, but, independently from their origins, they contribute to the affirmation and consolidation of an image of knowledge that can effectively contrast the hermetic–magical tradition.

Reason is complete in each one of us

The method of interpretation of nature that I propose (Francis Bacon wrote around 1603) must be compared with the preceding forms of knowledge. My method has a fundamental characteristic: 'doth in sort equal men's wits and leaveth no great advantage or preminence to the perfect and excellent motions of the spirit'. The method of the new science tends to eliminate the differences: in drawing a straight line or making a perfectly round circle 'by aim of hand only, there must be a great difference between an unsteady and unpractised hand and a steady and practised, but to do it by rule or compass it is much alike' (Bacon 1887–1892; III, pp. 250, 607). The expression *to equal men's wits* is translated in Latin (in 1608) as *ingenia et facultates fere aequare*. The comparison with the ruler and compass will be taken up again. The new method — this is now the conclusion — does not leave inequalities among human intellects greater than those that exist among the senses (*non multo maior in hominum intellectu eminet inaequalitas, quam in sensu inesse solet*). More incisively, in the *Novum Organum* 'My way of discovering sciences goes far to level men's wits, and leaves but little to individual excellence; because it performs everything by the surest rules and demonstrations' (Bacon 1887–1892; III, pp. 638, 572–3; IV, p. 109).

For many exponents of the new philosophy, the equality of intelligences is not only an end which can be reached, and it does not derive solely from the application of the method. It appears as a starting point and as a presupposition to the construction of the method. The intellectual differences among people do not depend on reason (which is equal in all persons and in which all are equally gifted), but on the passions or the conditioning exerted by education, culture, and the absence of methodological rules.

The truths that are called common notions (*notiones communes*), Descartes wrote in his *Principia Philosophiae*, are the ones that many people are capable of perceiving clearly and distinctly. Nevertheless, to some people, these truths are not sufficiently self-evident — it was not because 'one man's faculty of knowledge extends more widely than another's'. Inability to perceive truth was caused by prejudices acquired in childhood that were extremely difficult to shake off. I hardly need recall the famous beginning of the *Discourse sur la méthode*, which affirms that 'good sense is the best distributed thing in the world'. The power of judging well and the faculty of distinguishing truth from falsehood 'is by nature equal in all men'. Reason or good sense, which distinguishes us from animals, 'is complete in each one of us'. The diversity of our opinions did not arise 'because some of us are more reasonable than others', but 'because we direct our thoughts along different paths and do not attend to the same things' (Descartes 1897–1913; IX, pp. 46, 58, 60; Descartes 1952, p. 116).

Every person, according to Hobbes, 'brought philosophy, that is, Natural Reason, into the world with him'. Errors and deviations depend only on the lack of the right method. The *recta ratio* is present in all persons and makes them equal. Differences in understanding derive from the passions, that is to say from the body and from customs. Reason, Hobbes affirmed in another text, 'is no less natural than passion, and is the same in all men'. In the first lines of the *De corpore*, Hobbes had opposed his philosophy to that 'which is found in the metaphysic codes' and to that 'by which philosophers' stones are made'. All knowledge that is acquired by divine inspiration or that comes to us not by reason, but by divine grace, in an instant, and, as it were, by some supernatural sense, is strictly excluded from philosophy (Hobbes 1839–1877; XIII, pp. 1–2; IV, p. 87).

The more a person stands for genius and intellectual activity (*ingenio et studio maxime valet*), Bacon affirmed, the more the person runs the risk of being closed in the dark and tortuous recesses of reveries. A cripple who follows the right path, according to Bacon, arrives before a runner who follows the wrong path. Since the problem does not regard the forces that individual persons use, but the path they follow, men of understanding are more subject to error than others. The human understanding, according to a well-known formula, must not be supplied with wings 'but rather hung with weights, to keep it from leaping and flying'. Excessive vanity is destructive of all greatness of mind, and no excessive grandeur should be attributed to the discoveries. In the *Novum Organum*, the same new logic was attributed 'rather to good luck than to ability', and was presented as 'a birth of time rather than of wit' (Bacon 1887–1892; III, pp. 604, 572; I, pp. 205, 217; IV, pp. 109, 97).

Speaking of himself, Descartes stated that he had 'never presumed my mind to be in any way more perfect than that of ordinary man'. The notions in his writings were 'simple' and in accordance with 'good sense', and his method followed 'simple and easy reasoning'. He assumed very hard positions on the theme of the profane: very often, he wrote in the *Regulae*, those who have never occupied themselves with letters are able to judge whatever presents itself to them; and learned men employ such subtle distinctions that they 'find obscurities in matters of which even the rustic is never ignorant' (Descartes 1952, pp. 116, 160–3, 15, 89).

Hobbes thinks that most people, in regard to science, 'are like children, that having no thought of generation, are made to believe by the women that their brothers and sisters are not born, but found in the garden'. Notwithstanding this, they who have not science 'are in better and nobler condition with their natural prudence, than men that by mis-reasoning or by trusting them that reason wrong, fall upon false and absurd general rules'. The situation is such that 'they who content themselves with daily experience [. . .] and either reject, or not much regard philosophy' are people of sounder judgement than those who are full of refined opinions, but full of uncertainty and who do nothing but dispute and wrangle (Hobbes 1839–1877; I, p. 2).

The new method is presented by Descartes as a set of rules which are certain and easy, and which do not require that a person 'uselessly waste his mental efforts. If the person deserves them, Descartes wrote, he 'will never assume what is false as true'. The fundamental operations of the mind are 'the simplest of all mental operations'. The human mind 'has in it something divine' because 'the first seeds of useful modes of knowledge' are scattered in it and 'spontaneously bear fruit'. Algebra and geometry are two of these fruits. The method must contain 'the primary rudiments of human reason' and must extend to 'the eliciting of truths in every field whatsoever'. The doctrine exposing the rules of method must not be veiled or covered 'to keep it far from the common people', but must be adorned and garbed so as 'to seem pleasing to human intelligence'. Since 'all the things which come within the scope of human knowledge are interconnected', if one began with the simplest notions and proceeded step by step 'it does not take great skill and capacity to find them'. The exposition of the method must proceed by 'clear and common' arguments; when it did, the truths reached 'will have course in the world in the same fashion as coins, which are of no less value when they come out of a peasant's purse'. If not many people devoted themselves to the search for wisdom, it was because they 'do not hope to succeed and do not know what they are capable of' (Descartes 1952, pp. 15–18, 43–4, 45–50).

Through 'its native force', Spinoza says in the *Tractatus de intellectus emendatione*, intelligence 'provides itself with intellectual tools from which other forces for other intellectual activities derive'. In this way 'it discovers other tools or powers for further investigations and thus proceeds step by step until it reaches the summit of wisdom'. The *summit of wisdom*, which Spinoza mentions in this text, contains nothing that transcends normal human faculties. Indeed, the construction of intellectual tools is a gradual process that reaches greater and greater perfection and seems to require less and less effort.

The few and first elements of philosophy, wrote Hobbes in the *De corpore*, are 'the seeds' out of which a true philosophy can be developed. Those seeds, or first principles, seemed to Hobbes to be 'poor, arid, and, in appearance, deformed'. Addressing his reader as a friend, Hobbes wrote that 'philosophy, the child of the world and your own mind, is within yourself'. The method he had constructed could be used by all: 'If it like you, you may use the same' (Hobbes 1839–1877; I, XIII, XIV, p. 2).

Hermetic tradition and Scientific Revolution

It is well known that, in defending the central position of the Sun, Copernicus calls upon Hermes Trismegistus. William Gilbert also refers to Hermes when he links his doctrine of magnetism with universal animation. Francis Bacon talks of the desires and aversions of matter, and he is influenced by the language and models prevalent in the alchemical tradition. It is from the world of magic that he derives his definition of the human as the servant and interpreter of nature, so replacing the venerable definition of the human as a rational animal. Kepler displays a profound knowledge of the *Corpus hermeticum*, and his conviction that there is a secret correspondence between the structures of geometry and those of the universe, as well as his theory of a celestial music of the spheres, is imbued with Pythagorean mysticism. Tycho Brahe persists in considering astrology as the legitimate and practical application of his science. 'I am used', he writes in 1589, 'to calling alchemy the terrestrial astronomy since the subjects under examination bear analogy to the celestial bodies and to their influence'. Galileo himself, always so clear and rigorous, and in whose writings there are no concessions to mysticism or magic, mentions in a letter Dionysius the Areopagite and speaks of 'an extremely spiritual substance that warms, gives new life to all living creatures and makes them fecund'. Descartes, who in his maturity rejected all forms of symbolism and whose philosophy became a byword for rational clarity, placed, in his youth, the works of imagination before those of reason. Like so many magicians in the sixteenth century, he enjoyed constructing automatons and 'shadow gardens'; like so many followers of Raymond Lull, he insisted on the unity of the cosmos: 'There is one active force, love, charity, harmony in things . . . Every corporeal form works by harmony'. These themes reappear in different key in Leibniz, whose *ars characeristica* blends theories taken from the Lullian tradition of hermeticism and Cabalism, and the dreams of Comenius' *Pansophia*. William Harvey's praise of a unique and central government of life (where the heart plays the role of the Sun in the microcosm) is compounded of heliocentric astronomy and cardiocentric physiology. Even the Newtonian concept of space as the *sensorium Dei* can be traced to Neo-platonic influence and the Judaic Cabala. Recent studies of Newton's manuscripts reveal his faith in an *ancient theology* (this is a central theme in hermeticism), the truth of which had to be established with the aid of the new experimental science (Rossi 1968, 1970, 2001*a,b*).

Political implications

The elements of continuity between the so-called hermetic tradition and the natural philosophy of the seventeenth century should not lead us to neglect the difference between the new image of the person of science and that of the magician–priest theorized by Ficino, or that of the magician as titanic being presented by Agrippa.

It is hardly accidental that the attack on the obscurities of magic, the illusions of the alchemists, the deception of astrology, are to be found in all those writers who, for various reasons, may be numbered among the champions of the scientific revolution. The scornful silence of Galileo and Descartes, Bacon's aggressive attack, Gassendi's opposition to Robert Fludd, Mersenne's long struggle against the practitioners of the occult, Boyle's ironic comments on Paracelsus' followers, Pierre Bayle's invective against the 'shameful superstition' of astrology are revealing. Different people from varying points of view all cry out against a mystical world picture and appeal for greater linguistic clarity, for models that can be checked and experiments that can be repeated (Rossi 1975, 2001*b*).

Marine Mersenne, the indefatigable 'secretary of cultivated Europe', put the radical antimagic and antioccult idea of equality of intelligences into a striking maxim (Mersenne 1634, pp. 135–6):

> A man can do nothing that another man cannot also do, and each man contains within himself all that is needed to philosophize and reason on all things

Even though historians of political thought have not always realized it, the thesis of equality of intelligence in the face of scientific truth had strong political implication. The distinction between masters and servants is, according to Hobbes, completely artificial and does not derive from a difference in intelligence. Many philosophers have transformed a factual difference into an ontological one (Hobbes 1839–1877; III, pp. 140–1):

> The inequality that now is, has been introduced by the laws civil. I know that Aristotle . . . maketh men by nature, some more worthy to command, meaning the wiser sort, such as he thought himself to be for his philosophy; others to serve, meaning those that had strong bodies, but were not philosophers as he; as if master and servant were not introduced by consent of men, but by difference of wit: which is not only against reason; but also against experience.

All human beings, Samuel Pufendorf said, have within them a principle for self-government, and all people are intelligent beings in their susceptibility to obligations (Pufendorf 1672; I, p. 2):

> I cannot be persuaded that the mere face of natural excellence is sufficient to give one being the right to impose any obligations on other beings, who have, just as he does, an internal principle for governing themselves.

The notion of equality of humans before the truth implied a renunciation of the image of a clear separation between philosophers and vulgar people, like beasts, for whom tales of miracles, angels, and devils were appropriate. Such people required fables, as Pietro Pomponazzi wrote, 'to induce them to good and preserve from evil, as one does with children with the hope of rewards and the fear of punishment' (Pomponatius 1567, pp. 200–8).

After the age of Bacon and Descartes, Hobbes, Mersenne and Galileo, all forms of knowledge that theorized secrecy in the name of inaccessibility, that envisaged 'superhuman difficulties' on the path to knowledge, or that stated that only initiates could know the truth and only the few could reach the *episteme*, became irremediably and structurally connected with the political notion that the commonality were unable to govern themselves unaided and, like children, needed fables that kept them from the truths.

When ambiguity and enigmatic language become essential to a philosophy, or when philosophy painstakingly avoids linguistic clarity or explicitly condemns clear expression as superficial or mere good sense, when the affirmation of a Hidden Wisdom of the Origins and the image of a Truth at the Beginning of Time become major guiding ideas in a philosophy, when philosophers theorize a difference of essence between the *Shepherds of Being* and those who remain forever confined within the temporality of daily experience, capable of intellect, but totally incapable of Thought, when, finally, all this occurs at one time (as, in our century, among many of Heidegger's followers), then the hermetic tradition reveals its unspent force and celebrates a belated triumph.

Against new magic

Some cultural anthropologists, as well as some philosophers of science of our century, have accepted the idea of an absolute *equivalence*, not only of all forms of culture but of all possible world pictures as well. Today, enthusiasm for the new magic is rampant. Many authors contrast the extraordinary possibilities of a new magical world picture with the narrow rationality of science, because science 'blunts our sense of marvellous', while shamanism offers a new, freer culture. A return to the archaic phase of magical experience is today accepted by many of our students as a valid method of freeing ourselves from the sins of our civilization.

The study of interconnections between hermeticism and modern science have greatly enlarged our historical horizon. However, I think it is one thing to become aware of the origins of our own civilization, and another to renounce our intellectual faculties, praise shamanism, and cultivate the occult and the prophetic as a new and superior form of knowledge.

The history of science, and more explicitly the history of the first scientific revolution, can help us to understand how logical rigour, experimental control, the public character of results and methods, and the very structure of scientific knowledge are not perennial facts of the history of humankind, but historical advances that can easily be lost.

A recognition of the troubled waters at the origins of the modern science, an awareness that the birth of scientific learning is not quite as aseptic as the men of Enlightenment and the positivists naively assumed, does not imply a surrender to primitivism and the cult of magic.

Only if we are ready to renounce a portion of our childish longings, as Freud observes, can we learn to accept that some of our aspirations will turn out to be mere illusions. It seems to me that some students of the hermetic tradition have undergone a process not unlike that of many readers of Freud who, once they learn of the existence of the unconscious and the influence of aggressive drives at work behind the respectable veneer of civilization, come to the conclusion (unlike Freud himself) that neither reason, nor civilization, nor science exists.

Must disillusionment necessarily coincide with a desire for regression?

References

Agrippa, H. C. (1967). De occulta philosophia, *herausgegeben und erläutert von Karl Anton Nowotny*. Graz: Akademische Druck.

Bacon, F. (1887–1892). *Works* (ed. R. L. Ellis, J. Spedding, and D. D. Heath). London: Longman.

Bonus P. Ferrarensis (1602). *Introductio in artem chemiae integra ab ipso authore inscripta Margarita Preciosa Novella*. Montisbeligardi: apud Jacobum Foillet.

Della Porta, G. (1607). *Magiae naturalis libri viginti*. Francofurti.

Descartes, R. (1897–1913). *Oeuvres* (ed. C. Adam and P. Tannery). Paris: Cerf.

Descartes, R. (1952). *Descartes' Philosophical Writings* (ed. N. K. Smith). London: Macmillan.

Eliade, M. (1956). *Forgerons et Alchimistes*. Paris: Flammarion.

Fludd, R. (1659). *Mosaicall Philosophy*. London: H. Moseley.

Garin, E. (1976). *Lo zodiaco della vita: la polemica sull'astrologia dal Trecento al Cinquecento*. Roma-Bari: Laterza.

Hobbes, T. (1839–1877). *English Works* (ed. W. Molesworth). London: John Bohn.

Mersenne, M. (1634). *Questions inouyes ou récréation des sçavans*. Paris: J. Villery.

Nock, A. D. and Festugière, A.-J. (ed.) (1945–1954) *Corpus Hermeticum*. Paris: Les Belles Lettres.

Paracelsus, T. (1584). *De summis naturae mysteriis commentarii tres*. Basileae, ex officina Pernaea per C. Waldkirch.

Perrone Compagni, V. (1975). Picatrix. *Medioevo*, **I**: 278–337.

Pomponatius, P. (1567). *Opera . . . de naturalium effectuum causis sive de incantationibus*. Basileae.

Pufendorf, S. (1672). *De jure naturae et gentium*. Londini Scanorum, sumptibus Adami Junghans imprimebat Vitus Haberegger.

Rossi, P. (1968). *Francis Bacon: From Magic to Science*. London: Routledge and Kegan Paul.

Rossi, P. (1970). *Philosophy, Technology and the Arts in the Early Modern Era*. New York: Harper and Row.

Rossi, P. (1975). Hermeticism, rationality, and the Scientific Revolution. In: *Reason, Experiment, and Mysticism in the Scientific Revolution* (ed. M. L. Righini Bonelli and W. Shea), pp. 247–274. New York: Science History Publications.

Rossi, P. (2001a). *The Birth of Modern Science*. Oxford: Basil Blackwell.

Rossi, P. (2001b). *Logic and the Art of Memory: A Quest for a Universal Language*. Chicago: University of Chicago Press.

Tommaso d'Aquino (1984). La somma teologica, *traduzione e commento a cura dei Domenicani italiani, testo latino dell'edizione leonina*. Bologna: Edizioni Studio Domenicano.

Walker, D. P. (1958). *Spiritual and Demonic Magic: From Ficino to Campanella*. London: The Warburg Institute.

Index